SMALL ANIMAL REPRODUCTION AND INFERTILITY

A Clinical Approach to Diagnosis and Treatment

Edited By
Thomas J. Burke, DVM, MS

Associate Professor
Department of Veterinary Clinical Medicine
College of Veterinary Medicine
University of Illinois
Urbana, Illinois

Lea & Febiger   1986   Philadelphia

Lea & Febiger
600 Washington Square
Philadelphia, PA 19106-4198
U.S.A.
(215) 922-1330

Library of Congress Cataloging-in-Publication Data

Small animal reproduction and infertility.

Includes bibliographies and index.
1. Dogs—Reproduction. 2. Cats—Reproduction.
3. Dogs—Infertility. 4. Cats—Infertility. 5. Dogs—
Breeding. 6. Cats—Breeding. 7. Generative organs—
Diseases. I. Burke, Thomas J. [DNLM: 1. Infertility—
veterinary. 2. Reproduction. SF 887 S635]
SF992.U75S63 1986   636.7′089′6692   86-10519
ISBN 0-8121-1042-0

PRINTED IN THE UNITED STATES OF AMERICA

Print number: 5 4 3 2 1

Dedication

To my mother and late father, Barbara and Fred,
for the genetics *and* the environment,

and

to my wife, Jane, a superb practitioner, for love,
support and helping keep this book "honest."

Preface

There exists today a dichotomy concerning canine and feline reproduction—too little and too much. Increased leisure time and disposable income have allowed owners of companion animals, many of them novices, to enter their charges in more exhibitions. This has resulted in an increased number of animals whose physical or performance traits are deemed desirable. Many of them have failed to reproduce, however, and thus pressure has been placed on veterinarians to find solutions. We also are aware of the surplus population of dogs and cats, and have become involved in solving this problem.

This book was designed to provide practitioners and students with up-to-date, practical information about normal and abnormal reproduction in the dog and cat. The contributors were chosen because of their expertise in this field and their willingness to share their knowledge. To be sure, there are some omissions and some information may quickly become dated—such is the nature of any textbook.

The publishers are to be commended for their support of this project since its inception (seemingly eons ago) and we hope that the somewhat prolonged gestation and mild dystocia have been worth it.

Thomas J. Burke, DVM
Editor

Acknowledgments

The editor is personally grateful to each contributing author; to the publishers; to his many patients and their very patient owners who have allowed him to work with their animal-breeding programs—especially Herb and Betty Holmes and the late C. L. Owens, Kennelmaster (Gunsmoke Kennels) and Joe and Mary Speiser (Speis-O-Life Kennels) who taught as well as learned; to the many veterinarians who have shared their cases; and, lastly, to my mentors who are to be blamed for fostering my interest in canine and feline reproduction—Drs. Harry Reynolds and Jim Sokolowski.

Thanks also to Dr. Joe Catcott, who did a fair amount of the technical editing and provided the initial impetus for this project.

Contributors

Jeanne Barsanti, DVM, MS, Diplomate ACVIM
Department of Small Animal Medicine
College of Veterinary Medicine
University of Georgia
Athens, Georgia

Robert R. Badertscher, II, DVM, MS, PhD, Diplomate ACVR
Associate Professor
Department of Veterinary Clinical Medicine
College of Veterinary Medicine
University of Illinois
Urbana, Illinois

G. John Benson, DVM, MS, Diplomate ACVA
Associate Professor, Veterinary Clinical Medicine
College of Veterinary Medicine
University of Illinois
Urbana, Illinois

Jenaay M. Brown, DVM
Technical Services Veterinarian
The Upjohn Company
Kalamazoo, Michigan

Thomas J. Burke, DVM, MS
Associate Professor
Department of Veterinary Clinical Medicine
College of Veterinary Medicine
University of Illinois
Urbana, Illinois

Leland E. Carmichael, DVM, PhD
John M. Olin Professor of Virology
New York State College of Veterinary Medicine
Cornell University
Ithaca, New York

P.K. Chakraborty, PhD
Department of Obstetrics & Gynecology
Uniformed Services University of Health Science
Bethesda, Maryland

Thomas R. Christie, DVM, Diplomate ACVS
Staff Surgeon
Burleigh Road Animal Hospital
Brookfield, Wisconsin

Emerson D. Colby, MS, DVM
Director, Animal Research Facilities
Dartmouth Medical School
Hanover, New Hampshire

Patrick W. Concannon, PhD
Senior Research Associate, Department of Physiology
New York State College of Veterinary Medicine
Cornell University
Ithaca, New York

Lloyd E. Davis, DVM, PhD
Professor of Clinical Pharmacology
College of Veterinary Medicine
University of Illinois
Urbana, Illinois

Gina B. DiGregorio, BS
Department of Physiology
New York State College of Veterinary Medicine
Cornell University
Ithaca, New York

Delmar Finco, DVM
Professor
College of Veterinary Medicine
University of Georgia
Athens, Georgia

Mary A. Herron, DVM, PhD
Professor
College of Veterinary Medicine
Texas A&M University
College Station, Texas

8

Stephen K. Kneller, DVM, MS, Diplomate ACVR
Associate Professor, Veterinary Clinical Medicine
College of Veterinary Medicine
University of Illinois
Urbana, Illinois

Rolf E. Larsen, DVM, PhD
Assistant Professor, Department of Reproduction
College of Veterinary Medicine
University of Florida
Gainesville, Florida

Flora E.F. Lindsay, MRCVS
Department of Veterinary Anatomy
University of Glasgow Veterinary School
Bearsden, Glasgow, Scotland

Jacob E. Mosier, DVM
Professor
College of Veterinary Medicine
Kansas State University
Manhattan, Kansas

John D. Rhoades, DVM, MS, PhD
Professor
School of Veterinary Medicine
Louisiana State University
Baton Rouge, Louisiana

Robert C. Rosenthal, DVM, MS, Diplomate ACVIM
Assistant Professor, Medicine/Oncology
School of Veterinary Medicine
University of Wisconsin
Madison, Wisconsin

Stephen W.J. Seager, MA, MVB, MRCVS
Department of Veterinary Physiology & Pharmacology
College of Veterinary Medicine
Texas A&M University
College Station, Texas

Frances O. Smith, DVM, PhD
Clinical Assistant Professor
Department of Clinical Sciences
College of Veterinary Medicine
University of Minnesota
St. Paul, Minnesota

Nickolas J. Sojka, DVM, MS
Professor & Chairman
Department of Comparative Medicine
University of Virginia Medical Center
Charlottesville, Virginia

James H. Sokolowski, DVM, PhD
Manager, Gaines Nutrition Center
Gaines Food, Incorporated
St. Anne, Illinois

John C. Thurmon, DVM, MS, Diplomate ACVA
Professor & Head of Anesthesiology Section
College of Veterinary Medicine
University of Illinois
Urbana, Illinois

Gregory C. Troy, DVM, MS, Diplomate ACVIM
Associate Professor
College of Veterinary Medicine
Texas A&M University
College Station, Texas

Grant H. Turnwald, BVSc, MS, Diplomate ACVIM
Associate Professor, School of Veterinary Medicine
Louisiana State University
Baton Rouge, Louisiana

David E. Wildt, PhD
Department of Animal Health
National Zoological Park
Smithsonian Institution
Washington, District of Columbia

Contents

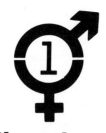

Physiology
of Reproduction

FELINE PHYSIOLOGY OF REPRODUCTION
BY MARY A. HERRON

Introduction

Feline reproduction has attracted relatively little attention until the last 2 decades. The increase in interest in registered cats and in cats as household pets has sparked interest in improving the reproductive performance of the species. The practicing veterinarian must combine an understanding of reproductive physiology with knowledge of the cat's estrous cycle and sexual behavior to answer routine inquiries about reproduction and to assess more complex problems.

THE QUEEN

Although feline reproductive physiology is basically similar to that of other domestic species, one element is unique — the queen requires the stimulus of copulation to ovulate. In all other domestic species (spontaneous ovulators), ovulation is not dependent upon copulation. Induced ovulation is a neuro-endocrine phenomenon involving a neural signal (initiated by stimulation of the anterior vagina) that ascends to the hypothalamus where gonadotropin releasing hormone (GnRH) is released. GnRH, in turn, stimulates the hypophysis to secrete luteinizing hormone (LH). LH is carried to the ovary in the blood and induces the release of ova from mature follicles.

Estrous Cycle

The average age of cats at puberty is 10 months, but the first estrus may occur as early as 4 months or as late as 12 months of age.

Persian females tend to mature late; some may not cycle until they are 1 to 1½ years old. The cat is seasonally polyestrous. In the US the season extends roughly from March to September. Exposure to light controls the seasonality of the cycle. With increasing daily photo-periods in the spring estrus is induced; with decreasing daylight in the late summer estrus is terminated. The late fall and winter months are a period of natural anestrus. By artificially controlling the queen's exposure to light, however, this anestrous period can be converted to a sexually active one. Exposure to approximately 50 foot-candles of light for 12 to 14 hours daily will cause many queens to cycle in the winter months.[1] Many cats exposed to normal household photoperiods receive enough light to stimulate cycling in the winter. The highest efficiency of the estrous cycle in terms of productivity is achieved by providing 12 hours of dark and 12 hours of light each day throughout the year. This exposure to light has resulted in an average of 2.2 litters per queen annually.[2]

Though the average length of the estrous cycle is 14 to 21 days, queens do not display estrous behavior at regular intervals throughout the season. They usually have several contiguous estrous cycles in early spring, followed by a period of acyclic behavior in the late spring. A queen may repeat this pattern once or twice before the end of the breeding season. The cause of the acyclic behavior between normal cycles is unknown. The quiescent periods may represent "silent heats" because it has been reported that follicular development and regression may occur at 14- to 19-day intervals without overt sexual behavior.[3] A form of "silent" or depressed heat may also occur in the initial estrus of the season. This estrus may be either shorter or less obvious than subsequent ones.

Among cats kept in groups there may be a tendency for many of the females to have synchronized estrous cycles. This suggests that

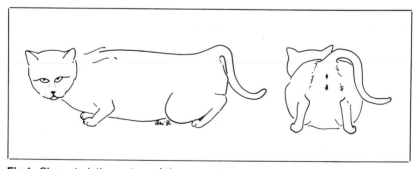

Fig 1. Characteristic posture of the queen during estrus.

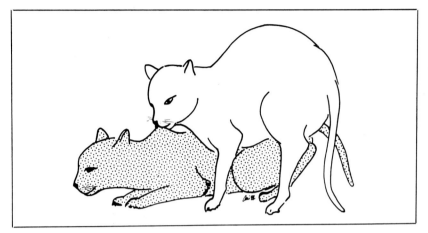

Fig 2. Position of male and female during mounting and copulation.

cycling in the cat, as in some other mammals, may be influenced by olfactory stimuli emitted by cohabitants.

Onset of cycling after parturition may occur between 2 weeks following parturition and 2 weeks after weaning. Even though the cycle may occur during lactation, the queen will breed and may conceive.

Each estrous cycle consists of 3 sequential periods: proestrus, estrus, and metestrus. Each period is distinguished by certain behavior that reflects hormonal changes. The duration of proestrus is 1 day or less. It is characterized by one or more of the following actions: rolling, head rubbing, vocalizing, crouching often with the rear quarters elevated (Fig 1), treading movement of the feet and, importantly, rejecting a male. Estrus, which averages 6 to 7 days, is characterized by intensification of proestrous behavior, but is marked by the female's willingness to accept a male. Acceptance consists of deviation of the tail to one side and permitting the male to grasp the dorsum of her neck and mount to copulate (Fig 2). The behavior during proestrus and estrus may be such a radical change that the inexperienced owner may suspect that the cat is having "fits." Metestrus is a period of follicular regression following a non-ovulatory estrus. It usually lasts 1 to 2 weeks and terminates with the onset of proestrus. There is no sexual behavior during metestrus.

During proestrus and early estrus, follicles mature under the influence of follicle stimulating hormone (FSH). Mature follicles appear as 2.5- to 3.5-mm, blister-like areas on the ovarian surface.[4] Estrogen produced by the growing follicles is the principal steroid hormone

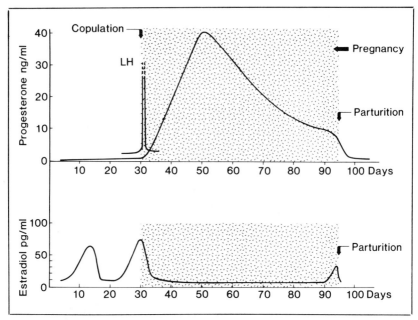

Fig 3. Graphic representation of progesterone, estradiol, and luteinizing hormone levels during the estrous cycle and pregnancy.

during proestrus and estrus. It is responsible for the characteristic behavior as well as cornification of the vaginal epithelium. Estradiol rises from base levels of about 8 pg/ml to 50 or 70 pg/ml at the peak of estrus.[5,6] After reaching the peak level, estradiol drops precipitously for 2 to 5 days to base levels (Fig 3). With this decline in estrogens the characteristic behavior of estrus ceases and metestrus ensues until onset of the next proestrus in 1 to 2 weeks.

If breeding is prevented, LH is not released from the hypophysis, ovulation does not occur, and follicles regress during the first week of metestrus. Progesterone remains at low levels (less than 1 ng/ml) throughout the non-ovulating cycle. If breeding is permitted, the serum level of LH rises within an hour after copulation.[4,7] The concentration is at its peak 20 minutes or 3 to 9 hours after copulation and it returns to baseline levels of 2 to 3 ng/ml 24 hours after copulation.[4] Peak levels of serum LH for individual queens vary widely in response to a single copulatory stimulus, ranging from 37 to over 200 ng/ml (Fig 3).[4,7,12]

Some queens have no rise in serum LH level following a single mating and their LH levels are greater and more prolonged when multiple matings are permitted.[4,7] Therefore, queens that require a greater stimulus to induce an increase of LH and subsequent ovulation should be allowed to mate repeatedly with a vigorous male.

Ovulation has traditionally been accepted as occurring between 24 to 32 hours after copulation; it recently was reported that ovulation occurs approximately 50 hours following the LH peak.[8] Corpora lutea appear as 4.0- to 4.5-mm masses in the ovaries. Along with development of corpora lutea, serum progesterone levels begin to rise 3 to 5 days after mating and they usually peak at 30 to 80 ng/ml between days 11 to 23 of pregnancy (Fig 3).[5,8] Levels gradually decline to 10 ng/ml by day 60 and fall below 1 ng/ml just after parturition.[5] During pregnancy, estradiol remains low and rises sharply to 20 to 40 pg/ml just before parturition.

Prolactin level increases gradually in the latter half of pregnancy and there is a significant rise (43.5 ng/ml) 3 days prepartum. It remains close to 40 ng/ml during the first 4 weeks of lactation. During the last 2 weeks of lactation, the prolactin level declines to less than 30 ng/ml; basal levels are reached 2 weeks after weaning.[9]

Ova are fertilized in the ampulla of the uterine tube and transported to the uterus before the 6th day after copulation.[10] Implantation occurs at 11 to 13 days. The embryo and fetal membranes grow in the uterus as a well-defined spherical mass (10 to 20 mm in diameter) that may be palpated abdominally as early as the 18th day of gestation (Fig 4). Pregnancy may be identified in radiographs after the 42nd day. Average duration of gestation in cats is 65±3 days.

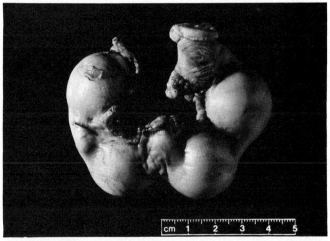

Fig 4. This uterus was surgically removed from a queen on the 24th day of gestation. Fetal membranes of the 4 embryos are well-defined and easily palpable enlargements.

Pseudopregnancy

Owners of cats may regard the continuous calling and posturing associated with the animals' estrus both inconvenient and irritating. They may wish to eliminate the objectionable behavior by temporarily ending cycling with a pseudopregnancy. This term (pseudopregnancy) refers to an interval in which corpora lutea are present and functioning but fetuses are not present in the uterus. It is not the equivalent of the familiar false pregnancy observed in bitches. The false pregnancy (often interchangeably called pseudopregnancy) in dogs is a pseudopregnancy accompanied by physical and behavioral changes that mimic the signs of true pregnancy, including mammary enlargement, lactation, and nesting activity. Feline pseudopregnancy is seldom accompanied by such physical and behavioral changes.

Pseudopregnancy can be induced in the cat by stimulation of the anterior vagina, coitus with a vasectomized male, or injections of human chorionic gonadotropin and, potentially, GnRH (25 μg IM). A glass rod or well-lubricated, cotton-tipped swab is used to stimulate the anterior vagina. The manipulation should simulate natural breeding. During vaginal stimulation the queen often cries sharply as during natural breeding. Vasectomized males may be used when ovulation is being induced in a large number of females.[11] Although some castrated males may breed, their use to induce ovulation is limited because the testosterone-dependent penile spines that provide vaginal stimulation become smaller in castrated cats. Human chorionic gonadotropin (250 to 500 IU) has been administered SC to induce ovulation.[12] Although induced ovulation has not been associated with adverse effects, no studies have evaluated the effect of induced ovulations on reproductive organs or reproductive performance.

The progesterone levels during pseudopregnancy rise similarly to those described for pregnancy, but decline to <1 ng/ml by day 40 or 42.[5,8] Therefore, regardless of the method used to induce ovulation, the pseudopregnancy will terminate as the corpora lutea regress and cycling normally resumes between 42 and 71 days following the induced ovulation.[8] Estrogen levels are low during pseudopregnancy, but periodic elevations have been demonstrated. This suggests that follicular activity continues even during the luteal phase.[8]

THE MALE

The following discussion of the male reproductive system in cats emphasizes factors that are known to or have the potential of adversely affecting reproductive performance. The collection and evaluation of semen are common in research laboratories, but they are seldom performed by practitioners. As a consequence there are few reports about the details of feline spermatogenesis. The basic hypothalamo-hypophyseal-gonadal axis is apparently similar to that of other domestic animals, but there have been no reports about the levels of the male cat's steroid hormone, gonadotropic hormone, or releasing hormone. In addition, there are only a few case reports that deal with the reproductivity of male cats.

Male Sexual Organs

Testicles

The testicles of male kittens are descended at birth and they may be palpated in the scrotum. The testes and epididymides gain most markedly in size and weight when the kitten is 3 to 5 months of age. Lipid-containing interstitial cells and seminiferous tubules with diameters of 70 to 110 microns are present. A testis of a 5-month-old male may have mitotic figures in the spermatogonia, but spermatozoa are not present until the cat is 7 to 9 months old.[13] Although males in late adolescence may fertilize a queen, the quality and concentration of their semen are inferior to that of adult males. To protect a male cat's breeding record, he should not be used for breeding until after he is 1 year of age. The weight gain of the male cat's testes parallels his gain in body weight.[11] In the same way that body weight may be lowered by poor nutrition or illness, maturation of the testes may be slowed by the same factors.

Although female cats cycle seasonally, males are fertile and will breed throughout the year. Semen quality declines with advancing age, but the rate of change is unknown.

The male cat ejaculates semen with low volume and high sperm concentration. A normal healthy male can breed as frequently as 3 times a week or daily for 3 days without seriously depleting the concentration of sperm.[14] More frequent breeding may result in smaller litters or conception failure. Feline spermatozoa must be in the uterus for 2 to 24 hours before they are capable of fertilizing ova.[15]

Anything that increases testicular temperature will depress spermatogenesis. Local infections of the scrotum or testis, scrotal dermatitis, and pyrexia may temporarily depress production of sperm. If the condition is corrected, sperm quantity and quality should improve within 30 to 60 days.

Both bilateral and unilateral cryptorchidism occur in the cat. The retained testicles produce testosterone, but not sperm. Bilaterally affected males are sterile. Though unilateral cryptorchids are fertile, breeding of these animals is discouraged because cryptorchidism can be inherited.

Inadequate libido is occasionally a breeding problem, especially in tomcats with little breeding experience. Although testosterone defi-

ciency is not known to be the cause of depressed libido, injections of
this hormone (0.25 to 0.5 mg/kg) are given as treatment. Excessive
use of testosterone should be avoided because it may suppress gonadotropin secretion. Hypothyroidism and other endocrine diseases are
also potential causes of depressed libido and fertility.

Cats with tricolor haircoats, tortoiseshell or calico, are usually
females because the genes for orange and black haircoat colors are
alleles on the X chromosomes. Therefore, 2 of these chromosomes
must be present to have a tricolor haircoat and males have only one.
A few tortoiseshell or calico males have been found. Some arise
through aneuploidy and have sex chromatin of XXY. This abnormality resembles Klinefelter's syndrome in human males, in which the affected humans are sterile. Other tricolor males may arise through
mosaicism or chimerism with sex chromatin of XY/XXY or XX/XY,
XY/XY respectively.[16] Males in which all or part of the cells contain
XXY chromatin are sterile. A few chimeric male cats have been
reported to be fertile.

Penis
The feline penis is conical and the glans penis is covered with
epithelial spines. The spines' development parallels the secretion of
testosterone. In the adult male cat the penile spines regress to half
their original size within 2 months after castration.[17] The spines
stimulate the vaginal mucosa and thus serve to induce ovulation. The
feline penis contains a bone that is 3 to 4 mm in length. Unlike the
canine os penis, this bone in cats does not surround the urethra. The
urethral diameter was once believed to decrease following prepubertal castration and thus be a factor in the urethral blockage caused by
calculi. It has been demonstrated, however, that castration does not
affect the urethra's diameter.[18]

The pain and discomfort of urethritis will inhibit breeding performance. After removing the cause of urethritis and preventing sexual
activity for 1 or 2 months, the cat can be used for breeding again.
Long-haired male cats may occasionally have hair wrapped around
the penis, which could inhibit breeding. Such rings of hair should be
carefully removed.

Acessory Sex Glands
The male cat has bulbourethral glands that secrete sulfated
mucopolysaccharides. The prostate gland is similar in shape to the
dog's, but the cat also has a poorly developed prostate composed of
isolated lobules disseminated along the urethra. The epithelium of the
bladder neck contains glycogen and is probably the origin of seminal

fructose.[19] Unlike the dog, which has a relatively high incidence of prostatic hyperplasia, neoplasia, and infections, the cat's prostate is seldom the site of disease.

Natural Mating

The cat is more nocturnal and secretive about breeding than the dog and thus the mating ritual is not frequently observed. Clinicians should be aware of natural breeding behavior so that they can evaluate failures in breeding.

In the mating ritual the male approaches the female cautiously and they rub their heads and bodies. Both animals may vocalize during this period. The female assumes a crouching position, frequently treads the ground, and may roll and stretch repeatedly (Fig 1). She may rebuff the male when he approaches; an indication of acceptance is the position of her tail. The queen will elevate the tail and deviate it to one side (Fig 1). Dog breeders refer to this tail gesture as "flagging". To facilitate coitus the female places her hindlimbs in a position that causes the vulva to be rotated horizontally with the ground. The male eventually grasps the dorsum of the female's neck in his teeth and then mounts (Fig 4). The grasp automatically positions the male for coitus and aids in restraint of the female. Male cats that quickly learn to grasp the female's neck securely usually become good breeders. Tomcats that do not grasp the queen correctly may lack adequate control of the female. Copulation lasts only a few seconds and is manifested by a series of sharp pelvic thrusts by the male. At the termination of breeding the queen usually screams sharply. The male quickly dismounts and retreats to some distance from the queen. During the first 10 to 20 minutes after breeding, the queen will stretch and roll, and lick her vulva. The queen may breed again within an hour with either the same or another male. Therefore, a multiple-sire litter is possible and breeders of cats should be cautioned to prevent another mating after the intended sire has bred the queen.

Copulation Failure

Although most breedings are uncomplicated, veterinarians occasionally must deal with complaints of copulation failure. Most reasons for a delay in or failure to breed are related to animal behavior and they may become apparent by taking a thorough history. For example, it is customary to transport the female to the male cat for breeding because the male prefers to breed in a familiar area that he has marked with his scent. Forcing a tomcat to breed in unfamiliar territory may not preclude breeding, but it may take the male some time to adjust to the unfamiliar environment. Occasionally the pairing of a short-bodied male with a long-bodied female will delay breeding. If such a tomcat instinctively grasps the queen's neck in the proper place, his genitalia will not be located properly for copulation. In such cases the male may adjust his position voluntarily, but it may be necessary for the owners to reposition the tomcat. Human intervention, however, often terminates any further effort by the cats to breed.

The female cat may also be responsible for delay or failure in copulation. Overanxious owners may attempt to breed cats during the queen's proestrus and she will not accept the male at this time. When this occurs, the owners should be advised to wait for 1 or 2 days and then to reunite the pair. A queen may occasionally reject a specific male. The reasons might be related to the male's haircoat color or pattern, body size, or odor. When this occurs, other males should be tried. Some females appear to be in estrus when in their regular environment, but when they are transported to the male all signs of estrus disappear. Queens that react in this manner are often sheltered animals with little contact with other cats. Their behavior during estrus may be subdued by fear associated with a change in environment or transportation. In such cases several compensatory approaches are possible. The queen might be left in the male's breeding area because she may relax enough to resume normal behavior and mate. Alternatively, she might be placed in the breeding environment several days in advance of estrus to allow time for adjustment.

It is sometimes helpful to pair a novice breeding animal with an experienced male for the first breeding. Though 2 novice breeders will probably mate eventually, experience will usually hasten breeding. Novice breeders should be protected from males that are known to be very aggressive or vicious. An initial breeding experience that is injurious or intimidating may interfere with an animal's future performance as a breeder.

References
1. Scott, PP and LLoyd-Jacob, MA: Nature (London) **184** (1959) 2022.
2. Hurni, H: Lab Anim **15** (1981) 229.
3. Wildt, DE et al: Hormones and Behavior **10** (1978) 251.
4. Wildt, DE et al: Endocrinology **107** (1980) 1212.
5. Verhage, HG et al: Biol Reprod **14** (1976) 579.
6. Shille, VM et al: Biol Reprod **21** (1979) 953.
7. Johnson, LM and Gay, VL: Endocrinology **109** (1981) 247.
8. Wildt, DE et al: Biol Reprod **25** (1981) 15.
9. Banks, DR and Stabenfeldt, GH: Biol Reprod **24** (1981) Suppl 1, 63A.

10. Herron, MA and Sis, RF: Amer J Vet Res **35** (1974) 1277.
11. Herron, MA and Herron, MR: MVP June (1972) 41.
12. Wildt, DE and Seager, SWJ: Hormone Res **9** (1978) 144.
13. Scott, MF and Scott, PP: J Physiol **136** (1957) 40.
14. Sojka, NJ *et al:* Lab Anim Care **20** (1970) 198.
15. Hamner, CE *et al:* J Reprod Fert **23** (1970) 477.
16. Certerwall, WR and Benirschke, K: Amer J Vet Res **36** (1975) 1275.
17. Aronson, LR and Cooper, ML: Anat Record **157(1)** (1967) 71.
18. Herron, MA: JAVMA **160** (1972) 208.
19. Aitken, RN and Aughey, E: Res Vet Sci **5** (1964) 268.

CANINE PHYSIOLOGY OF REPRODUCTION
BY PATRICK W. CONCANNON

Introduction

This review is based extensively on observations made in the author's laboratory during the last 10 years as well as on previous reviews of the topic.[1-29] It also includes observations made of a colony of Beagles and experiences of colleagues in the Small Animal Clinic at the New York State College of Veterinary Medicine. The review also refers to recently published reports based on research of canine reproduction during the last several years.[30-35]

Much of the following information has been incorporated into veterinary teaching programs and may be merely a review and update for recent graduates. Some of the material, however, may represent entirely new viewpoints or information for veterinarians who have been in practice for several years and to breeders or pet owners. In some instances the observations may not be consistent with previously-held assumptions or viewpoints. For that reason and despite the redundancy, this review is divided into overlapping sections. The follicular and luteal phases of ovarian activity will be considered first; then the other genital changes during proestrus, estrus, metestrus, and anestrus; and finally the secretion patterns of individual hormones associated with different stages of the estrous cycle. This is followed by a review of the fertile cycle, events during gestation, and pregnancy-specific alterations in hormone levels, ovarian activity, and maternal physiology.

Though reproductive physiology of the ovarian cycle and pregnancy has not been studied as extensively in the bitch as in

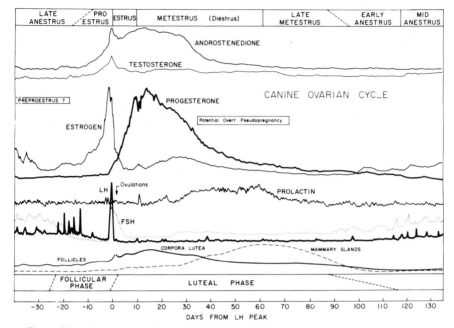

Fig 1. Typical endocrine changes reported or presumed to occur during the non-pregnant ovarian cycle in dogs, and their relation to observable stages and functional phases of the cycle.[29]

larger domestic animals or the more common species of laboratory animals, a considerable amount of new information has been reported in the last 10 years. It still is important, however, to recognize some of the pioneering and landmark studies in this field.[36-41]

Phases of the Ovarian Cycle

The changes in hormone levels associated with the follicular phase, ovulation, and luteal phase of the nonfertile canine ovarian cycle are shown in Figure 1. The extent of follicle development is often not readily apparent on the canine ovary because the ovary is nearly completely enclosed in a bursa. In adult bitches the bursa is usually not transparent due to fat content and the bursal slit is normally too small to enable a clear view of the ovarian surface (Fig 2a). Furthermore, the follicles do not bulge above the ovarian surface until just prior to ovulation. They remain below the ovarian surface throughout most of their development, appearing as grayish, semitransparent foci on the surface of the ovary (Figs 2a, b).

Follicular phase

Bitches ovulate spontaneously at the end of a 1 to 3 week follicular phase. As follicles develop in the ovaries they produce

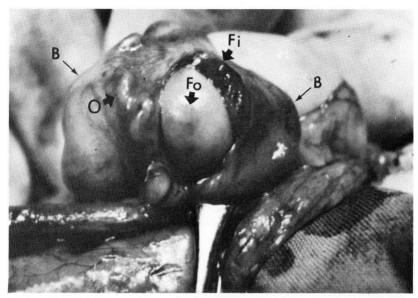

Fig 2a. Ovary of a bitch in proestrus exposed by cutting the bursa (B) which normally encloses the ovary completely except for a small slit through which the fimbriated end of the oviduct normally protrudes during proestrus and estrus. Fo-follicle is beginning to show as a darker area on surface of the ovary. Fi-part of the fleshy, hyperemic fimbriated end of the oviduct. O-portion of the oviduct prominent on the surface of the bursa.

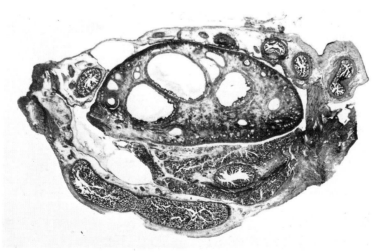

Fig 2b. Histologic section of an ovary removed from a bitch in proestrus reveals the ovary entirely surrounded by the bursa. Cross sections of oviduct with proliferated epithelium protruding into the lumen can be seen throughout the bursa. The rippled surfaces of 3 largest ovarian follicles are areas of proestrus luteinization prior to the LH surge.

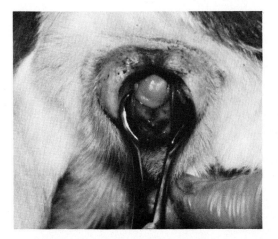

Fig 3. Hypertrophy of floor of vagina often seen during proestrus or estrus. In extreme cases, area can become tumescent and protrude from vulva as a large spherical mass up to 10 cm in diameter, which regresses at end of estrus.

estradiol that progressively increases serum estradiol from basal levels of 2 to 10 pg/ml to peak levels of 50 to 120 pg/ml.[1,35] Concurrent increases in estrone, testosterone, and androstenedione have also been found. The increased estrogen causes external signs of proestrus to become increasingly evident. These include vaginal discharge of

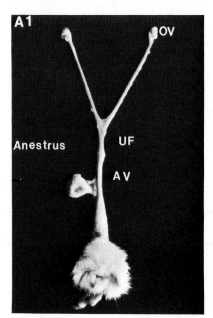
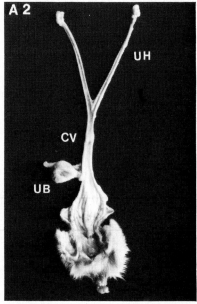

Figs 4a-c. Ventral views of reproductive tracts removed from bitches during (A) anestrus, (B) late proestrus, and (C) early metestrus (day 15) of nonpregnant cycle, shown intact (left), and cut open dorsally to expose the vaginal mucosa and endometrium (right). OV-ovary. UH-uterine horn. UF-uterine fundus. CV-cervix. B-urinary bladder. AV-anterior vagina in which the natural lumen is usually occluded by the dorsal median fold-DMF.

uterine blood; enlargement, edema, and hyperemia of the vulva and perineum; and hypertrophy of the floor of the posterior vagina (Fig 3), all of which can be observed by direct inspection. Increased estrogen causes the uterine horns to lengthen and begin to form folds and it also causes the cervix to enlarge until it is readily palpable and the entire vaginal wall is thickened (Figs 4a-c).

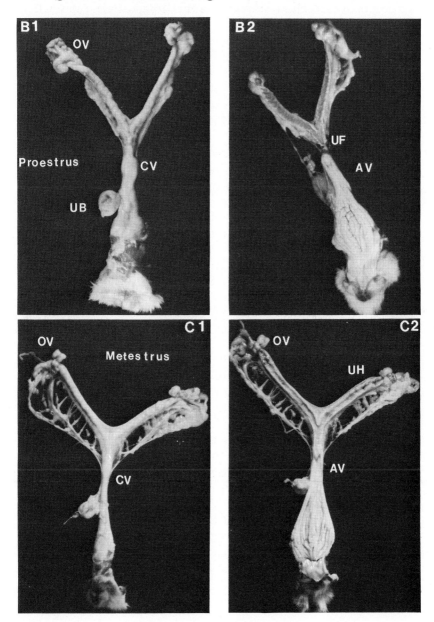

The rise in estrogen level also promotes secretion of sex phero-
mone(s) and attraction of males. During proestrus, however, the bitch
will not permit mounting and intromission. Behavior associated with
proestrus usually lasts 5 to 10 days but can be observed for 2 to 22
days. The transition from proestrus to estrus occurs when the bitch
permits copulation and stands firmly for the stud. In most instances,
this occurs in association with events that comprise the culmination
of follicle development: a decline in estrogen secretion and in serum
estrogen levels; a rapid increase in previously initiated follicle luteinization; a corresponding increase in serum progesterone levels;
and the occurrence of the preovulatory surge release of luteinizing
hormone (LH) from the anterior pituitary.[1,4] The LH release is the
trigger for ovulation. Ovulation occurs about 2 days later.[4] The histologic details of preovulatory follicular development and ovulation are
shown in Figures 5-10.

The change from refusal to acceptance of the male in the transition from proestrus to estrus may occur rapidly (within 8 to 12 hours)
or slowly (1 to 3 days). Though it usually occurs synchronously with
the preovulatory LH release, it can also occur out of synchrony with
the LH surge. It is not uncommon for the onset of estrus (and potential first day of mating) to occur as early as 2 to 3 days before the LH
peak or as late as 4 to 5 days after the peak. Therefore, the first day of
estrus (the first day that the bitch stands firmly for the male with
steady tail deviation and presentation of the vulva to allow intromission) may commonly occur as early as 5 days before ovulation or as
late as 2 to 3 days after ovulation. There are more detailed descriptions of sexual behavior in the bitch throughout the ovarian
cycle.[1,4,9,42]

Preovulatory Luteinization and Ovulation
The hormonal changes during the LH surge in late proestrus or
early estrus reflect the transition from the follicular phase to the
luteal phase of the cycle. Corpora lutea are strictly defined as histologically transformed, progesterone-secreting structures that form
from follicles after ovulation. In the bitch, however, follicles slowly
begin to luteinize during mid-proestrus before estrogen secretion is
maximal, and then undergo a more rapid, extensive luteinization during the preovulatory LH surge. The ovulating follicles thus have
many of the characteristics of, and in fact are, rapidly developing corpora lutea (Figs 9, 10). Serum progesterone levels during proestrus
rise from 0.4 to 0.6 ng/ml to reach 0.8 to 1.2 ng/ml at the time of peak
estrogen levels. Progesterone then increases rapidly throughout the

Figs 5 to 10. Stained sections of ovaries (Beagle) removed during proestrus and estrus. Each section reproduced (a) at 5X and (b) at 55X.
Biol Reprod **17** (1977) 604.

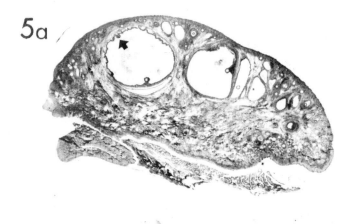

Fig 5. Ovary removed on day 3 of proestrus prior to preovulatory LH
surge. Plasma progesterone was 0.9 ng/ml. a. Two growing
preovulatory follicles with membrana granulosa thrown into slight
folds (arrow).

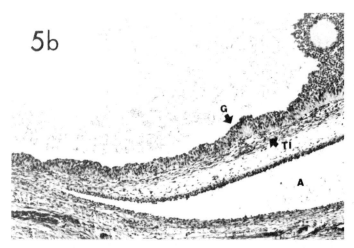

b. An atretic follicle (A) is compressed by a growing preovulatory follicle with an oocyte attached to cumulus. Granulosa cells (G) are
elongated and theca interna (TI) contains many hypertrophied cells.

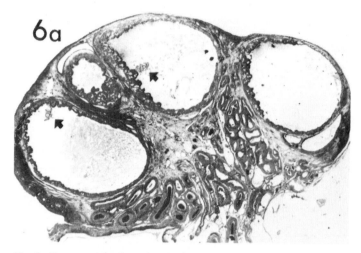

Fig 6. Ovary removed on day 5 of proestrus 8 hours after LH peak, when plasma progesterone was 2.8 ng/ml. a. Four preovulatory follicles with infolded walls containing detaching oocytes (arrows). Crescent-shaped vesicular follicles are atretic.

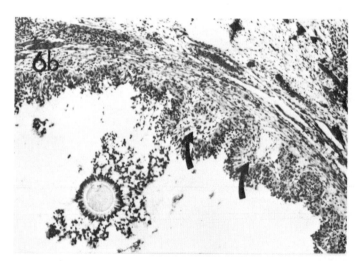

b. Cumulus cells are dispersed between detaching oocyte and follicle wall. Hypertrophied thecal cells and thecal blood vessels are incorporated into mural folds (arrows).

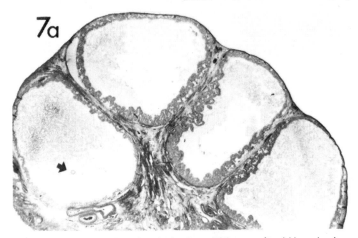

Fig 7. Ovary removed on day 4 of estrus, 36 hours after LH peak when plasma progesterone was 3.3 ng/ml. a. Free-floating antral oocyte (arrow) is seen in one of the 4 preovulatory follicles.

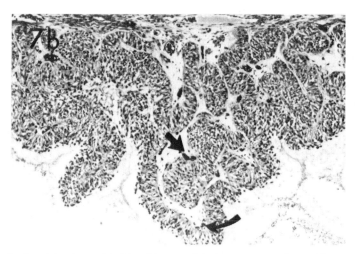

b. Luteinized mural folds with vacuolated secretory cells and incorporation of thecal blood vessels (arrows).

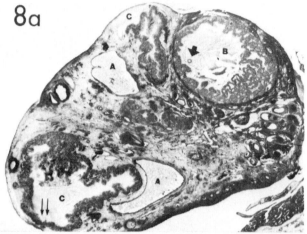

Fig 8. Ovary removed on day 4 of estrus, 44 hours after LH peak when plasma progesterone was 4.4 ng/ml. a. Atretic follicles (A), preovulatory follicle (B) containing free-floating antral oocyte (arrow) and 2 recently ovulated developing corpora lutea (C). Double arrows indicate wall of corpus sectioned 1 mm from rupture site.

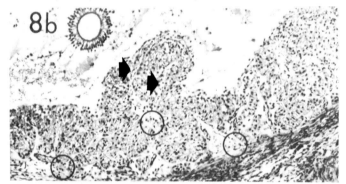

b. Details of preovulatory follicle showing ingrowth of thecal blood vessels (arrows) deeply into mural folds of vacuolated luteinized cells. Except for a few isolated nests of theca interna cells (circles), theca-derived cells are not readily distinguishable from granulosa-derived cells within the mural folds.

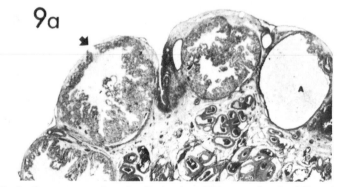

Fig 9. Ovary removed on day 2 of estrus 50 hours after the LH peak when progesterone was 6.9 ng/ml. a. Three recently ovulated developing corpora lutea and a partially luteinized atretic follicle (A); arrow indicates rupture site of one of the corpora.

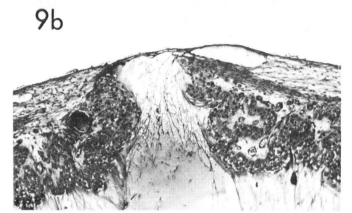

b. Detail of rupture site.

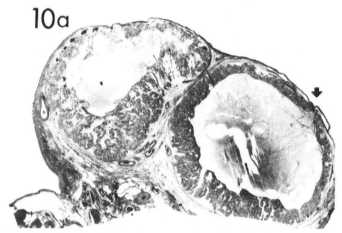

Fig 10. Ovary removed on day 3 of estrus 96 hours after the LH peak when progesterone was 9.4 ng/ml. a. Two developing corpora lutea, in one of which the rupture site was still unrepaired (arrow).

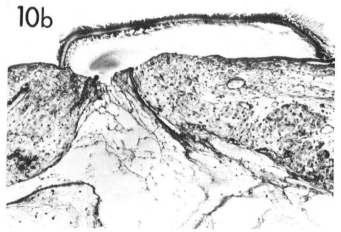

a. Details of rupture site with luteal cells lining the antrum and with a bleb of congealed follicular fluid on the outer surface of ovary (top).

LH surge as estrogen levels decline. Serum progesterone levels are usually 2 to 4 ng/ml at the time of the LH peak, and 4 to 8 ng/ml at the time of ovulation 2 days later.

Luteal Phase

Serum progesterone levels continue to increase throughout the 5 to 15 days during which estrous behavior is usually observed. They reach a peak of 15 to 80 ng/ml between 15 and 25 days after the LH peak as the corpora lutea become fully developed (Fig 11). Corpora lutea continue to secrete progesterone and serum progesterone levels are usually above 1 ng/ml for 2 months or more after the LH peak and onset of estrus.

The pattern of secretion and the variation in duration of secretion differ, however, in pregnant and nonpregnant bitches. In nonpregnant bitches progesterone levels slowly decline, reach 1 ng/ml between 55 to 110 days after ovulation, and may not reach basal levels of 0.3 to 0.4 ng/ml until 120 to 150 days after the LH peak.

Duration of the luteal phase, and thus of the post-estrus or metestrus period of ovarian activity, is variable and any stated duration would depend on what criterion is being considered. The luteal phase in the nonpregnant bitch can be stated to last "about" 2 months, as in pregnancy; 2-3 months when mammary development associated with overt or covert pseudopregnancy subsides; about 80 days when average progesterone levels fall to 1 ng/ml; 100 to 160 days when progesterone levels reach anestrous basal values of <0.5 ng/ml; or 120 to 140 days when the effect of progesterone on the endometrium is no longer evident.[39] The transition from metestrus (the end of a nonpregnant luteal phase) into anestrus thus involves progressive changes that are variable within and among bitches. Likewise, the transition from anestrus into the subsequent proestrus also involves slow progressive changes associated with the onset of the next follicular phase.

New Follicular Phase

The possibility that a "pre-proestrus" period of follicular activity may occur regularly should be acknowledged. Anestrous bitches whose ovaries and uterus were removed between 150 and 180 days following the onset of estrus exhibited no external signs of impending proestrus but did exhibit evidence of ovarian follicular activity, including gross uterine and oviductal hyperemia, enlarged oviductal fimbria protruding through the bursal slit, and a markedly sanguine endometrium. Perhaps the period of "anestrus" is a physiological

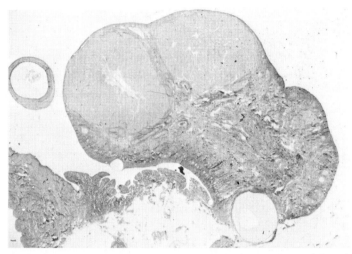

Fig 11a. Section of canine ovary with fully developed corpora lutea at day 20 of a nonpregnant cycle.

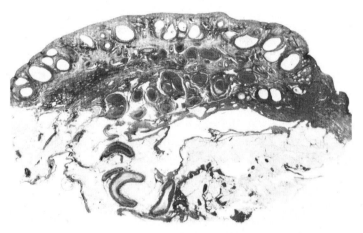

Fig 11b. Section of an ovary from an anestrous bitch showing follicles in various stages of development and atresia.

"nonevent," at least following a nonpregnant cycle, and represents the transition from the late luteal phase of one cycle to the early follicular phase of the next cycle.

Antral follicles in various stages of development and atresia are always present on the ovary (Fig 11) and a basal estrogen secretion

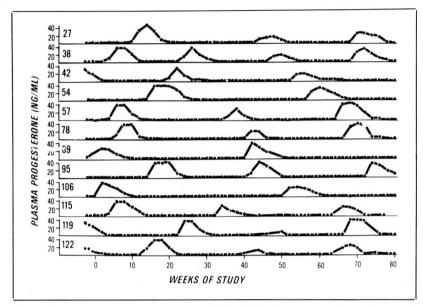

Fig 12. Plasma progesterone levels in 12 Beagle bitches over an 18-month period, during which the number of complete ovarian cycles, as represented by luteal phase increases in progesterone, ranged from 2 (bitch #54) to 4 (bitch #38).

always keeps secretion of LH below levels seen in ovariectomized bitches.[2] Variable elevations in serum estradiol levels observed during anestrus may indicate that, especially when the interestrus interval is greater than 7 months, the ovaries may make several "attempts" to develop vesicular follicles before emergence of synchronous follicles that are able to mature normally.

Cycle Intervals

The interval from one estrous cycle to the next can range from 3.5 to 13 months and it may be consistent or variable within individual bitches. In our Beagle colony the shortest and longest intervals consistently recorded for individual bitches have been about 4 months and 10 months, respectively. The longest interval that could be verified by serial measurement of progesterone was 13 months. Intervals between subsequent estrous periods that were longer than 13 months have always included an intervening ovulatory cycle and luteal phase for which external signs were not observed (Fig 12). The mean interval between cycles is about 7 months. Though studies of differences in mean interestrous intervals among breeds have involved too few animals to be meaningful, there is some evidence that it may be only 5 to 6 months in German Shepherds.[44] Some breeds have only one estrous cycle a year.

Environmental factors can also affect the interval between estrous cycles. In large commercial kennels it is common practice to place an anestrous bitch with or next to a bitch in estrus to induce a premature cycle. The anestrous bitches will often show signs of proestrus within 1 or 2 weeks. Similarly, bitches that are housed together often have synchronous cycles. The response is assumed to be pheromone-induced and olfaction-dependent.

Seasonality

The interestrous interval can vary considerably within as well as among bitches, even when they are housed in similar environments. Estrus is observed at all times of the year in outdoor kennels, although there can be a tendency for a greater incidence in the late winter or early spring and again in the late summer or early autumn.[38] This tendency usually disappears when bitches are kept under artificial lighting for 12L:12D or 14L:10D. When artificial lighting is supplemented by natural light, the incidence of cycles at the solstices may then decrease. The tendency for some dogs to cycle at nearly 6-month intervals, spring and autumn, is thus likely to be influenced by the annual photoperiod.

The annual change in the daily photoperiod must likewise be a major factor in regulation of the single annual or circannual estrous cycle observed in Basenjis and also, apparently, in Tibetan Mastiffs. These 2 breeds routinely cycle during the autumnal equinox or shortly thereafter. These photoperiod effects are probably mediated via modulation of pineal secretions. Indolamines, including melatonin, and argine vasotocin have been shown to have an inhibitory effect on LH release in the dog.[45]

It is possible that unnatural light exposure in homes or small kennels might contribute to apparent infertility or prolonged anestrus. There are no data, however, that enable prediction of the probable effects of persistent "long days" or "short days" or of inconsistent light schedules on canine ovarian cycles.

Stages of the Estrous Cycle

The ovarian cycle of the bitch is best considered in terms of follicular and luteal phases and the corresponding changes in circulating levels of estrogen, LH, and progesterone. Most observations are usually restricted, however, to externally visible criteria when recording the reproductive history or status of a bitch. It thus is necessary to refer to the classical stages of the canine cycle and to appreciate the extent to which their meaning and usage can and do vary.

Estrus is a behavioral term that has an etymological history of meaning gadfly, sting, frenzy, female sexual frenzy, and presentation to males or acceptance of a male. Estrus in the bitch lasts about a week and is the period during which the bitch will accept mounting by a male and assume an obvious sexual posture while doing so. This includes standing steadily with marked extension of the hindlimbs, raising the perineum, and deviating the tail to one side. In contrast, during the preceding week or so of proestrus the bitch resists attempts at mounting or intromission initially by confronting the male and later by retreating, sitting, or crouching. In late proestrus the bitch may stand passively without a positive sexual posture.

Metestrus is the period after estrus during which there is evidence of progesterone secretion. The subsequent anestrus is usually described as a period of ovarian quiescence because there is no external evidence of ovarian activity.

Proestrus

Details of endocrine, behavioral, and vaginal changes during proestrus and estrus are shown schematically in Figure 13. The first evidence of proestrus may be vulval enlargement or bloody vaginal discharge. One may precede the other by 1 to 4 days or they may occur simultaneously. Some bitches may be so fastidious in cleaning the vulva that the bloody discharge is not observed even though it is present in the vagina. This blood originates in the uterus and is the result of diapedesis.

Proestrus lasts an average of 5 to 9 days, but it may be as short as 2 to 3 days or as long as 3 to 4 weeks. Vulval tumescence increases throughout proestrus and reaches maximal size and turgidity in late proestrus at the peak level of estrogen.

During proestrus the bitch is attractive to males because of the secretion of one or more sex pheromones, an active component of which has been reported to be methyl-hydroxybenzoate.[46] In early proestrus the bitch is antisexual and she will growl, retreat, or fight in response to attempts by males to mount. As proestrus progresses the increasing level of estrogen causes the bitch to become more passive or confused and results in playful and teasing behavior, but this behavior is generally asexual. In late proestrus, this behavior may continue, though the bitch is often passive to attempts at

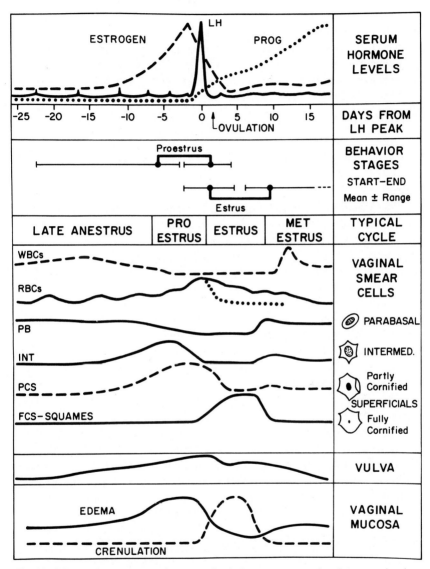

Fig 13. Schematic summary of temporal relations among periovulatory endocrine events, behavioral and vulval changes, and general changes in vaginal exfoliate cytology associated with proestrus and estrus in the bitch.[27]

mounting and will either stand without promoting intromission or will sit, crouch, or lie down when mounted.

During the middle or late stages of proestrus, a bitch may display masculine behavior, mount other dogs (both males and females) and even exhibit pelvic thrusting while maintaining a firm grasp on her partner with the forelimbs. Such masculine behavior could be related to increased secretion of androgen at the end of the follicular phase; testosterone and androstenedione have been observed to increase at this time.[23,47] In our Beagle colony we have observed masculine behavior during proestrus that was induced in bitches by injecting estrogen alone. It thus appears that male behavior by bitches in proestrus is due to the action of estrogen on the central nervous system.

Estrus

The transition from the passive or confused behavior of a bitch during late proestrus to the positive sexual behavior during estrus can be observed by testing daily the bitch's response to a male. During estrus the bitch continues to display playful and teasing behavior, but will stand steadily and deviate the tail to one side when the male prods her, licks at her vulva, or starts to mount. The sexually aggressive and experienced bitch will often turn her perineum towards the male, back into him, and even pout her vulva at him, especially if he is not steady and aggressive in his attempts to mount. Some bitches will often show a preference for one male over another and one male may elicit a full display of estrous behavior while another may not.

The onset of estrus often occurs rapidly over 8 to 32 hours within 1 day of the LH surge. In ovariectomized bitches given sex steroids, proestrous behavior was associated with continuous increases in blood levels of estrogen. Estrous behavior was triggered by a subsequent fall in estrogen level and could be facilitated by a simultaneous increase in progesterone.[9] Similar experiments indicated that a rapid decline in the estrogen:progesterone ratio will also produce a preovulatory-like surge in LH. The onset of estrus in normal bitches, however, may be asynchronous with the LH peak.[4,16] It can be as early as 3 days before the LH surge, especially in sexually experienced bitches. Such an "early" onset of estrus is probably caused by a transient decline in estrogen or a rise in progesterone prior to the final peak in estrogen. The onset of estrus can also be as late as 4 to 6 days after the LH surge and 2 to 4 days after ovulation, especially in pubertal bitches. This may indicate a relative insensitivity of behavioral centers to the initial decline in the estrogen:progesterone ratio at the time of the LH peak.

Abnormal Estrus: A transition from proestrous to estrous behavior may not occur and what appears to be a prolonged proestrus slowly subsides. This may be due to a failure in LH release and subsequent failure of mature follicles to luteinize and ovulate though they continue to produce diminishing amounts of estrogen for some time without an acute fall in estrogen level. More often, however, prolonged proestrus and failure of estrus occur when behavioral centers fail to respond to normal hormonal levels.

Another type of "false heat" can also occur. A bitch can exhibit signs of a normal proestrus during follicular development and then, in the absence of an LH surge or ovulation, display an apparently normal estrus or intermittent periods of estrous behavior. This presumably occurs in response to the decline in estrogen levels during atresia of the nonovulating follicles.[48] A false proestrus or false estrus related to failure to ovulate is often followed by a normal cycle within 3 to 4 weeks. Such a false estrus is not uncommon in anestrous bitches that fail to ovulate in response to FSH or gonadotropin-releasing hormone given to induce ovulation.[24]

Duration of Estrus: Estrous behavior in a typical cycle lasts 6 to 12 days. It may be abbreviated to 2 to 3 days when the onset of estrus is delayed in relation to the LH peak and ovulation. It can also be protracted as long as 3 weeks and in some cases estrus may ocur intermittently or variably for even longer periods. A bitch in our Beagle colony exhibited estrous behavior almost daily through the 40th day of her pregnancy. Even in normal estrous cycles the end of estrus may not be acute but extend for 3 to 6 days of less intense estrous behavior.Studies of vaginal cytology and morphology provide better evidence about the end of the fertile period of estrus and the beginning of metestrus. They should be performed to determine the end of the fertile period or to estimate retrospectively the time of previous matings in relation to ovulation.

Copulation: Following a variable period of pelvic thrusting, complete insertion of the penis is followed quickly by ejaculation of a small (1 to 5 ml) sperm-rich fraction of semen and dismounting by the male. The male dismounts by lifting one of his hindlimbs over the back of the bitch, thereby causing an 180° torsion of the base of the penis just behind the bulbus. Due to the torsion and lateral deflection of the penis at the same point, it remains within the vagina throughout the coital lock, which usually lasts for 5 to 30 minutes. During the coital lock or "tie" a large volume of prostatic fluid (5 to 30 ml) is ejaculated, presumably facilitating the passage of semen through the cervix (Fig 14). Though the physiology of penile erection and the coital lock have been studied, the mechanics of the lock are poorly understood.[34]

Period of Fertility: Such nonspecific terms as "in heat" or "in season" cause an unfortunate but unavoidable problem when discussing with pet owners the condition of a bitch for which there is concern about her fertility or reproductive status. Though such terms can be useful in reporting much of the reproductive history of the bitch, they are useless when used in reference to the actual events and course of an individual cycle or attempts to breed. It is important that the owners understand that a bitch's normal "heat" or period of attractiveness to males consists of 2 distinct parts — a preparatory phase (proestrus) of variable length in which she will not allow copulation followed by a receptive period (estrus) of variable duration during part of which fertility is maximal.

Single matings as early as 3 days before the LH peak (5 days before ovulation and 6 to 7 days before ovum maturation) can be fertile. Though not routinely, matings initiated as late as 8 days after the LH peak can also be fertile. In rare instances, matings as late as 9 to 10 days after the LH surge (and thus 7 to 8 days after ovulation) may be fertile and result in birth of the litter 55 to 57 days after mating. Peak fertility is associated with matings 0 to 5 days after the LH peak. Because of the variability in the onset of estrus and potential time of first mating, it thus is advisable to recommend matings as early as possible in estrus, followed by 2nd and 3rd matings at 2-day intervals. Such a schedule enables early mating of a bitch that doesn't "stand" until after ovulation and provides a late mating for a bitch that starts accepting the male 5 or more days before she ovulates.

In the absence of a sexually aggressive male or when the bitch has a history of conception failure or abnormal estrous behavior, scheduling of breeding or artificial insemination can be a problem. Nonbehavioral criteria can be used to estimate the time of ovulation or to monitor the transition from the follicular phase to the luteal phase. Because of the variability associated with normal proestrus and estrous behavior, serial assessment of vaginal cytology, vaginal morphology and vulval swelling should be routinely considered when giving advice about breeding.[49,50]

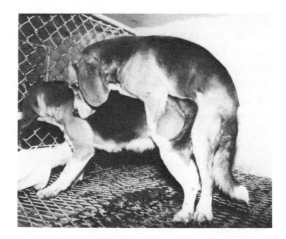

Fig 14. Copulation.
a. Coital lock maintained
after dismount may last
from 5 to 30 minutes.

b. Close up view of coital
lock in which the shaft of
the penis is held in the
vagina and bent over the
pelvic brim. The enlarged
bulbus glandis is held in
the vestibule and the base
of the penis behind the
bulbus is twisted 180° on
its axis and 180° laterally,
permitting the penis to
maintain its normal orientation within the vagina.

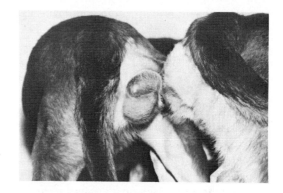

c. Dorsal view of the penis
with prepuce deflected
back and held manually in
same posterior direction to
collect semen. The enlarged
glandis is in collector's
hand and the collector's
fingers are constricting at
ring or preputial attachment
and point of torsion. The
urethral process projecting
in front of the slightly ex-
panded corona is maintained in its normal ventral
position.

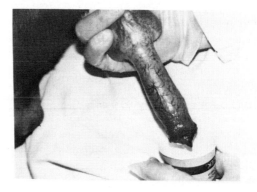

Vaginal Smears: Examination of vaginal smears at 1 to 2 day intervals can reveal the progression or not of proestrus to the completion of vaginal cornification indicative of follicle maturation. The expected changes in vaginal exfoliated cells are shown in Figure 13. When partially or fully cornified superficial cells comprise 95 to 100% of the cells in a smear and there is concomitant loss of leukocytes and nonsuperficial epithelial cells, it is an indication that estrogen secretion and follicle maturation have reached the point at which an LH surge will result in ovulation. A distinct, readily discernible change in the smear that reflects the occurrence of the LH surge, ovulation, or preovulatory progesterone secretion has not been found, however. Within 3 to 4 days after the LH peak fully cornified superficial cells often completely replace the partially cornified cells and dominate the smear from middle to late estrus. In some cases, partially cornified or even some intermediate cells may persist. Near the time of the LH peak a clearing of the background of a vaginal smear, possibly related to a decrease in mucoprotein content of the vaginal mucus, occurs in some but not all bitches. When this is observed in serial vaginal smears of an individual bitch, it probably reflects the decline in the estrogen:progesterone ratio near the LH peak and thus indicates the beginning of the optimal period to begin breeding.

The extent of vaginal cell cornification may not be as reliable an index of the onset of the occurrence of the estrogen peak as some reports would suggest. Furthermore, the cornification will vary with the fixation and staining methods used. When Shorr's trichrome stain or the rapid hematology stain from Harleco (Diff-Quik) is used, for example, fully cornified cells usually do not have discernible nuclei, but nuclear elements usually are visible in cornified cells stained with the Sano-Pollack trichrome method.[49] The hematology stain from Harleco is fast and easy to use, inexpensive, and useful for routine examination of progressive changes in vaginal smears.[50] A decrease in red blood cells in the vaginal smear, as well as a decrease in the vaginal discharge of blood, often but not routinely occurs in early estrus during preovulatory secretion of progesterone. A delay in breeding in anticipation of its occurrence is not recommended. In many cases the bloody discharge will continue throughout and beyond estrus and the fertile period; it can persist into metestrus.

Examination of vaginal smears on a daily or every other day basis may be helpful after full vaginal cornification has occurred or after breeding. An abrupt decrease in superficial cells and increase in nonsuperficial cells usually occurs about 7 or 8 days after the LH peak. It can be used to retrospectively determine the time of breeding in relation to the LH peak or ovulation. This reappearance of intermediate and parabasal cells in vaginal smears appears to occur at a rather consistent time after the abrupt preovulatory decline in estrogen. It probably indicates the last day that a previously unmated bitch is likely to be fertile. This shift in the vaginal smear can be considered the start of metestrus, independent of estrus behavior.

The reappearance of intermediate or parabasal cells among the superficial cells can occur as soon as 6 days and as late as 10 days after the LH peak. In most bitches it occurs on the 7th or 8th day and is usually unmistakable 9 to 10 days after the LH peak. This change in the vaginal smear in late estrus has also been termed the onset of diestrus.[51,52]

The term diestrus has been suggested as a replacement for metestrus in the canine ovarian cycle on the concept that diestrus is more appropriate for indicating the period of luteal activity and is more compatible with descriptions of the cycles of several other species. Because estrus lasts for some time during the beginning of the luteal phase in the bitch, however, metestrus (literally the period after estrus) seems to be an appropriate term for the remainder of the long luteal phase in the dog.

The reappearance of leukocytes in vaginal smears towards the end of estrus has also been used to indicate the end of the fertile period. This change may occur at a more variable time, however, in relation to prior endocrine events than does the abrupt reappearance of non-superficial epithelial cells. Though the reappearance of leukocytes may coincide with the shift in epithelial cells, it may also occur 1 to 2 days earlier or 2 to 4 days later and in some cases may not be abrupt.

Vaginal Endoscopy: Visualization of gross changes in the vaginal mucosa may also be helpful. As estrogen increases during proestrus the vaginal mucosa is initially pink and then pink-white and progressively more edematous, rounded, puffy, and turgid. Near the LH peak the white, rounded, smooth mucosal prominences initially become slightly shrunken, sacculated, or folded and then the mucosa rapidly develops a more wrinkled surface that is markedly peaked or crenulated. These gross changes probably reflect an abrupt withdrawal of the water-retention effects of estrogen during the hormone's preovulatory decline. The crenated, dehydrated appearance of the vaginal mucosa persists for 5 to 6 days and then disappears at about the same time as the metestrus-shift in the vaginal smear. Low, flaccid vaginal folds are then formed.[53,54] The appearance of the vaginal mucosa can be inspected best with a fiberoptic endoscope, and it is also seen satisfactorily with a small, light-fitted proctoscope.

Vulval Swelling: The vulva and adjacent perineum become progressively enlarged and turgid throughout proestrus. The swelling is maintained to a considerable degree throughout proestrus and estrus, but in many bitches there is a distinct softening and decrease in swelling following the LH surge and just before ovulation. This softening has also been used as an indication of the appropriate time for artificial insemination of bitches in which the cycle was induced by giving gonadotropins.[55]

Metestrus

The onset of metestrus will vary with the criteria used and is characterized by the loss of estrous behavior, loss of vaginal cornifi-

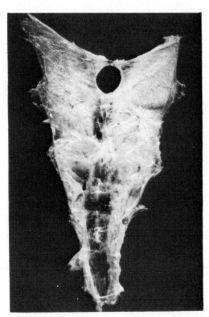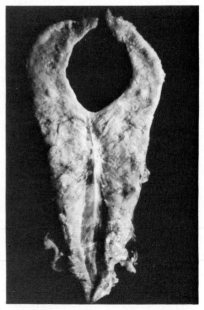

Figs 15a,b. Normal canine mammary gland (a) at day 20 of nonpregnant cycle, near time of peak progesterone levels. It has moderate duct and tubule development, but little glandular alveolar development within connective tissue fascia. b. Mammary gland at day 80 from a nonpregnant bitch that was not overtly pseudopregnant. Glandular alveolar development is at a peak, and the increase in size detectable in nearly all nonpregnant bitches around day 35 of the cycle is evident.

cation, loss of vaginal crenulation, and reappearance of leukocytes in the vaginal smear. Duration of metestrus will likewise vary depending on criteria used. It lasts until the effects of the remaining 2 to 3 months of luteal progesterone secretion are no longer evident.

During early metestrus, progesterone levels continue to increase and a peak level is reached 20 to 30 days after the LH peak. Throughout the remaining 30 to 100 days of metestrus, progesterone levels decline at variable rates within and among bitches. During the period of declining progesterone and about 35 days after the LH peak, there is an obvious increase in mammary development that can be detected by serial palpation; the posterior 1 or 2 pairs of glands have greater development than the anterior pairs (Fig 15). Such mammary development occurs routinely even in bitches that show no gross signs of pseudopregnancy (Fig 16).

The concomitant prolonged period of progesterone secretion and mammary alveolar development has prompted the use of the term "physiologic pseudopregnancy" for the luteal phase in the nonpregnant bitch. It apparently is during the same period of declining pro-

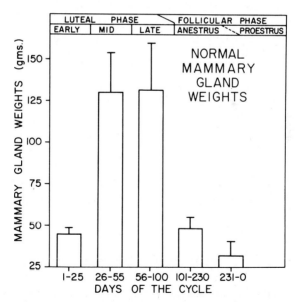

Fig 16. Weights of mammary gland removed from Beagle bitches at known stages of nonpregnant cycles are given as mean ± standard error for 5 groups of 6 bitches each. Notice increase in size of the mammary glands that occurs normally during the middle and late luteal phase in the absence of any overt signs of pseudopregnancy.

gesterone secretion that the secretory activity of the uterine endometrium is greatest because it is at this time that the events leading to mucometra are usually first noted. In many cases, however, clinical signs do not become severe until much later in metestrus after several weeks of progressive uterine changes. For these reasons affected bitches are usually presented after serum progesterone levels are below 1 ng/ml.

The increases in mammary size and uterine secretion in the second half of metestrus may be related to modest increases in serum prolactin levels. Both the mammary gland and endometrium have prolactin receptors, and preliminary studies in our laboratory suggest that prolactin receptors increase in proestrus, decrease in early metestrus, and increase again later in metestrus apparently in concert with the estrogen:progesterone ratio (Fig 17).

Overt Pseudopregnancy in Metestrus: Overt pseudopregnancy probably represents the extreme in the hormonal changes possible during middle to late metestrus or in the response of individual bitches to those changes, especially the abruptness in the decline of progesterone and the resulting increase in prolactin secretion. In overt pseudopregnancy the mammary enlargement may be as great as that seen during late pregnancy and lactation. There is usually some lactation and release of milk and moderate to extreme behavioral changes similar to those associated with pregnancy, parturition, and lactation. The behavioral changes may include restlessness, an increase in demand for affection, nesting, reclusiveness, and gathering of inanimate objects. The indictment of declining progesterone and elevated prolactin is supported by alleviation of clinical signs following administration of a progestin such as megestrol acetate, or of an inhibitor of prolactin secretion, such as the ergot alkaloid, bromergocryptine. The administration of the androgen mibolerone, has also been reported to be effective as a treatment for pseudopregnancy.[56]

Anestrus

Representing the transition of one cycle to the next, anestrus is characterized by low serum progesterone levels (<1.0 ng/ml); it may last 1 to 6 months. Elevations of both FSH and estrogen have been observed during anestrus.[43] The absence of external signs of estrogen activity may be due to the absence of a progressive increase in estrogen levels, as seen in proestrus, and the occurrence of only sporadic rises in estrogen levels.

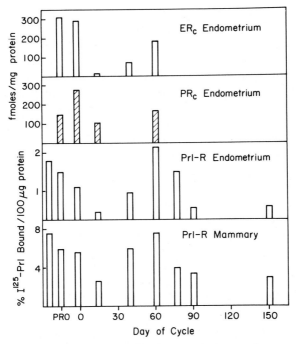

Fig 17. Amounts of specific estrogen- and progesterone-binding by cytosolic receptors in the endometrium of individual bitches at various stages of the cycle are recorded in relation to amounts of prolactin-binding by endometrial and mammary gland membranes.

REPRODUCTIVE HORMONES AND ENDOCRINE REGULATION OF THE OVARIAN CYCLE

Anterior Pituitary Hormones

Hormones of interest include LH (luteinizing hormone), FSH (follicle stimulating hormone), prolactin, and GH (growth hormone). As its name implies, FSH promotes the growth and development of antral follicles in the ovary. It also is required for synthesis of estrogen. LH is required for normal follicle growth and steroidogenesis, being responsible for conversion of cholesterol to progesterone, the precurser of androgen and estrogen. LH is also the ovulatory hormone, a large surge being required for ovulation. In the process the follicles are luteinized and transformed into progesterone-secreting corpora lutea. Both LH and prolactin are needed for normal luteal secretion of progesterone in the dog.

LH

Secretion of LH during the follicular and luteal phases of the cycle has been monitored and reported, but detailed analyses of subtle changes in basal levels or of pulsatile release throughout the cycle have not been reported. Mean serum levels of LH during anestrus are variable and slightly elevated above the decrease reported during proestrus and prior to the preovulatory surge at the end of proestrus or in early estrus.[43] Recent studies in our laboratory have revealed that LH release in the dog, as in other species, is pulsatile and that the interval between pulses can range from 1.5 hours to more than 7 hours. Pulse frequencies greater than once every 3 hours usually occur during early proestrus or the preceding week. They may represent the stimulus for development of a competent wave of follicles. In early and mid-anestrus and during mid-proestrus, LH pulse frequencies are usually less than once every 3 hours.

The mechanisms regulating LH release in the dog appear similar to those reported for other species. A hypothalamic decapeptide, gonadotropin releasing hormone (GnRH), stimulates release of LH (and FSH) from the pituitary. Exogenous GnRH causes LH release within minutes. LH release is suppressed by ovarian estrogen through a negative feedback mechanism. LH levels are chronically elevated after ovariectomy and can subsequently be suppressed by administration of estrogen. Studies in our laboratory have revealed that continuous increases in estradiol will keep LH at basal levels in ovariectomized bitches and that a subsequent decline in estrogen causes a surge in LH that can be facilitated by a simultaneous increase in progesterone. Thus, in the normal transition from proestrus to estrus the decline in the estrogen:progesterone ratio that occurs as the follicles reach maturity is probably the trigger for the preovulatory surge release of LH. The preovulatory surge in LH lasts 24 to 72 hours and causes accelerated enlargement of follicles, luteinization, and ovulation. Ovulations occur 36 to 50 hours after the LH surge.[4] LH is luteotrophic and basal LH levels are required for progesterone secretion during the luteal phase of the cycle.[10,13]

Recent studies have revealed that the pulsatile administration of exogenous GnRH at a rate of once every 90 minutes can induce follicular development, estrogen secretion, and proestrous activity followed by either estrus and ovulation or by a false estrus and subsequent rebound proestrus and estrus.[24]

Unlike estradiol, progesterone alone does not appear to exert any significant negative-feedback effect on LH secretion in the bitch. In ovariectomized bitches given large doses of medroxyprogesterone acetate, serum LH levels remained elevated.[58] In the intact bitch, however, progesterone may interact with estrogen to maintain LH secretion at basal levels.

FSH

Secretion and regulation of FSH have not been extensively studied in the bitch. It has been shown that FSH is released simultaneously with LH following administration of GnRH and during the preovulatory surge of LH.[59] The preovulatory rise in serum FSH lasts longer than that of LH because the circulating half-life of FSH is longer. It has recently been observed that FSH levels are elevated above baseline during anestrus and subsequently depressed during proestrus.[43] Apparently follicles for the next cycle are recruited by elevated FSH secretion and, once recruited, they selectively regulate FSH secretion by a negative feedback mechanism. FSH inhibition may be caused by elevated estrogen and/or, as proposed for several other species, by elevated serum levels of inhibin, a follicular peptide that selectively inhibits FSH secretion.

Prolactin

Secretion of prolactin has been studied in the bitch, but primarily in relation to pregnancy, parturition, and lactation. Besides being a metabolic and lactogenic hormone, prolactin is also part of the pituitary luteotropic requirement along with LH. Prolactin may be required to provide luteal cells with cholesterol as a precursor of progesterone. Its secretion also seems to be inversely proportional to secretion of progesterone. Serum prolactin levels surge prepartum as progesterone levels decline.[7] Transient rises in prolactin also were observed in a few bitches during the early luteal phase, shortly before implantation when progesterone levels decreased transiently.[60]

Prolactin is released following injection of the hypothalamic tripeptide, TRH (thyrotropin releasing hormone).[59] Thus factors that affect endogenous TRH release probably affect prolactin as well as thyroid function. Hypothyroidism has been associated with chronic anestrus and infertility.

Secretion of prolactin is normally held to basal rates by a hypothalamic prolactin-release inhibitory factor, probably dopamine. Bromergocryptine, a plant alkaloid derivative, is a dopamine agonist and reduces prolactin secretion in the dog as in other species. Its administration will also reduce the severity of overt pseudopregnancies that can occur during the 2nd or 3rd month of the luteal phase. It thus appears likely that prolactin plays a major role in the development of overt pseudopregnancy. Differences in prolactin levels during metestrus may be the basis for the variation in the extent that pseudocyesis is observed among individuals or breeds. In nonpregnant bitches, at least moderate increases in prolactin have been reported to occur late in normal metestrus during or shortly after the period of declining progesterone levels.[59,61] Though prolactin levels in overtly pseudopregnant bitches have not been reported, they are assumed to be higher than in normal metestrus.

GH

Growth hormone is primarily a metabolic hormone, but it is also lactogenic in some species. GH secretion is regulated, at least in part, by the tetradecapeptide somatostatin, an inhibitor of growth hormone secretion, and by GH-releasing factor activity found in hypothalamic extracts of dogs as well as other species. In addition, however, secretion of growth hormone in the dog can be affected by secretion of progesterone during the ovarian cycle as well as by treatment with medroxyprogesterone acetate (MPA). Pharmacologic doses of MPA have resulted in elevated GH levels early in the course of treatment and after 6 to 18 months caused acromegaly-like changes (Fig 18), including overgrowth of skin and alterations in glucose and insulin levels.[11,12,17] More recently it has been reported that elevated GH levels and acromegaly-like signs may occur following contraceptive doses of MPA in some bitches. Some bitches may undergo such changes spontaneously and transiently in response to the secretion of progesterone during the luteal phase of the cycle.[62,63] Such findings may be relevant to the etiology of mammary gland tumors in older bitches. In one study the bitches that developed the most severe mammary neoplasms in response to high doses of MPA did so only following elevations in serum GH levels.[12]

Ovarian Steroid Hormone Secretion

Estrogen

During proestrus, follicles increase from 1 or 2 mm to 3 or 4 mm in diameter. The estradiol secreted by proestrous follicles is first reflected externally by vulval swelling and the discharge of blood originating in the uterus. The pituitary gonadotropin needed for follicle maturation and estradiol secretion in the dog has not been studied in detail. As in several other species, however, it probably includes FSH to induce aromatase activity in granulosa cells and LH to induce production of progesterone and consequently androgen. The androgen serves as aromatase substrate for estradiol synthesis in the

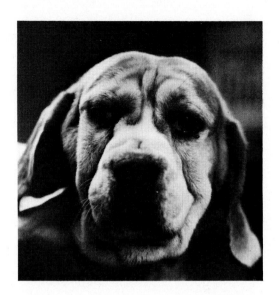

Fig 18. Acromegaly due to hypersecretion of GH that developed in a Beagle bitch during 15 months of treatment with medroxyprogesterone acetate (MPA) at 3 times the contraceptive dose. A similar response has been reported in bitches treated with progesterone alone or with low contraceptive doses of MPA, and spontaneously in untreated older bitches during nonpregnant cycles.

granulosa cells. It has been demonstrated that levels of estrone, a weakly estrogenic steroid, are also elevated during proestrus and generally parallel those of estradiol before and after the LH surge.[64] Estrone appears to be a less reliable indicator of follicular development than is estradiol. Serum estradiol reaches peak levels (50 to 120 pg/ml) in late proestrus or early estrus, 1 or 2 days before the LH peak, and decreases sharply thereafter. The sharp decline in estradiol during and following the LH peak probably reflects an aromatase-inhibiting effect by LH on fully matured follicles. In response to the LH surge the follicles rapidly enlarge and bulge from the surface of the ovary. They are about 8 to 10 mm in diameter at ovulation.[65]

During proestrus estradiol induces vaginal cornification, edema, and elongation; hyperemia and elongation of the uterine horns with concomitant folding or flexing of the horns along their length; enlargement of the oviduct; and proliferation of the fimbriated end of the oviduct through the bursal slit. Except for minor elevations in mid-metestrus, estrogen remains near baseline level (5 to 15 pg/ml) during the nonpregnant luteal phase. We have found, however, that estrogen levels are increased during the last third of pregnancy, but then are not as high as levels observed during proestrus.

Androgens

Serum testosterone levels are about 0.1 ng/ml during anestrus and they increase slightly, along with estradiol, during proestrus to reach peak values of about 0.3 to 1.0 ng/ml shortly after the estradiol peak

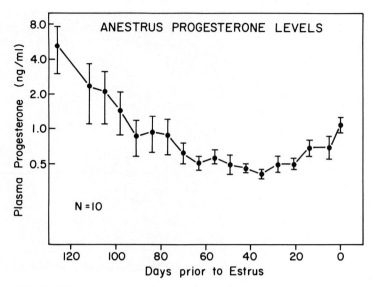

Fig 19. Plasma progesterone levels during anestrus shown on a logarithmic scale to emphasize the protracted decline to basal levels by 40 days prior to next estrus, and the slight increase in levels associated with follicle development prior to and during proestrus.

and coincident with the preovulatory LH peak.[47] Testosterone levels then decline and remain below 0.2 ng/ml throughout the luteal phase. Serum androstenedione levels are less than 0.2 ng/ml during anestrus.[23] They increase during proestrus and reach levels of 0.6 to 2.3 ng/ml at the time of the LH peak. During the luteal phase in both pregnant and nonpregnant cycles, androstenedione levels remain elevated and follow the pattern of luteal progesterone secretion, with mean levels of 0.7 ng/ml at day 20, slowly declining to 0.5 ng/ml near day 40 and to lower levels during the progression into anestrus. Elevated androgen levels during proestrus probably reflect excess production by follicles beyond that needed to provide androstenedione as the substrate for aromatase enzymes and synthesis of estrogens. The significance of luteal production of androstenedione in preference to testosterone during the luteal phase and pregnancy is unknown, but the levels produced are considerably lower than in several noncarnivore species.

Progesterone
    Secretion of progesterone declines slowly throughout early and mid-anestrus following a nonpregnant cycle (Fig 19). At about 40

days prior to the next estrus, serum levels are the same as in ovariectomized bitches and the 0.2 to 0.5 ng/ml probably represents adrenal
secretion of progesterone.[66] Administration of ACTH to ovariectomized bitches can cause an elevation of progesterone up to 2 ng/ml
(Fig 20). From late anestrus through the onset of proestrus, serum
progesterone levels remain low, fluctuate between 0.4 and 0.8 ng/ml,
but generally tend to increase slightly. This increase as well as the
further increase to 0.6 to 1.0 ng/ml observed during proestrus is probably due to secretion by developing ovarian follicles.

During the 2nd half of proestrus, follicles undergo partial luteinization prior to the LH surge.[4] In late proestrus and concomitant with
the beginning of the LH surge, progesterone levels increase sharply,
reaching 2 to 3 ng/ml at the time of the LH peak and 3 to 8 ng/ml at
ovulation 2 days later. A pause in the rate of increase often occurs in
association with ovulation. Levels then rise to maximum concentrations of 15 to 80 ng/ml 15 to 25 days after the LH peak. A brief fall in
progesterone and rise in prolactin 8 to 12 days after the LH peak has
been observed in a limited number of bitches.[60] After reaching a peak

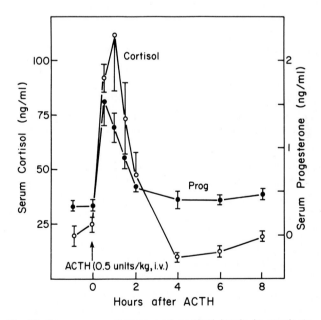

Fig 20. Serum progesterone and cortisol levels in ovariectomized bitches administered ACTH. They show that basal progesterone levels in anestrus represent adrenal progesterone
secretion that can be stimulated by ACTH.

level around day 25, progesterone levels slowly decrease over the remainder of a nonpregnant metestrus and fall below 1 ng/ml by day 55 to 90 and reach 0.3 to 0.6 ng/ml by day 100 to 160. Structural regression of the corpora lutea appears to parallel the decline of the progesterone level.

Luteal secretion of progesterone depends on pituitary LH and prolactin for support throughout the luteal phase and ceases following hypophysectomy.[10] Administration of anti-LH serum causes a dramatic decline in progesterone secretion, as does the administration of bromergocryptine.[13,67]

No significant difference in progesterone levels was found in overtly pseudopregnant bitches and bitches having a normal metestrus.[68] The possibility that the rate of decline in progesterone is a significant factor, with more abrupt declines causing greater elevations in prolactin, could be relevant to the etiology of pseudopregnancy. This could explain the rapid onset of overt pseudopregnancy in some bitches following ovariohysterectomy during metestrus and the temporary amelioration of pseudopregnancy following short-term treatment with megestrol acetate.

The rapid increase in progesterone that occurs at the start of the preovulatory LH surge and concomitant with the fall in estrogen facilitates the completion, if not the start, of the LH surge.[8] This rapid withdrawal of estrogen at the LH peak may be the basis for the consistency of the subsequent loss of vaginal cornification in relation to the LH peak. The continued rise in progesterone during the first part of the luteal phase promotes the growth and development of the endometrium and mammary epithelium, although neither shows significant secretory activity until the phase of declining progesterone levels.

Rising progesterone levels also cause the uterine horns to elongate and coil (actually fold) so that by day 12 to 18 the turns of the horns may be mistaken for early implantation swellings. By day 25 the elongated uterine horns no longer appear so coiled and have become accommodated by the mesenteries. The endometrium is then obviously secretory for 1 or more months, during which time cystic endometrial hyperplasia may develop and promote a long-lasting mucometra or pyometra. In normal bitches, obvious secretory activity slowly subsides as the progesterone levels decline to 1 ng/ml. Complete return of the endometrium to the anestrous state has been reported to occur rather consistently between day 120 and 130 of the nonpregnant cycle.[39]

The protracted period of luteal retrogression and decline in serum progesterone, together with the absence of any dramatic or consistent effects of hysterectomy on luteal function, suggests there is no uterine luteolytic mechanism involved in canine luteolysis.[69] Other observations indicate that the dog does not possess the intimate relationship between the uterovarian vein and ovarian vein seen in species in which hysterectomy prolongs luteal function and in which the transfer of uterine prostaglandin to the ovarian artery has been proposed as the basis of the uterine luteolytic mechanism.

Prostaglandin $F_2\alpha$ is luteolytic in the bitch. Relatively large doses must be administered repeatedly, however, for several days to obtain complete luteolysis. The developing corpora lutea are resistant to $PGF_2\alpha$, but after day 30 doses of 30 to 50 $\mu g/kg$ administered 2 or 3 times a day will cause complete luteolysis in nonpregnant bitches.[3]

Mechanism of Hormonal Action and Interaction

In target tissues of sex steroids there are specific cytoplasmic and nuclear receptors for both estrogen and progesterone. Each hormone acts on target cells by binding to its specific receptors in the cytoplasm and causing their translocation to the nucleus. Interaction of hormone-receptor complexes with the genome then results in hormone-specific modulation of subsequent nuclear-directed events, including cytoplasmic protein synthesis.

Each of the 2 hormones can regulate the synthesis of not only its own receptors but those of the other steroid as well. Increasing estrogen causes increased synthesis of estrogen and progesterone receptors. These effects are reversed by estrogen withdrawal. Increasing progesterone causes suppression of estrogen and progesterone receptor synthesis and these effects are reversed by progesterone withdrawal. Thus, estrogen facilitates subsequent progesterone action, progesterone facilitates estrogen withdrawal, and progesterone withdrawal facilitates estrogen action.

Limited observations of estrogen and progesterone receptors in the canine endometrium at different stages of the estrous cycle are similar to observations made in more extensive studies of other species (Fig 17).

PREGNANCY AND PARTURITION

Length of Gestation

Pregnancy in the bitch is often reported to last 63 to 64 days without reference to the variation that can occur. The interval from a fertile mating to parturition can range from 56 to 68 days; the

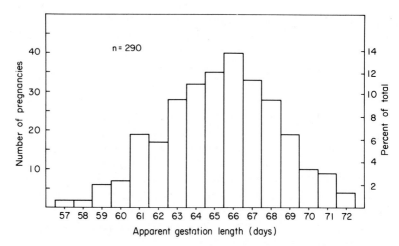

Fig 21. Distribution of apparent gestation lengths in a colony of Beagles. In a subset of these pregnancies the day of the preovulatory LH peak was determined and parturitions occurred on 64, 65, or 66 days after the LH peak.[18]

average is 64 days (Fig 21). Parturition may not occur until 71 or 72 days after the first of a series of matings in bitches that are forced to mate 5 or 6 days before the LH peak or display receptive behavior that early. Such variation is not due to any great inconsistency in the timing of the physiologic events of pregnancy. It results from the large variations that exist in the time from mating to ovulation, to oocyte maturation, and to passage of blastocysts through the tubo-uterine junction, and the fact that canine sperm can retain the ability to fertilize for 6 to 7 days after mating.[18] The onset of behavioral estrus can vary considerably in relation to the LH peak and fertile matings can occur as late as 5 days after ovulation or as early as 5 days before ovulation.

Ova are released as primary oocytes about 2 days after the pre-ovulatory surge of luteinizing hormone (LH) and they do not undergo maturation until 2 or 3 days later. Starting 4 to 5 days after the LH peak and ending with degeneration of oocytes in the oviduct 3 to 4 days later, there is a period in which canine oocytes can be fertilized by either previously deposited or freshly deposited spermatozoa. Thus the high incidence of mixed litters in bitches bred at random. Because of the limited period for fertilization and the apparently consistent time for opening of the tubo-uterine junction late in estrus, the events in canine pregnancy and the length of gestation vary little related to the time of ovulation or of the preovulatory LH surge. For

Table 1. Timing of Various Events of Canine Pregnancy in Relation to the Preovulatory LH Peak and to Potential Times of Fertile Matings.

Event of Pregnancy	Days After LH Peak[a]	Days After Fertile Mating[b]
Proestrus onset	−25 to +3	
Maximum vaginal cornification	−3 to +3	
Estrus onset	−4 to +5	
Estradiol peak	−3 to −1	
Preovulatory LH peak	0	−9 to +3
First of multiple matings	−5 to +9	−12 to 0
Fertile mating	−3 to +9	0
Ovulation of primary oocytes	2	−7 to +5
Oocyte maturation	4	−4 to +7
Fertilization	4 to 9	0 to 7
Vaginal cornification reduced	6 to 10	0 to 12
Reappearance of WBCs in smear	6 to 12	
Morulae in distal oviducts	8 to 10	2 to 13
Blastocysts enter uterus	9 to 11	2 to 14
Zonae pellucidae shed	15 to 17	8 to 20
Attachment sites established	16 to 18	9 to 21
Swelling of implantation sites	18 to 20	11 to 23
Palpable 1-cm swellings	22 to 24	15 to 27
Pregnancy anemia onset	27 to 29	20 to 31
Uterine swellings detectable in radiographs	30 to 32	23 to 35
Reduced palpability of 3-cm swellings	32 to 34	25 to 37
Hematocrit below 40% PCV	38 to 40	31 to 43
Fetal skull and spine radiopaque	44 to 46	36 to 49
Earliest pregnancy diagnosis by radiography	45 to 47	39 to 50
Hematocrit below 35% PCV	48 to 50	41 to 53
Fetal pelvis is radiopaque	53 to 57	45 to 60
Fetal teeth are radiopaque	58 to 63	50 to 66
Prepartum luteolysis and hypothermia	63 to 65	55 to 68
Parturition	64 to 66	56 to 69

a — Estimates based on published and unpublished observations.

b — Based on single fertile matings as early as 3 days before or as late as 8 or 9 days after the LH peak.

nearly all normal pregnancies parturition occurs 64, 65 or 66 days after the LH peak.[18]

Based on a consistent gestation length of 65 ± 1 days relative to the LH peak, it is possible to time with a reasonable degree of accuracy some of the individual events of pregnancy relative to one another. Many aspects of pregnancy in the dog, however, have only been studied in relation to the time of mating or onset of estrus, including implantation and development of the fetus, placenta, and fetal membranes. For these events, estimates must be made based on the fact that the average breeding date is about 1 day after the LH peak and 1 day before ovulation.

The timing of many of the clinically relevant events of pregnancy in the dog is given in Table 1 and discussed in more detail subsequently.

Endocrinology of Pregnancy

The patterns of hormonal levels during pregnancy are not unlike those observed during nonpregnant cycles except for the dramatic changes in hormones associated with parturition. Hormone profiles during pregnancy and the timing of various events of gestation are summarized in Figure 22.

Serum estradiol levels increase during pregnancy to 20 to 30 pg/ml prior to parturition. These levels are considerably below those that occur in late proestrus (50 to 100 pg/ml).[1,5] The changes in secretion and/or metabolism of estrogen responsible for its rise in late pregnancy are probably greater than what is reflected by peripheral serum levels because the latter are "dampened" by an increase in volume of distribution associated with increased body weight and decreased packed cell volume.[5] Estradiol falls abruptly to basal levels (5 to 10 pg/ml) following parturition. Levels throughout lactation and postlactation anestrus have not been determined, but a considerable elevation in estradiol level has been reported during anestrus following nonpregnant cycles.[43] Estrogen metabolites, such as estrone sulfate, have not been studied intensively during canine pregnancies.

In fertile cycles as in nonfertile cycles, progesterone levels continue to increase throughout estrus to reach initial peak levels of 15 to 85 ng/ml by 15 to 30 days after the LH peak. Throughout the period of elevated progesterone levels, considerable fluctuations can occur from day to day, and even within days. In pregnant bitches, however, following implantation and placental development, when progesterone levels are either near their initial apex or declining, there is a 2nd increase in progesterone levels that either rises to a 2nd peak or

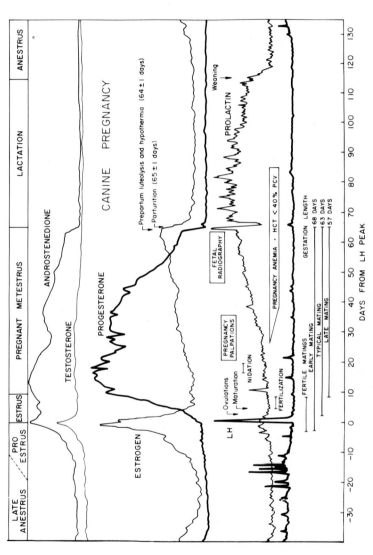

Fig 22. Schematic representation of typical endocrine changes reported or presumed to occur during the course of a fertile canine ovarian cycle, including pregnancy and lactation.[29]

causes a broadening of the ongoing decline during the 4th and 5th weeks of gestation.[1,5,68] During the last third of pregnancy, progesterone levels decline slowly to a plateau of 4 to 16 ng/ml that is maintained for 1 to 2 weeks until the abrupt decline to 1 to 2 ng/ml that occurs 1 to 2 days before parturition. Following parturition, progesterone levels are usually below 1 ng/ml. A transient rise to 2 to 3 ng/ml may occur 2 to 3 days postpartum.[7]

Though progesterone levels are generally higher during the 2nd half of pregnancy than during the comparable period in nonpregnant bitches, serum progesterone levels cannot be used to diagnose pregnancy because the range in absolute progesterone levels in both pregnant and nonpregnant bitches is quite large. The magnitude of specific changes in progesterone secretion or metabolism during the 2nd half of gestation, as those of estrogen, are apparently reflected poorly in peripheral serum due an increased volume of distribution associated with the progressive, postimplantation anemia characteristic of canine pregnancy.[5] Actual increases in blood volume during canine pregnancy have not been determined.

LH levels continue to fluctuate near basal levels throughout pregnancy and dramatic changes in either LH or FSH have not been reported. Following implantation, however, FSH levels are somewhat higher than in nonpregnant cycles and apparently remain so throughout gestation. This increase in FSH has been suggested to be the basis for elevated estrogen levels in late pregnancy.[59]

Serum prolactin levels fluctuate somewhat during proestrus and estrus and prior to implantation. A transient surge in prolactin levels during a concomitant decline in progesterone levels has been observed in some bitches shortly prior to implantation.[60,61] As in nonpregnant cycles, prolactin levels increase during the protracted period of declining progesterone levels after day 35 to 40 of pregnancy. The broad rise in prolactin levels during the 2nd half of pregnancy appears to be clearly greater than that in most nonpregnant cycles.[61] It terminates with a transient, large surge during the rapid decline in progesterone 12 to 36 hours prior to parturition.[7,61] Prolactin levels are usually reduced for 1-2 days postpartum, possibly because of a transient depletion of pituitary prolactin. Levels then become elevated and fluctuate during lactation in response to prolactin release induced by suckling. Prolactin levels decline slowly during the 2nd half of lactation and fall abruptly following weaning.[7]

Preimplantation Events

The timing of pre- and post-implantation events appears to be relatively consistent among bitches when viewed relative to the preovulatory LH peak and ovulation, which are considered herein as day 0 and day 2, respectively, of the pregnant cycle. Under clinical conditions the expected times of various events of gestation can be reasonably estimated in bitches in which the late-estrus decrease in vaginal cornification is monitored by daily vaginal cytology or daily vaginal endoscopy.[51,53,54] The initial, discrete reappearance of noncornified cells in the vaginal smear and the late estrus regression of the vaginal mucosa occur 7 to 8 days after the LH peak in the majority of bitches.

Fertilization is probably limited to a 3 to 4 day period between day 4 and day 8 after the LH peak, ie, 2 to 6 days after ovulation, because oocyte maturation probably occurs 2 or 3 days after ovulation (day 4) and most unfertilized oocytes degenerate by day 9. These estimates are based on the following observations. Canine oocytes require 48 to 72 hours to mature spontaneously in vitro.[70] Fertilization by extremely short-lived, previously frozen sperm is limited to the 3 days prior to the late-estrus decrease in the number of cornified cells in vaginal smears, ie, around day 8 of the cycle.[71,72] The in vivo requirement for sperm capacitation in the dog is not known. It has been shown that dog sperm can penetrate oocytes after 7 hours of incubation in vitro and they can penetrate immature or degenerated oocytes as well as mature oocytes.[70]

Embryos accumulate as morulae in the distal segments of the oviducts and develop there into 32 to 64 cell blastocysts.[41] Passage of blastocysts into the uterine horns after opening of the tubo-uterine junctions has been estimated to occur around day 10 or 11. This is followed by 3 days in which 1-mm blastocysts are floating freely in their ipsilateral uterine horns and another 3 days in which 2-mm blastocysts migrate freely from one horn to another. The zonae pellucidae are then shed and rather equally spaced attachment sites are established around day 16. Distinct swellings of implantation sites are evident by day 18 during formation of the embryonic primitive streak and initial development of the placenta.

Postimplantation Events
Uterine swellings at implantation sites are about 1 cm in diameter by day 20. They reflect localized uterine edema, expansion of the embryonic membranes, and early placental development. The canine placenta is endotheliochorial in composition, zonary, and circumferential (Fig 23). The girdle of fetal trophoblast tissue develops marginal hematomas, but the chorioallantoic poles remain thin and transparent. The marginal hematomas contain large pools of stagnant maternal blood from which the extraembryonic circulation absorbs various

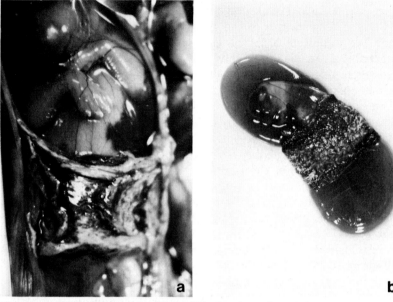

Fig 23a. Third trimester canine fetus within the circumferential placenta and chorioallantois membrane is exposed *in vivo* by removal of a portion of the uterine wall.

Fig 23b. Canine fetus within the zonary placenta and the nonvillous poles of the chorionic sac. The variegated surface of the maternal side of the placenta reflects tearing of chorionic villi during separation from the uterine endometrium.

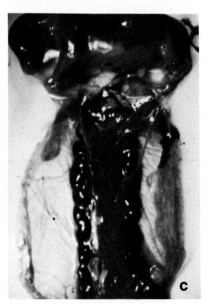

Fig 23c. Canine fetus covered by amniotic membrane is attached by the umbilicus to the inner surface of the placental girdle with its marginal hematomas. It is exposed by cutting through and unwrapping the placental girdle and poles of the chorioallantois.

metabolites, especially iron. In the dog there is also the somewhat unique persistence of an elongated yolk sac often attached to both ends of the paraplacental zones and not attached to the zonary placenta. The ultrastructure of the placenta and fetal membranes including the yolk sac has recently been described.[73]

The maternal hematocrit slowly declines following implantation and is usually below 40% (PCV) by day 35 and below 35% at term. It has been suggested that a major cause of the anemia in canine pregnancy is the hemodilution effects of increased plasma volume.[5] If this is so, the potential increase in blood volume must be considered when measuring peripheral levels of hormones or metabolites during late pregnancy.

Total body weight of a bitch may increase 20 to 55% during gestation; in one survey the average increase was about 36%.[5] During the second half of pregnancy there is also a decrease in hemoglobin levels and an increase in sedimentation rate. There is also a potential for development of moderate immunosuppression during pregnancy, as reflected in serum IgG levels below 500 mg/dl.[74]

Plasma levels of fibrinogen and other proteins involved in coagulation increase following implantation. Fibrinogen increases rapidly and becomes maximal at day 30, declines near term, and increases again at parturition.[75] Pregnancy has also been associated with an increase in systemic and pulmonary vascular resistance in the dog.[76] Related to this observation is the fact that during late pregnancy the canine uterus produces large amounts of prostacyclin, which may act as a circulating vasodepressor substance.[77]

The extent to which pregnancy alters general metabolism or the efficacy of metabolic hormones in the bitch has not been studied extensively. The effects may be considerable because as early as midpregnancy (day 30 to 35) at least minor alterations in metabolic hormone responses have been demonstrated relative to anestrus and/or the comparable period in the luteal phase of nonpregnant bitches.[21,79] Serum concentrations of thyroxine (T_4) but not T_3 were somewhat elevated, both before and after TSH injection. Basal cortisol levels were normal, but post-ACTH were higher than those in anestrous and nonpregnant metestrous bitches.

Pregnancy will aggravate pre-existing subclinical diabetes in dogs. Sensitivity to insulin, but not glucagon, is reduced as early as day 35 of pregnancy.[19] Insulin requirements in pregnant bitches is thus increased for management of diabetes.[80] Prolactin does not appear to be involved in this change because it does not alter glucagon tolerance or insulin responses in dogs.[81] The rise in prolactin during late pregnancy probably affects lipid metabolism, but the direct effects of prolactin have only been studied in nonpregnant dogs.[81]

The requirement for available carbohydrate in the diet is also increased in pregnancy. Bitches maintained on a carbohydrate-deficient diet during pregnancy became hypoglycemic during the last 2 weeks of gestation, had a 7-fold increase in dead pups in litters, and had an abnormally high incidence of mortality among their pups during the first 3 days postpartum.[82]

Pregnancy Diagnosis

Palpation

By day 20 to 25 uterine swellings at placental sites are usually detectable in all but obese bitches by digital palpation as 1- to 2-cm enlargements along the uterine horns. These swellings remain readily palpable, however, for only about 10 days (Fig 24). By then the horns have dropped to a more ventral position and the cranial ends are pushed forward under the caudal ribs. By day 35 the fetal swellings are over 3 cm in diameter, elongated, nearly confluent, and pliable rather than firm; in most bitches they become difficult to palpate as distinct structures associated with pregnancy. At about the same time, mammary gland development becomes evident, but no more so than in many nonpregnant cycles. When diagnosis of pregnancy is important, the bitch's abdomen should be palpated weekly or more frequently starting on day 20 after breeding. The observations should be interpreted with an appreciation of the potential range in the time of implantation relative to the time of mating (Table 1).

The use of ultrasonography to detect pregnancy has been compared to manual palpation.[83] In that study, A-mode ultrasound and

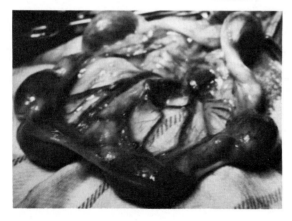

Fig 24. Canine uterine horns and fundus exposed via mid-ventral laparotomy near day 28 of pregnancy and just prior to period when palpation becomes difficult due to further vesicle enlargement and confluence of uterine swellings.

Doppler-ultrasound instruments were no more effective than manual palpation in detection of pregnancy prior to midgestation (day 32). They were especially effective, however, after day 35 to 40, and gave accurate results in 85 to 100% of the cases depending on the instrument used and stage of pregnancy. They were also effective when palpation of implantation vesicles became difficult. More sophisticated and expensive ultrasound equipment enables direct visualization of vesicles and/or fetal heart movement. Such devices enable diagnosis of pregnancy throughout the post-implantation period (after day 20).Information on the methodology used with this equipment has not been published in detail for the bitch.[84]

Radiography

Conventional radiography can be used to distinguish pregnancy from pseudopregnancy or uterine disease, or to evaluate fetal development, during the last 3 weeks of gestation. The fetal skeletons do not become radiopaque until after day 44 (21 days prepartum) and only become distinct after day 46 (18 days prepartum). However, because of variable intervals between mating and implantation, the fetal skeleton in some bitches may not be distinct until 50 days after mating; in others it may be distinct by 39 days after mating.[16] The stage of fetal development during the last 2 weeks of gestation can be assessed with radiographs on the basis of the sequence and timing of the appearance of distinct calvaria, proximal and then distal limb bones, pelvis, caudal ribs, and finally the teeth (Table 1).

Radiographic analysis has been made of changes in uterine morphology throughout canine gestation.[20] It is important to note, however, that the fetal skeleton must be evident after day 45 for an unequivocal diagnosis of pregnancy because earlier radiographic changes in uterine morphology may be similar to changes that occur in various uterine diseases. Enlargements of implantation sites seen in conventional radiographs appear small and ovoid on day 30, larger and spherical on day 35, and then large and ovoid on day 40. The spherical shapes seen around day 35 are usually, but not necessarily, distinct from irregular enlargements observed in bitches with mucometra or pyometra. In late pregnancy fetal death can be recognized in radiographs that reveal abnormal calvaria, intra- or peri-fetal gas spaces, and abnormal fetal postures including excessive flexion of the body or extension of the hind limbs.

Pregnancy Tests

There are no validated assays for the diagnosis of pregnancy in bitches either before or after implantation. The existence of any placental gonadotropin or feto-placental protein on which such a test might be based has not been demonstrated. The anemia of late pregnancy might be useful for differentiation of pregnancy from overt pseudopregnancy, but this has yet to be demonstrated by evaluation of hematocrits during pseudopregnancy. Concomitant decreases in serum creatinine and gammaglobulin (IgG) levels 21 days after breeding have been described as useful indicators of pregnancy in the bitch.[74]

Maintenance of Pregnancy

Progesterone is required for maintenance of pregnancy throughout gestation and the circulating levels normally present are probably well in excess of the minimum amount required. The corpora lutea are the major if not only source of progesterone. Ovariectomy at any time during pregnancy results in either resorption of fetuses or abortion.[86]

Progesterone appears to be the only sex steroid required for maintenance of pregnancy in the bitch. The synthetic progestin medroxyprogesterone acetate (MPA) can maintain pregnancy in an ovariectomized bitch.[5] The presence of low but detectable levels of estrogen during pregnancy may contribute to the synthesis or availability of intracellular progesterone receptors. It is probably critical that estrogen levels do not increase to any great extent during pregnancy in the bitch. Abnormally high levels of estrogen can not only prevent nidation but also terminate a postimplantation pregnancy.[5] During pregnancy, progesterone probably supports endometrial development, promotes placental integrity, and reduces myometrial activity and sensitivity to oxytocin.

The secretion of progesterone depends on pituitary secretion of luteotrophic hormones; pregnancy at any stage is terminated by hypophysectomy.[10,87] Both LH and prolactin appear to be required by the pregnant bitch. Administration of anti-LH serum dramatically reduces progesterone levels.[13] Bromergocryptine can cause complete luteolysis and subsequent abortion in bitches after day 40 when injected once daily at a dose of 100 μg/kg for 6 or more days (Fig 25).[13,88] Oral administration of bromergocryptine at doses of only 20 to 30 μg/kg twice daily for 4 days has also been reported to cause abortion within 3 to 5 days in bitches during the 6th or 7th week of pregnancy. Abortion did not occur in pregnant bitches treated earlier.[89] Elevated prolactin levels may serve to promote progesterone synthesis during the 2nd half of pregnancy in the bitch because this hormone can antagonize the response to bromergocryptine.[90]

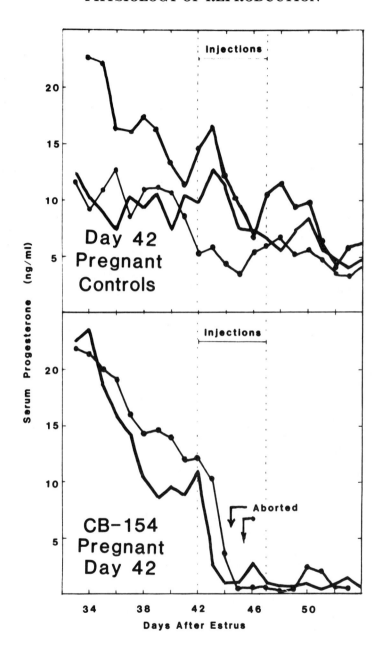

Fig 25. Serum progesterone levels in 2 pregnant bitches that aborted during the course of daily injections of bromergocryptine given at a dose of 0.1 mg/kg/day.

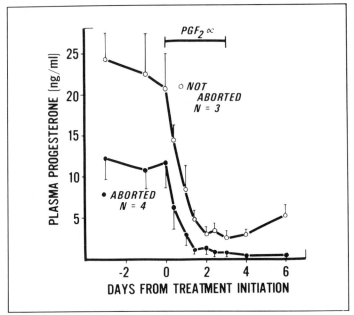

Fig 26. Serum progesterone levels in pregnant bitches that aborted or failed to abort in response to treatment with prostaglandin $F_2\alpha$ administered in doses of 20 or 30 µg/kg every 8 to 12 hr for 3 days.[3]

The corpora lutea of pregnancy are sensitive to the luteolytic effects of prostaglandin F2α (PGF). Repeated administrations of PGF are required, however, to induce complete luteolysis and abortion, even after day 30 when the corpora lutea are more sensitive than during early pregnancy (Fig 26). Administration of 30 to 50 µg/kg body weight 2 or 3 times daily, or of 100 µg/kg or more daily for 3 to 6 days, can cause luteolysis after mid-pregnancy, with resorption or abortion occurring after suppression of progesterone levels to below 1 to 2 ng/ml for 3 or more days.[91] A slow-release formulation of prostaglandin has been reported to induce abortions routinely after day 25 of pregnancy.[92] A single administration of a long-acting PGF analog has been reported to terminate pregnancy at any stage of gestation.[93] Pregnancy could also be terminated by administration of a steroidal competitive inhibitor of the enzyme (d5, 3B hydroxysteroid dehydrogenase) that converts pregnenolone to progesterone. Such a compound might become useful as an abortefacient in the bitch. The fact that PGF is luteolytic in the bitch is important because uterine release of PGF_{2a} during late pregnancy is negligible while that of other products of arachidonic acid, PGE_2 and PGI_2

(prostacyclin), is considerable.[77] The high PGE_2 to PGF_{2a} ratio may be important for maintenance of luteal function and also help to maintain myometrial and uterine vascular tone during gestation.

In a study of early pregnancy in bitches, endometrial and uterine vein plasma levels of PGE_2 were no different than those of PGF.[78] Endometrial PGE_2 concentrations were higher, however, shortly after implantation than they were in nonpregnant bitches at the same stage of the cycle. This suggests that uterine PGE_2 has a role in nidation and placental development.

Parturition

Delivery of an average or large litter can be rapid and completed within 4 hours or may take up to 18 hours for completion. Delivery of the 1st pup nearly always occurs 64 to 66 days after the preovulatory LH peak, but this can range from 57 to 72 days after the first of multiple matings. Gestation is reportedly longer in bitches bearing small litters, but supporting evidence of this is lacking. There is evidence that bitches can actively postpone the delivery of pups for as long as 1 day when stressed.

The mechanisms of parturition in the bitch are not completely known, but available data indicate they are not unlike the mechanisms proposed for several other species. The major endocrine event is a rapid and considerable increase in the peripheral and/or local estrogen:progesterone ratio. In the bitch this occurs with a rapid decline in progesterone levels, starting 24 to 36 hours prepartum, and moderately elevated levels of estrogen remaining unchanged until after parturition when they decline. The fall in progesterone is due primarily to lysis of the corpora lutea, although alterations in progesterone metabolism may also be involved. Because exogenous PGF_{2a} is luteolytic in the bitch, it has been suggested that the prepartum feto-placental unit releases luteolytic amounts of PGF_{2a}.[5] Direct evidence of this is lacking, however, because prepartum changes in PGF levels or secretion rates have not been determined for the bitch.

Maternal cortisol levels are variable, but within the normal range during the last week of gestation (15 to 25 ng/ml) and, in most bitches, are clearly elevated (40 to 80 ng/ml) on the day prior to parturition and then reduced (10 to 25 ng/ml) at the time of parturition.[5,7] As suggested for several other species, the trigger for the timing of parturition in the dog likely involves the maturation of the fetal pituitary-adrenal axis at the completion of fetal development. The increase in maternal cortisol levels may represent a far greater increase in fetal cortisol secretion acting locally to promote the release of luteolytic amounts of PGF.

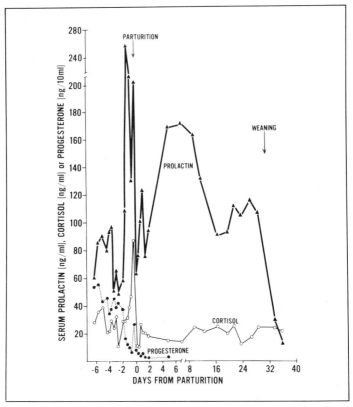

Fig 27. Serum concentrations of progesterone, cortisol, and prolactin during peripartum period and lactation, in an individual bitch. Notice rapid decline in progesterone and rise in cortisol and prolactin during the 24 to 36 hours prior to parturition, and subsequently reduced level of cortisol at time of parturition.[7]

Prolactin increases to peak levels shortly prior to parturition. It has been suggested that the rise in prolactin occurs in response to the simultaneous decline in progesterone. PGF could also be involved because PGF can cause release of prolactin in other species. The extent to which the rise in prolactin is incidental to the events of parturition or plays a role in accelerating the mechanism of parturition has not been evaluated, but its potential to stimulate fetal corticoid secretion has been observed. Maternal serum levels of progesterone, cortisol, and prolactin near parturition and during lactation in an individual bitch are shown in Fig 27.

The prepartum decline in progesterone levels is required for normal parturition. Its prevention by administering exogenous progesterone prevents parturition and results in death of the pups *in situ.*[5] Decline in progesterone level and the resulting increase in the estrogen:progesterone ratio is probably the major cause of placental dislocation, dilation of the cervix, and increased uterine contractility; other factors are most likely involved. As myometrial sensitivity to oxytocin is increased during progesterone withdrawal, basal oxytocin levels would be expected to play an increasingly important role in uterine contractions as would any increases in oxytocin released reflexly in response to fetal pressure on the cervix or vagina. There have been no reports, however, of measurements of oxytocin or relaxin levels around the time of parturition. Increases in relaxin and its contribution to dilation of the cervix and relaxation of the pelvis have been documented for several species. Synthesis of prostaglandin in the cervix may also be important in cervical dilation.

The occurrence of prepartum luteolysis can be monitored by observing the prepartum decline in the bitch's rectal temperature (Fig 28). The hypothermia parallels the decline in progesterone with a delay of about 12 hours, with rectal temperature falling about 1 C between 12 and 24 hours prior to the onset of parturition.[5] The hypothermia is transient and the body temperature rises during or imme-

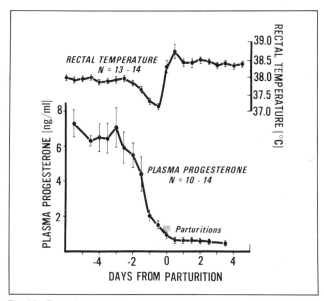

Fig 28. Transient prepartum hypothermia shown in relation to prepartum decline in plasma progesterone levels.[5]

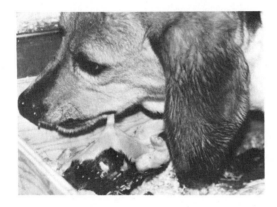

Fig 29. Bitch shortly after delivery of a pup is vigorously chewing on the umbilicus after having eaten the placenta.

diately after parturition and remains slightly above normal for several days. Because of the known hyperthermic effects of exogenous progesterone and the transient hypothermia observed during PGF-induced luteolysis, it has been suggested that the prepartum hypothermia represents a transient failure in temperature compensatory mechanisms during the rapid withdrawal of the hyperthermic effects of progesterone.[3]

For 2 to 3 days prior to parturition, bitches usually become restless, seek seclusion, and eat less food, possibly in response to elevated levels of prolactin. Restlessness, panting, scratching, chewing, and nesting are usually noticed during the 12 to 24 hours prior to parturition when prolactin levels are highest. This is stage 1 of labor, during which uterine contractions increase but are not accompanied by voluntary abdominal contractions. During stage 2 the fetuses are delivered through the cervix and vagina. Individual pups may be delivered with or without rupture of the membranes.

In pregnancies that are not equilateral, the 1st delivery is usually from the horn containing the most pups. The incidence of alternation between uterine horns in the delivery sequence is relatively high in the bitch.[94] Although usually completed within 6 hours, delivery of the entire litter can extend to 24 hours without complications. The intervals between delivery of individual pups may be 2 to 3 hours, especially between the 1st and 2nd pups; subsequent intervals are usually shorter.

Normal maternal behavior includes breaking of intact fetal membranes, intensive licking of the pups, and obsessive chewing of the umbilicus (at times resulting in perforation of the fetal abdomen), and eating the placentae (Fig 29). Placentae are delivered attached to the umbilical cords or, when detached, within 5 to 10 minutes after the delivery of individual pups. Endocrine factors affecting peripartum and postpartum behavior of the bitch have not been determined, but they probably involve elevations in prolactin and oxytocin. Normal uterine involution in the postpartum bitch has been described in detail.[95]

Runts of litters are apparently not merely the tail-end of the normal distribution in pup size. The results of a recent study suggest that in the dog and other species the growth-retarded neonates represent a distinct, separate class of offspring.[96] Whether they result from delayed implantation, genetic defect, or unequal competition for uterine support is unknown. In my experience, underdeveloped implantation sites observed after laparotomy are often associated with close proximity to normal-sized vesicles or with a cranial location in the horn.

References

1. Concannon, PW et al: Biol Reprod **12** (1975) 112.
2. Concannon, PW and Hansel, W: Fed Proc **34 (3)** (1975) 323.
3. Concannon, PW and Hansel, W: Prostaglandins **13** (1977) 533.
4. Concannon, PW et al: Biol Reprod **17** (1977) 604.
5. Concannon, PW et al: Biol Reprod **16** (1977) 517.
6. Hansel, W et al: In: *Pharmacology of Steroid Contraceptive Drugs.* Raven Press, New York, pp 145-161, 1977.
7. Concannon, PW et al: Biol Reprod **19** (1978) 1113.
8. Concannon, PW et al: Biol Reprod **20** (1979) 523.
9. Concannon, PW et al: Biol Reprod **20** (1979) 799.
10. Concannon, PW: J Reprod Fert **58** (1980) 407.
11. Concannon, PW et al: Endocrinology **106** (1980) 1173.
12. Concannon, PW et al: Fertil Steril **36** (1981) 373.
13. Concannon, PW: Ann Conf Soc Study Fert, Edinburgh, 1981.
14. Reimers, TJ et al: JAAHA **18** (1982) 923.
15. Reimers, TJ et al: Proc Soc Exp Biol Med **170** (1982) 507.
16. Concannon, PW and Rendano, V: Amer J Vet Res **44** (1982) 1506.
17. Scott, DW and Concannon, PW: JAAHA **19** (1983) 523.
18. Concannon, PW et al: Amer J Vet Res **44** (1983) 1819.
19. McCann, JP and Concannon, PW: Biol Reprod **18 (suppl 1)** (1983) 41.
20. Rendano, VT et al: Vet Radiol **25** (1984) 132.
21. Reimers, TJ et al: Biol Reprod (In press, 1984).
22. Concannon, PW et al: Unpublished data.
23. Concannon, PW and Castracane, VD: Biol Reprod **16** (1986) 1.
24. Vanderlip, S et al: Unpublished data, Univ Calif, San Diego, 1983.
25. Concannon, PW: Proc Voorjaarsdagen, Royal Netherlands Vet Assn and Netherlands Small Animal Assn. Publ #13, pp 21-26, 1981.
26. Concannon, PW: Proc Voorjaarsdagen, Royal Netherlands Vet Assn and Netherlands Small Animal Vet Assn. Post Academisch Onderwijs Pub #13, pp 117-124, 1981.
27. Concannon, PW: In: *Current Veterinary Therapy, Small Animal Practice VIII.* WB Saunders, Philadelphia, pp 886-901, 1983.
28. Concannon, PW: In: *Current Veterinary Therapy, Small Animal Practice, VIII.* WB Saunders, pp 901-909, 1983.
29. Concannon, PW: Vet Clin No Amer **16** (1986) 1.

30. Nett, TM and Olson, PN: In: *Textbook of Veterinary Internal Medicine,* ed 2, vol 2, p 1698. WB Saunders, 1983.
31. Shille, VM and Stabenfeldt, GH: Adv Vet Sci Comp Med **24** (1980) 211.
32. Johnston, SD: JAVMA **127** (1980) 1335.
33. Sokolowski, JH: Vet Clin No Amer **12 (1)** (1982) 99.
34. Hart, BL: In: *The Beagle As An Experimental Dog,* p 296. Iowa State Univ Press, 1970.
35. Wildt, D *et al:* J Anim Sci **53** (1981) 182.
36. Evans, HM and Cole, HH: Memoirs Univ California **9 (2)** (1931) 65.
37. Hancock, J and Rowlands, IW: Vet Res **61** (1949) 771.
38. Andersen, AC: In: *The Beagle As An Experimental Dog,* pp 31-39. Iowa State University Press, Ames, Iowa, 1970.
39. Anderson, AC and Simpson, ME: *The Ovary and Reproductive Cycle of the Dog (Beagle).* Geron-X, Los Altos, CA, 1973.
40. Phemister, RD: Biol Reprod **8** (1973) 74.
41. Holst, PA and Phemister, RD: Biol Reprod **5** (1971) 194.
42. Beach, FA *et al:* Horm Behavior **16** (1982) 414.
43. Olson, PN *et al:* Biol Reprod **27** (1982) 1196.
44. Sokolowski, JH *et al:* JAVMA **171** (1977) 271.
45. Yamashita, E and Mieno, M: IRCS Med Sci **8** (1980) 652.
46. Goodwin, M *et al:* Science **203** (1979) 559.
47. Olson, PN *et al:* Amer J Vet Res **45** (1984) 145.
48. Renton, J *et al:* J Reprod Fert **61** (1981) 289.
49. Roszel, JF: Vet Scope **XIX (1)** (1975) 3.
50. Olson, PN *et al:* Compend Contin Educ **6** (1984) 288.
51. Holst, PA and Phemister, RD: Amer J Vet Res **35** (1974) 401.
52. Holst, PA and Phemister, RD: Amer J Vet Res **36** (1975) 705.
53. Lindsay, FEF: J Small Anim Pract **24** (1983) 1.
54. Lindsay, FEF: In: *Current Veterinary Therapy, Small Animal Practice, VIII* WB Saunders, Philadelphia, 1983.
55. Takeisi, M *et al:* Jap J Anim Reprod **22** (1976) 28.
56. Brown, JM *et al:* JAVMA **184** (1984) 1467.
57. Johnston, SD: In: *Current Veterinary Therapy VI.* WB Saunders, Philadelphia, 1977.
58. Concannon, PW: Unpublished data, 1977.
59. Reimers, T *et al:* Biol Reprod **19** (1978) 673.
60. Graf, KJ: J Reprod Fert **52** (1978) 9.
61. DeCoster, R *et al:* Acta Endocrinol **103** (1983) 473.
62. Eigenmann, JE and Venker-van Hagen, AJ: JAAHA **17** (1981) 813.
63. Eigenmann, JE *et al:* Acta Endocrinol **104** (1983) 167.
64. Wildt, DE *et al:* Biol Reprod **20** (1979) 648.
65. Wildt, DE *et al:* Anat Rec **189** (1977) 443.
66. Concannon, PW and Cowan, RG: Unpublished data, 1978.
67. Concannon, PW: Unpublished data, 1984.
68. Smith, MS and McDonald, LE: Endocrinology **94** (1974) 404.
69. Olson, PN *et al:* Amer J Vet Res **45** (1984) 149.
70. Mahi, CA and Yanagimachi, R: J Exper Zool **196** (1976) 189.
71. Smith, F and Graham, E: Proc 10th Intern Cong Anim Reprod Artif Insem, Univ Illinois, Urbana, Il, #216, 1984.
72. Smith, F and Johnston, S: Personal communication, 1983.
73. Lee, S *et al:* Amer J Anat **16** (1983) 313.
74. Fisher, T and Fisher, D: MVP **62** (1981) 466.
75. Gentry, PA and Liptrap, RM: J Small Anim Pract **22** (1981) 185.
76. Moore, LG and Reeves, JT: Amer J Physiol **239** (1980) 297.
77. Gerber, JG *et al:* Prostaglandins **17** (1979) 623.
78. Olson, P *et al:* Amer J Vet Res **45** (1984) 119.

79. Reimers, RJ *et al:* Biol Reprod **28** Suppl. 1 (1983) 41.
80. Siegel, ET: *Endocrine Diseases of the Dog.* Lea & Febiger, Philadelphia, 1977.
81. Renauld, A *et al:* Acta Diab Lat **10** (1973) 1286.
82. Romsos, D *et al:* Nutr **111** (1981) 678.
83. Allen, WE and Meredith, MJ: J Small Anim Pract **22 (9)** (1981) 609.
84. Taverne, M and deBois, C: Proc 10th Intl Cong Animal Reprod Artif Insem, Univ Illinois, Urbana, #113, 1984.
85. Rendano, V: In: *Current Veterinary Therapy, Small Animal Practice VIII.* WB Saunders, Philadelphia, pp 947-952, 1983.
86. Sokolowski, J: Lab Anim Sci **21** (1974) 696.
87. Votquenne, M: Hypophysectomie Cor Seanc Soc Biol **122** (1936) 91.
88. Concannon, PW: Rec Progr Horm Res **37** (1981) 287.
89. Conley, A and Evans, L: Proc 10th Intl Cong Anim Reprod Artif Insem, Univ Illinois, Urbana #504, 1984.
90. Migday, A: Proc Conf Res Workers Anim Dis, 59th ann mtg, Chicago, 1978.
91. Paradis, M *et al:* Canad Vet J **24** (1983) 239.
92. Jackson, P *et al:* J Small Anim Pract **23** (1982) 287.
93. Vickery, B and McRae, G: Biol Reprod **22** (1980) 438.
94. Van der Weyden, G *et al:* J Small Anim Pract **22 (8)** (1981) 503.
95. Albassam, MA *et al:* Canad J Comp Med **45** (1981) 217.
96. Wooton, R *et al:* J Reprod Fert **69** (1983) 659.

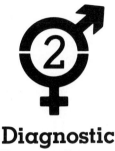

Diagnostic Procedures

OBTAINING A BREEDING HISTORY
BY NICKOLAS J. SOJKA

Introduction

The primary purpose of obtaining a history of an animal's reproductivity is to direct the clinician toward the most likely causes of infertility. The history should be of sufficient detail to also encourage investigation of less common conditions. Though the owners will not always be able to supply all the desired information about a patient, a partial answer may enable a valid assumption. The topics that should be covered in the history include the animal's age, weight, general condition, previous breeding performance, breeding environment, and familial background.

Age of Breeding Animals

Puberty

Clients attempting to breed young animals may be unaware that different breeds mature at varying ages and rates. Though feral and domestic shorthair cats may reach puberty as early as 4 months of age, long-haired cats may be 1½ years old. Similar variations occur among large and small breeds of dogs.

The season at birth can also affect the time of year at which an animal first comes into estrus.

The use of hormones to induce precocious puberty for the convenience of or economic gain for the owner should be discouraged because of the possible adverse effects of these agents on subsequent reproductive capacity.

79

Maturity

Another problem associated with the age of breeding animals occurs when clients attempt to breed mature animals that have been prevented from breeding during their prime reproductive years (generally from 2 to 5 years of age). Females may have difficulty related to reduced elasticity of tissues and increased variability of hormone levels. An inexperienced, mature male may have difficulty in copulating successfully. This may be due to the male's reluctance to approach the female in a normal manner and/or his inability to mount, intromit, and ejaculate successfully.

Excessive psychologic dependence on their owners can affect the breeding performance of cats and dogs of any age. This rarely occurs in animals that have previously bred successfully.[1,2]

Older Animals

Many cats and dogs continue to breed and produce litters when they are considered old. The litters of aged females may be smaller than average and less viable. There also is an increased probability of difficult deliveries and postpartum complications among older animals.

Weight and Reproductivity

Little is known about the direct effects of obesity on reproduction in dogs and cats. The general lethargy associated with obesity can be accompanied by decreased interest in sexual activity. There is some evidence that though fecundity among heavier queens (>3.5 kg) may be higher than average, the survival rate of their kittens to weaning is poorer than that observed in litters of queens that weigh less.[3] The cause of this apparent paradox is unknown, but it could result from factors related to fetal development, psychologic influences within large litters, or physiologic limitations on the quality or quantity of prenatal or postnatal nutrition.

Considerable loss of weight and chronic anorexia are usually indicative of disease. Severe parasitisms, infections, malnutrition, neoplasia, and metabolic disorders affect reproductive ability. Queens that weigh less than average (<2.88 kg) and have no identifiable disease have smaller litters than normal. There are no adverse effects on survival of kittens to weaning, however.[3]

General Condition

Recent surgery or serious illness accompanied by fever, dehydration, weight loss, or prolonged antibiotic therapy can adversely affect the gonads and the synthesis of reproductive hormones. Such damage is almost always reversible and normal function can be regained within several weeks to months if there is no additional impairment, such as adhesions obstructing or constricting the reproductive tract following abdominal surgery. Information from the owner concerning visible birth defects in a cat or dog should always be considered as possibly indicative of other internal defects. Obvious abnormalities may have been corrected surgically and not be apparent during a routine physical examination. Though some heritable anomalies, such as polydactyly, usually occur without accompanying defects, abnormalities that are exogenously induced during embryonic development often appear in more than one organ system.

Breeding Record

When there is a history of earlier successful reproductive behavior and function, a current problem may be traceable to injuries to the male genitalia during previous breeding, to injuries suffered by a female during her last parturition, or to injuries from accidents unrelated to reproduction. The use of drugs, especially hormones that directly affect reproduction, should be considered as a possible cause.

Excessive natural breeding is usually not considered a cause of reduced fertility. Males allowed to breed as often as they desire will rarely do so to the point of depleting their sperm count significantly. Bitches and queens that have 2 or 3 litters annually do not suffer adverse effects on their reproductivity if their increased nutritional needs are met. In a study of queens producing 3 litters per year under laboratory conditions, there was no reduction in either litter size or survival of kittens to weaning, and the queens had no unusual health problems.[3]

The fertility and fecundity of the sexual partners of the animal being examined should also be considered. It usually is advantageous to breed an inexperienced animal to an experienced one whose fertility has been demonstrated. Attempting to breed 2 sexually inexperienced animals can result in an unjustified bias against both. If the sexual partners of an animal in question have had prior successful matings, however, the responsibility for reproductive failure is more reliably assigned to the inexperienced partner.

Diagnosis of the exact nature of reproductive problems requires questioning about estrous behavior, length of estrous cycle, postcoital behavior, etc. It may be necessary for the owner to keep a log of such events. A diagnosis of infertility in a male should never be based on only one semen sample. At least 3 samples should be examined over a month or so. Individual semen samples vary so much that any one of them is almost worthless for definite diagnosis.

Environmental Influences

Cats and dogs that spend most of their lives outdoors and in contact with other animals can be expected to exhibit more normal sexual behavior than isolated or confined animals. Because both cats and dogs are inherently territorial animals, they can cause problems when they attempt to establish a territory for breeding or parturition indoors by urinating on furniture, etc.

Aberrant sexual behavior, such as persistent estrus, unusually shy or aggressive breeding postures, and mounting members of the same sex or other species or inanimate objects, is observed more frequently in animals kept indoors. Such behavior may occur in response to a combination of factors.

Use of disinfectants with strong odors to sanitize areas for breeding or birthing can have adverse results by blocking perception of pheromones. This can lead to unnatural aggressive behavior and cannibalism of newborn animals.

Identification of odors is essential for normal breeding behavior by both males and females. Females also identify their offspring by smell as they clean them after delivery and they may be inhibited from performing this natural function by strong odors. When several breeding animals are confined in an area, odors usually can be reduced by providing a constant exchange of air. Including some fresh air in each exchange will also dilute the number of airborne viruses and other pathogens in the environment.

The effect of prolonged exposure to light on reproductive function has been best identified in the feline species. When year-round estrous cycles are desired in cats kept in laboratories, they are exposed to artificial light for 12 to 14 hours per day. Such lighting is common in many homes and it can have the same effects on susceptible animals. Though breeding behavior and ovulation may not occur with every estrus, episodic restlessness, aggression, and vocalization will be apparent.

Another environmental influence that should be considered is the owner's behavior during a pet's estrus and pregnancy. The presence of humans, especially those with whom there is a close pet-owner bond, can be inhibitory to normal coital and parturitional behavior. An animal's emotional attachment to its owner may distract attention from the intended mate or newborn offspring to such an extent that even the strongest instinctive urges are overridden. When this occurs, the owner should be advised to keep away from the pet for the time required.

Male cats that do not readily breed females that are in estrus may become more sexually aggressive if they have a room or even a large cage where they can establish a territory. They should be allowed at least 2 weeks to establish this identification and then queens can be brought to this area for mating.

Familial History

A number of reproductive problems may be traced in a canine or feline family when information is available about prior generations. Reduced fertility or fecundity may be due to such heritable conditions as hypophyseal-hypothalamic dysfunctions, leukodystrophies, cryptorchidism, uterus unicornus, or osseous deformities of the pelvis or spine.[4] Production of poor-quality semen may be a heritable characteristic that is self-limiting.

In utero exposure to x-rays, especially during organogenesis, and transplacental exposure to fetotoxic substances can adversely affect the subsequent reproductivity of animals. Aberrant maternal behavior can have adverse effects on the reproductive capacity of the offspring. This has been observed in laboratory animals and may occur occasionally in cats and dogs.

References
1. Hart, BL: Feline Pract **5(12)** (1975) 12.
2. Mosier, JE: MVP **56** (1975) 699.
3. Cline, EM and Sojka, NJ: Manuscript in preparation, 1982.
4. Stein, BS: The Genital System. In *Feline Medicine and Surgery.* American Veterinary Publications, Santa Barbara, CA 1975.

PHYSICAL EXAMINATION
BY THOMAS J. BURKE

Introduction

A complete physical examination of breeding animals should follow or accompany the taking of the animal's breeding and medical history. All of the body systems should be examined because a disorder of any could affect reproductive efficiency.

Examination of the Female

The mammary glands should be inspected and palpated. The uterus can be palpated by locating the cervix and uterine body between the colon dorsally and urinary bladder ventrally. The cervix is readily identified as a firm fusiform mass. The bladder usually is relatively empty. A thermometer inserted in the rectum will aid identification of the colon. The uterine horns can then be palpated by moving the fingers cranially. Normal ovaries are not palpable, but some ovarian cysts and tumors can be felt just caudal to the kidneys.

After the vulva is inspected and palpated, the labia are parted and the caudal vestibule and clitoral fossa are inspected. The perineum should then be washed, rinsed, and dried. If material is to be taken for culture or cytology, it should be obtained at this time prior to application of a lubricant. One of the most important yet most frequently omitted examinations is digital palpation of the vestibule and vagina. A sterile glove and lubricant are used for this procedure and a gloved index finger is inserted into the vestibule in a dorsocranial direction until the urethral meatus is felt when the finger is advanced to a more horizontal plane. It is important to determine the vagina's size and to detect any strictures. Female cats must be sedated and an otoscope used for this part of the examination. If a mass or any abnormal contour is palpated, the free hand should be gloved, lubricated, and the index finger inserted per rectum to assist palpation of the abnormality. If necessary, a vaginoscopy can be performed.

Examination of the Male

The mammary glands should be inspected and palpated. After the scrotum is inspected, it should be palpated to detect abnormal thickness or enlargements. Both testes should be in the scrotum by the time decidual dentition is complete. The testes should be palpated to determine their size and consistency. Generalizations about normal size are impossible because of the wide variation in the size of dogs. The testicular contour should be smooth and its consistency should be firmly resilient.

Each epididymis should be palpated. The head of the epididymis is located on the dorsal craniolateral aspect of the testis. The body lies on the dorsolateral surface and extends to the caudal pole where the tail of the epididymis turns medially and then extends cranially as part of the spermatic cord. The surface of the epididymis is normally smooth, but there may be slight convolutions and sulci. Extreme firmness or a rope-like consistency is abnormal. If the testicle is undersized, the epididymis may feel enlarged.

The prostate can be palpated per rectum or per abdomen. This gland is bilobate with a prominent dorsal sulcus. The lobes are normally smooth, firm, and of equal size.

The prepuce should be inspected and the penis should be extended and examined as far caudally as possible. Sedation may be required to examine the penis back to the reflection of the penile mucosa onto the preputial mucosa. This area may also be inspected with an otoscope or cystoscope. Most cats must be sedated prior to examining the penis. The presence of penile spines is related to the androgen level and thus their presence or absence may be a clue about the endocrine function of the animal. Because excessive hair around the glans penis of cats may interfere with copulation, it should be removed if present. Rectal palpation of the prostate gland in cats is not feasible nor is it routinely necessary because diseases of this gland in cats are rare. It is best examined by radiography.

PREGNANCY DIAGNOSIS
BY THOMAS J. BURKE & ROBERT R. BADERTSCHER, II

Pregnancy diagnosis is not just a "nice thing for the owner to know." In many cases of so-called failure to conceive, the patient was not checked during the potential gestation period, and it is therefore impossible to rule out abortion or fetal resorption. The authors recommend that all mated females be examined for pregnancy as early as possible. If the animal has a history of infertility, appropriate determinations of pregnancy should then be performed weekly or biweekly. In addition, in certain competitions, the puppies are nominated prior to birth. The importance to the owner of an accurate diagnosis of pregnancy in these cases is obvious.

Palpation
Abdominal palpation remains the cheapest and easiest means of pregnancy diagnosis. It is most accurate early in gestation because the maternal-fetal swellings become less distinct in mid- to-late gestation. In late pregnancy, however, one may be able to feel the heads and rumps of the fetuses as well as fetal movement.

Palpation of the uterus is easiest when the patient is standing. A gentle, calm approach is necessary to keep the patient as relaxed as possible. It is advisable to have the patient urinate and defecate just prior to the examination; a full colon or bladder may hinder accurate palpation. The use of sedatives is to be avoided unless pregnancy must be determined and the patient refuses to allow her abdomen to be examined. In these cases, an intravenous dose of diazepam is usually sufficient. Such treatment has not, to the authors' knowledge, had adverse affects on fetal development. The duration of effect is brief enough that it may be performed as an outpatient procedure.

Implantation occurs about 16 to 17 days following conception in the bitch. In the queen, implantation occurs 2 to 3 days earlier. Within a few days, firm, equally spaced swellings are palpable. At 21 days, these swellings measure approximately 1 cm in diameter. By day 24 to 26, they are nearly 2 cm in diameter. The size is relatively constant among all breeds.[7] By day 32 to 35, the size of the dam begins to affect the size of the lumps, with smaller breeds averaging about 3 to 3.5 cm and medium breeds about 4 cm; giant breeds may approach 6 to 7 cm.[7] After day 35, the swellings become indistinct from one another, and palpation becomes nearly useless. Fetal heads and rumps are usually palpable during the last 2 weeks of pregnancy.

Radiography

Although ossification begins as early as day 28, it is not detectable by routine radiography until about day 42; it is prominent by day 45 to 47. Diagnostic radiology at this time is not teratogenic. The number of fetuses can usually be determined by this method, although it is difficult in large litters. The patient should be as calm as possible because movement may blur the fetal outlines and may "erase" them.

Ultrasound

Three types of ultrasonic instruments have been used for pregnancy detection in small animals: A-mode, B-mode, and Doppler-type devices.[1-3,5,6] Each mode produces pulses of high-frequency ultrasound waves and, between pulses, detects retrograde reflections. Variations in tissue density encountered and reflected (echogenic) are detected and displayed. A-mode units only display the amplitude of the returning echoes as peaks. on an oscilloscopic screen. The urinary bladder does not show peaks (anechotic) because the fluid transmits all sound to deeper tissues. The placenta also contains a significant amount of fluid and may give a signal similar to that of the bladder on A-mode.[1] Thus, the patient should have an empty bladder at the time of examination with an A-mode instrument.

B-mode ultrasound units display images, much like a radiograph, of the cross-sectional features of internal organs (Fig 1). The relative densities of internal organs are displayed as different shades of gray (gray scale). Commercial units are available that utilize multiple crystals (linear-array scanners) or moving crystals (sector scanners), to create the moving, two-dimensional image (real-time image). Thus, B-mode real-time ultrasound units allow noninvasive visualization of the uterus and fetus and can measure structures as small as a millimeter. Because fluid transmits the entire sound wave to deeper structures, it is helpful for the patient to have a partially distended urinary bladder when B-mode units are used to image the uterus. The animal is usually placed in dorsal recumbency, and the transducer is moved in both transverse and longitudinal planes over the abdomen. In cases of early pregnancy (less than 25 days), it is important also to scan the bitch in the standing position because the uterus may be located lateral, instead of directly dorsal, to the bladder.

Doppler-type instruments rely on the principle, first demonstrated

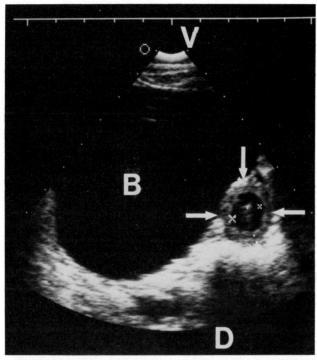

Fig 1. Cross-sectional image of anechotic urinary bladder (B) and enlarged uterus (arrows) in a Labrador Retriever bred 25 days before. The dog was standing, and a mechanical sector scanner was used to make this image. The diameter of the uterus measured 2.3 cm, and the inner chorionic vesicle measured 1.1 cm (between x and x). The fetus is represented by the faint internal echos. V, Ventral; D, dorsal.

by Christian Doppler, that the frequency of sound emitted or reflected from a moving object varies with the velocity of the object. Thus, when the object is moving toward the transducer, a rise in pitch is perceived; a fall is perceived as the object recedes. Transducers of Doppler instruments receive their reflections from moving objects in the abdomen. When the object moves rhythmically, like a blood vessel or heart wall, a pulsed signal is heard. Because the fetal heart beats 2 to 3 times as fast as the maternal heart, differences are readily detectable. In addition, the placenta produces a low, "wind-in-the-trees" sound.

For all instruments, the transducer must be placed in a relatively hairless area (umbilicus), or a small area of hair should be clipped. The skin must also be lubricated to eliminate an air interface between the skin and the transducer. Special lubricants are available for this purpose, but standard gels, such as K-Y, and corn oil have been used with good results. Once the transducer head is applied, the abdomen is scanned by slowly moving the transducer in a circular fashion. It may be necessary to scan all quadrants of the abdomen, if pregnancy is not detected in the caudal abdomen.

One study used A-mode ultrasound in 4 bitches, 3 of which were pregnant.[6] Pregnancy was detected as early as day 18 in 1 bitch, day 20 (but not 18) in the second, and day 23 (but not 21) in the third.[6] In another study comparing A-mode and Doppler units, the earliest correct positive results with A-mode devices were not obtained until day 26.[1] The greatest accuracy (90%) was obtained from day 32 to 62.[1] Much of the variability in accuracy can be attributed to the skill of the sonographer.

The use of B-mode units allows visualization of uterine enlargement as early as 7 days in gestation.[2] The embryo has been reported to be observed as early as gestational day 10.[2] In our experience, correct documentation of the chorionic vesicle with real-time units is difficult prior to 18 days, a difficulty also encountered by other investigators.[5] The resolution of commercial units varies and depends on the frequency and design of the transducer. Favorable resolution is obtained with either 5.0- or 7.5-megahertz (MHz) units. It is difficult to visualize the actual fetus prior to 28 days. At this time, fetal movements can often be observed, and the beating hearts can be easily detected by day 35.[5]

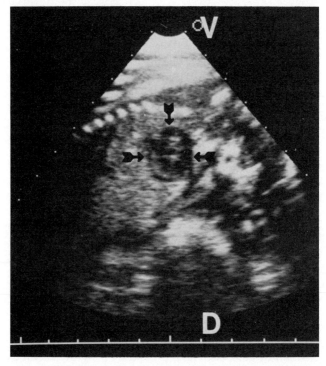

Fig 2. Sector image showing longitudinal section through the thorax of a 54-day embryo. The costal cartilages can be identified closest to the transducer (top), and the head is faintly visualized toward the right. The chambers and valves within the heart (arrows) can be identified, along with the fetal aorta. V, Ventral; D, dorsal.

Most rapid growth rate of the fetus occurs between the fourth and fifth weeks of gestation, with an increase in body length and width of over 150%.[2] Many internal organs, such as the heart, liver, bladder, and stomach, can often be identified by day 45 (Fig 2). The transverse measurements of the skull, the biparietal diameter (BPD), is commonly used to determine the gestational age of the fetus after 35 days (Fig 3). Earlier determinations of fetal age are difficult because of variability in the size of the bitch, variation in growth rate of individual fetuses, and fluid content of the chorionic vesicle.

Initial examination for pregnancy is usually performed between days 21 and 28; the accuracy rate is greater as the pregnancy develops. One report compared digital palpation techniques with ultrasonic detection of pregnancy in 33 Greyhounds. The accuracy was 15 to 25% higher during this period using a real-time linear-array unit than with

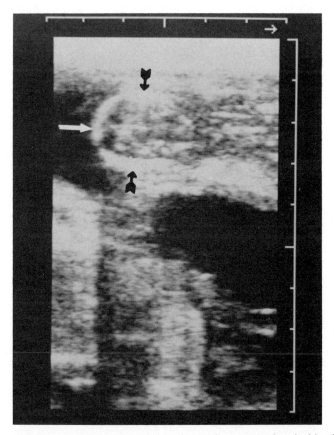

Fig 3. The skull (arrows) of this 42-day-old fetus is seen in cross-section; the biparietal diameter was 1.7 cm. A linear-array transducer was used to make this image. The black anechotic areas represent the amniotic fluid in 2 separate vesicles.

palpation methods.[5] These workers still reported that pregnancy was not diagnosed in 33% of the bitches even at 30 days in gestation. We have noted a greater accuracy using a sector scanner early in gestation, when compared to a linear-array unit. By scanning the animals both when they are in dorsal recumbency and while they are standing, pregnancy can almost always be detected by 30 days. Animals are often rescanned 7 to 10 days later when pregnancy is not detected at 21 days. Other reasons for failure to image the pregnancy include lack of distension of urinary bladder, excessive gas in colon and bowel loops, and inexperience of the sonographer. Internal organs with an appearance similar to that of the early, anechotic, chorionic vesicles include the abdominal aorta (pulsates), fluid-filled bowel loops, and pathologic uterine conditions (pyometra). See Figures 4 and 5 for examples of these structures and conditions.

An early study with a Doppler-type ultrasound unit in 30 bitches detected placental sounds as early as day 25 and fetal heart sounds by day 29 in one bitch; consistently positive results were found in all pregnant bitches by day 32.[3] The foregoing comparative study used 2 Doppler instruments and found one to be superior. Reliable positive results were consistently obtained by day 33 in this study; the rate of

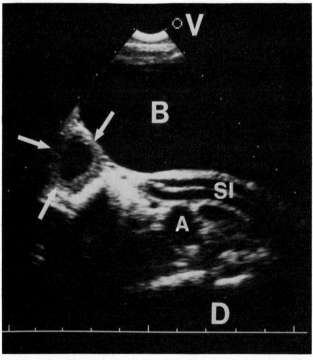

Fig 4. This transverse scan using a sector scanner again shows the anechotic urinary bladder (B) and thick-walled, enlarged uterus (arrows) with the chorionic vesicle. A longitudinal loop of small intestine (SI) is immediately dorsal to the bladder, and the circular, thin-walled aorta (A) is also imaged. V, Ventral; D, dorsal.

accuracy for both pregnant and nonpregnant bitches was 85% from day 36 to 42 and 100% from day 43 to 64.[1] These findings are in general agreement with other studies. It appears that the accuracy may be affected by the acoustic energy of the instrument because the inferior one had an energy rating of 10 Mw/cm², whereas the superior instrument was rated at 50 Mw/cm². One should select an instrument with relatively high energy output and a frequency between 2 and 5 MHz. The author's experience with so-called mini-Dops (low-power, handheld units designed for use in women) bears this out; these devices were much less accurate than conventional units.

The accuracy of ultrasonic determination of pregnancy is affected by abdominal motion caused by panting and movement of the patient. Tranquilization may be necessary in some animals. The patient should be as calm as possible. Because ultrasound techniques are operator dependent, accuracy improves with experience.

With A-mode ultrasound, one can detect pregnancy earlier than with Doppler-type devices.[1] One cannot detect fetal viability. A-mode units are generally more expensive than Doppler units, although neither can be considered inexpensive. Most Doppler units come with a speaker and earphones. Because the noise generated during the examination can produce apprehension in the patient, the authors first

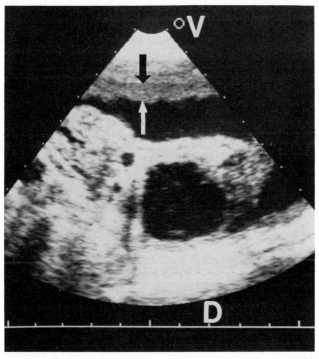

Fig 5. Longitudinal and transverse presentation of enlarged uterine horns. Note the thickened, irregular uterine wall (arrows) and the multiple echos within each lumen. Pyometra was confirmed during a surgical procedure. V, Ventral; D, dorsal.

use the earphones, so the room stays quiet. Once the diagnosis is made, the speaker is used, to allow the owner to hear the fetuses. The effect is dramatic, and in our opinion, many owners become more conscientious about the prenatal care of their animal after hearing or seeing the fetuses. Doppler ultrasound is also useful in animals with dystocia and apparent impending abortion, to determine fetal viability when formulating a therapeutic plan.[4] B-mode units are more expensive than A-mode or Doppler devices, but they are also more accurate and provide a dynamic image. Both fetal viability and size can be determined by B-mode ultrasound in animals with dystocia.

In queens, the authors have found Doppler ultrasound to be consistently accurate after day 31. B-mode units provide similar images for queens and bitches.

The ultrasonic energy used by diagnostic ultrasound instruments is safe for the dam and her fetuses.[3] No known harmful effects have been documented in humans or animals.

Biologic Tests

As of this writing, no biologic or chemical tests are available for pregnancy detection in the bitch or queen.

External Observations

Grossly visible changes are usually not detected until the second half of gestation and are more marked in the primipara. Teat enlargement may be seen as early as day 21, but it is more prominent after day 35. Some pigmentary changes may occur, with the teats becoming bright pink. Noticeable hypertrophy of the glands occurs after day 50. Milk letdown may occur as early as 36 hours prior to parturition, or even earlier in the multipara.

Weight gain and abdominal distension are not obvious until after day 35. Distension is frequently most pronounced just after eating.

References

1. Allen, WE and Meredith, MJ: J Small Anim Pract **22**(1981) 609.
2. Cartee, RE and Rowles, T: Amer J Vet Res **45**(1984) 1259.
3. Helper, LC: JAVMA **156**(1970) 60.
4. Jackson, PGG and Nicholson, JM: Vet Rec **104**(1979) 36.
5. Shille, VM and Gontarek, J: JAVMA **187**(1985) 1021.
6. Smith, DM and Kirk, GR: J Am Anim Hosp Assn **11**(1975) 201.
7. Whitney, LF: Vet Med **31**(1936) 216.

VAGINOSCOPY WITH ABNORMAL FINDINGS
BY THOMAS J. BURKE

Introduction

Vaginoscopy is a minor diagnostic procedure that requires little time, a moderate amount of equipment, and often provides useful information. Even negative observations are helpful because they direct attention to another area of the body.

Indications

Ideally vaginoscopy should be performed on all potential breeding females to search for congenital strictures, vaginal septa, and other congenital malformations (Fig 1). Unfortunately, in many cases such defects are discovered only after a problem has occurred. Most breeders are willing to accept vaginoscopy as part of the routine pre-breeding examination.

The most common indications for vaginoscopy are bleeding inappropriate for the stage of the estrous cycle, other abnormal vaginal discharge, dysuria, and pain at breeding. The procedure should be preceded by obtaining specimens for cytologic evaluation (before any lubricant is used) and then by digital palpation of the vagina if the patient is large enough. Suitable material for culture can be obtained during vaginoscopy if precautions are taken to avoid contamination.

Tractable animals may not require any chemical restraint. Mild to heavy sedation is usually sufficient for the remainder. General anesthesia is rarely required.

Instruments Used

The vestibule, clitoris, and caudal vagina can be examined with the aid of an anoscope or nasal speculum (Figs 2,3). Inspection of the middle and cranial vagina requires longer instruments.

The primary factor affecting the selection of instruments is cost. Flexible fiberoptic instruments are ideal because they can be used to

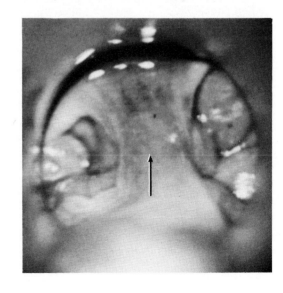

Fig 1. Vaginal septum (arrow) extends from floor of the vagina to the dorsal wall. Normal vaginal mucosa is on either side.

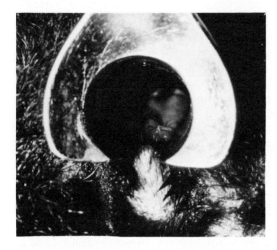

Fig 2. Examination of the vestibule and urethral orifice with an anoscope. Courtesy of Dr BC McKiernan, University of Illinois.

examine almost any animal and they provide cool lighting and excellent visualization. They are expensive, however. Rigid instruments are second choice. Instruments with front lights are preferred. Those with fiberoptic light sources are moderately priced and are preferred over incandescent lights. Proctoscopes and sigmoidoscopes designed for humans are often satisfactory for animals. They provide magnification and enable insufflation of the vagina with air to improve

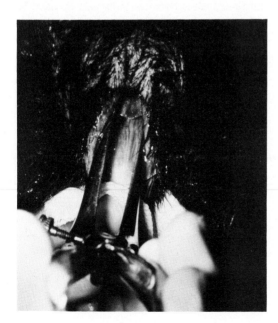

Fig 3. Examination of the clitoris with a nasal speculum. Courtesy of Dr BC McKiernan, University of Illinois.

visibility. Very small bitches and queens may be examined with an otoscope with a gas-sterilized cone of appropriate size. A cystoscope may also be used.

Other rigid instruments may be fashioned from plastic tubes or made from glass. I have a set of Pyrex glass specula that were made by a glass blower. They range in diameter from 0.5 to 4.0 cm and vary in length from 12 to 30 cm. They were inexpensive and proved quite useful until they were replaced by fiberoptic equipment. Such specially made specula should have slightly bevelled tips to facilitate their insertion and a flanged viewing end to assist in their manipulation.

Examination Procedures

All instruments used for vaginoscopy should be sterilized. Cold (chemical) sterilization is not recommended if swabs for culturing are to be inserted through or around the instrument. A sterile lubricant is applied to the animal's vulva and caudal vagina prior to insertion of

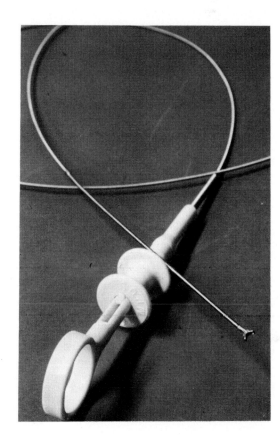

Fig 4. Flexible biopsy forceps for use through a flexible endoscope.

the instrument. If a proctoscope is being used, the obturator is held in place and the instrument is inserted as far cranially as it passes freely. The obturator is then removed and the viewing lens is secured. The vagina is viewed as the instrument is withdrawn. Lesions can be located precisely by the centimeter markings on the outside of the instrument. If resistance is encountered during insertion of the instrument, the obturator is removed and the area is examined closely before forceful attempts are made to pass the instrument further. When a flexible instrument is used, the vagina is inspected as it is inserted.

Either a proctoscope or fiberoptic instrument will usually enable inspection of the caudal vagina from the vestibule cranially to the posterior median vaginal fold (pseudocervix). An impression of the condition of the vaginal mucosa should be formed early in the examination because continued exposure of mucosa to air will cause mild erythema. The mucosa is normally smooth, white-pink, and may glisten slightly.

Because many vaginal lesions are similar in appearance, biopsy equipment should be available when performing a vaginoscopy. A vaginal or colonic punch biopsy forceps is satisfactory and little practice is needed to become proficient in its use. Most flexible instruments include a flexible biopsy forceps and, although the sample is smaller, it usually provides a piece of tissue sufficient for histopathologic examination (Fig 4). Tumors and other masses may be sampled with this instrument. Sliding knife biopsy capsules may be used to obtain samples of proliferative mucosal lesions.

CANINE VAGINAL CYTOLOGY
BY PATRICK W. CONCANNON & GINA B. DIGREGORIO

Introduction

Serial evaluation of the vaginal mucosa on a daily or alternate-day basis should be an integral part of the management of a bitch whenever there is concern about the appropriate time for breeding, the result of a breeding, the scheduling of pregnancy examinations, or the management of whelping. Changes in exfoliate vaginal cells observed in simply and rapidly prepared smears can provide direct evidence of the progression of follicular development and estrogen secretion during proestrus, a reasonable estimate of the fertile period during estrus, and fairly accurate estimations of the end of the fertile period and the timing of subsequent events of a resulting pregnancy.

Collection and examination of vaginal smears on a routine basis during proestrus and estrus also provide an opportunity to monitor the degree of vulval swelling and of reflex responses typical of estrus. Daily or alternate-day evaluation of perineal and/or tail reflexes, vulval turgor, and vaginal cytology is usually sufficient to monitor the progression of periovulatory events in most bitches. Whenever it is feasible, however, direct visualization of the vaginal mucosa can provide additional evidence of the approximate time of ovulation and/or the status of a bitch relative to the time of ovulation or oocyte maturation. Normal canine vaginoscopy is discussed on page 108.

Methods of collecting and preparing canine vaginal smears, along with their interpretation, have been reviewed by several authors.[1-17] There is no general agreement, however, about the best method of collecting samples, use of instruments, area of the vagina to sample, method of fixing and staining samples, or terms to be used for categories of cell types. The procedures to be described are used in the senior author's laboratory for routine, rapid evaluations of vaginal cytology during proestrus and estrus. There will be only limited commentary on other procedures.

Collection of the Sample

Smears are obtained from the mid- or cranial vagina while avoiding contamination with material in the clitoral fossa or vestibule. A moistened cotton-tipped swab is guided and protected by a previously inserted speculum to collect a sample of vaginal cells that is rolled onto a clean glass slide and fixed immediately to prevent air drying. The swabs are either cotton-tipped wooden applicators (Q-Tip: Chesbrough-Ponds) or cotton-tipped culture collection swabs (Culturettes: Marion Scientific Co). Both are 6 inches long. Either is satisfactory for bitches that weigh more than 4 kg. For smaller bitches, household-type swabs (Q-Tips), hand-prepared or modified swabs, or wire loops may be used or the collection may be accomplished by lavage, using a medicine dropper with a small volume of saline. Loose-packed swabs are moistened with a small amount of water or saline solution; excess fluid should be shaken from the swab prior to its insertion. Culture swabs are moistened with the fluid provided in individual sterile packs.

The preferred speculum is 2-bladed, 4 to 5 inches long, tapered, and spreadable. Such specula are also useful for examination of the clitoral fossa, vestibular mucosa, caudal vagina, and urethral meatus. The clean or sterile speculum is inserted into the vestibule with its tip pointed upwards 50 to 60 degrees or more from the horizontal. It is gently passed up the vestibule until the tip is felt to have entered the caudal vagina and/or passed over the pelvic brim. Any pressure against the mucosa should be directed dorsally to prevent the speculum's lodging in the anterior vestibule or entering the urinary meatus. The speculum is then gently passed forward and horizontally into the vagina as far as possible before the blades are spread and held open. The swab is inserted its full length along the inside of one of the blades, avoiding contact with the mucosa until it is in the vagina (Fig 1). Turning the swab on its axis will facilitate its entry.

The best smears are obtained with the swab at its full depth, wiping the vaginal mucosa with a combination of circular, twisting, and back-and-forth motions. The amount of circular motion needed will vary with the stage of the estrous cycle and size of the vaginal lumen. The motion should be vigorous enough to ensure good contact with the vaginal mucosa. The swab is then withdrawn within the speculum to avoid contact with the vestibule or vulva. The color and content of the swab's surface are noted and a smear is prepared immediately. The speculum is withdrawn in a half-open position to avoid pinching tissue. A tubular speculum with appropriate diameter can also be used.

Several authors have stressed the importance of obtaining smears from the cranial vagina and avoiding contact with the caudal portion.[14] Others have reported that it is not necessary to cover the swab for routine collection of samples.[11] In our experience the vestibule and clitoral fossa contain cells that are less representative of vaginal changes, and we believe that these areas are best avoided. Moistened swabs are preferred to dry ones because the latter may absorb both mucus and cells and prevent the transfer of a representative sample to the slide. The 6-inch swabs are used because they are available and are also suitable for large bitches in which the distance from the vulva to the vagina may be 3 to 4 inches and the vagina may be 8 to 10 inches long. A swab can be lengthened by attaching a piece of tight-fitting plastic tubing to it.

Preparation of Slides

The swab is rolled gently onto a clean glass slide, making 2 or 3 separate stripes that are each ⅓ to ½ the length of the slide. Any one area should not be smeared more than once, but rolling stripes close to each other in a limited area will facilitate microscopic scanning and examination. The smears should be made without applying much pressure on the swab. The purpose is to transfer representative material but not all of the material on the swab.

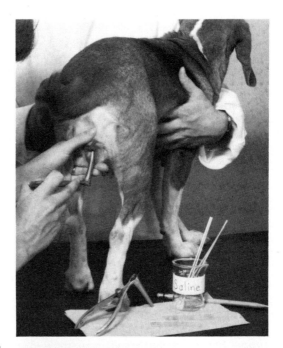

Fig 1. Collection of vaginal smear. A. Insertion of speculum in an upward (cranio-dorsal) direction for passage through vestibule and over pelvic brim.
B. Speculum is then advanced horizontally through cingulum into caudal mid-vagina to enable insertion of a moistened swab along the inner surface of one of the blades and avoid the labia and vestibular mucosa.

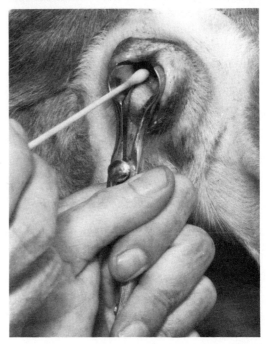

The smear can be fixed immediately (within 1 or 2 seconds) while it is still moist and before any appreciable air drying by immersing the slide into a liquid fixative or by spraying it with a commercial aerosol fixative (Spray-Cyte: Clay Adams; Cyto-Prep: Fisher Scientific). The aerosol fixative may be preferred because of its portability, accessibility, and ease of use and maintenance. Some believe that it is critical to fix slides while they are still moist and that air drying causes unacceptable deterioration and distortion of cells.[4,14,15] In contrast, other workers have routinely used air-dried preparations for detailed analysis of canine vaginal smears.[10] Though absence of a fixative should not deter performing vaginal cytology, the routine use of one will enhance the standardization of the procedure and the differences observed will more likely represent differences in the cells and not the methodology.

Staining the Slide

Stains and staining procedures used or recommended for vaginal cytology have ranged from use of polychromatic stains that require several minutes or hours for processing to use of simple staining methods requiring less than a minute.[4,11] One of the latter methods is probably preferable for routine clinical application. Examples include use of Wright's stain, Wright's-Giemsa stain, new methylene blue, and a modified Wright's-Giemsa (Diff-Quik).[11]

The modified Wright's-Giemsa stain has been satisfactory for routinely monitoring the progression of proestrus and estrus in the bitches of our Beagle breeding colony and in bitches of various breeds presented for fertility examinations or breeding management. The Diff-Quik staining set (distributed by American Scientific Products, McGaw Park, Illinois) consists of stock bottles of a fixative solution, an orange stain, and a blue stain. Suitable amounts of each are kept in screw-capped glass or plastic Coplin jars labeled as solution (or step) #1, #2, and #3, respectively. They are placed alongside a 4th jar or preferably a large beaker in which fresh rinse water is placed prior to each use (Fig 2). The manufacturer recommends 5 immersions of 1 second each, repeated for each of the solutions. After dipping a slide 5 times for 1 second each into the fixative (either air-dried or spray-fixed slides), we routinely dip the slide into the orange stain 2 or 3 times to wet the slide evenly before counting off the recommended 5 dips. The slide is then usually dipped 5 times into the blue stain although, in some studies and with some batches of stain, 4 immersions will result in better overall results. Proceeding too rapidly can be avoided by counting the second for each immersion. The stability

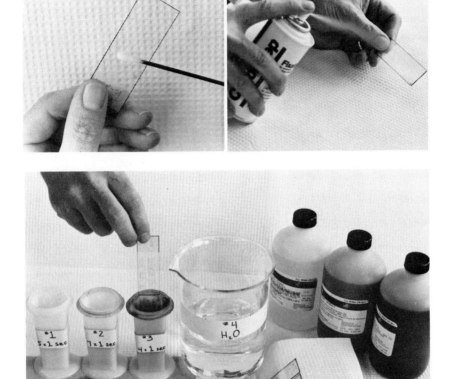

Fig 2. Procedures for preparation of vaginal smear, including gentle rolling onto slide, application of spray fixative, use of serial steps for Diff-Quik staining, rinsing by dipping in water, and setting on end to dry.

of the stains can be prolonged and the rinsing and drying times can be reduced by draining excess fluid off the slide after each step by touching the slide's end to absorbent paper.

Cell Types

With estrogen stimulation the vaginal mucosa becomes a stratified squamous epithelium comprised of many layers of cells pro-

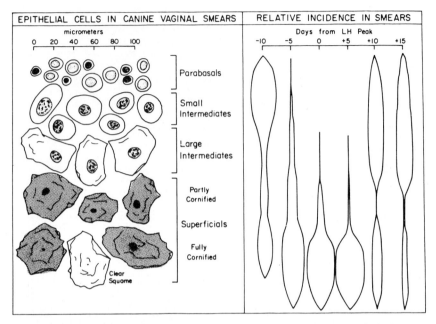

Fig 3. Epithelial cell types in canine vaginal smears drawn to scale on left. Balloon-figures on right indicate by changes in width the changes in incidence of different cell types at selected times relative to the preovulatory LH peak.

duced by the basal layers. Prior to puberty and during anestrus in the adult, the mucosa is only a few cell layers thick. It consists of a low cuboidal epithelium composed of the basal cells attached to the basement membrane and parabasal cells derived from the basal cells. The terminology for cell types found in vaginal smears is based on their position in the layers comprising the intact, fully developed mucosa at estrus, namely basal, parabasal, intermediate, and superficial cells. *In situ,* basal cells are cuboidal, small, and compactly arranged. Parabasal cells are polyhedral, larger than basal cells, and less orderly in arrangement. Intermediate cells are larger still, more ovoid, and slightly to obviously flattened. The superficial cells are squamous, arranged in irregular flat layers, and have lost normal nuclear detail due to insufficient nutrition and resulting keratinization. This division of cell types is somewhat arbitrary, however, in that there is a continuum of cell types from parabasals through cornified superficials.

The relative number of each cell type in the vaginal smear will vary with the extent of mucosal proliferation, the predominant surface cell type, and the number of cell layers removed in collecting the smear. The expected changes in a typical cycle are noted schematical-

Table 1. Characteristics of Commonly Observed Epithelial Cell Types in Canine Vaginal Smears

	Parabasals	Small Intermediates		Large Intermediates	Superficials		
Cell Type							
Alternate Terminology	None	Early Intermediate Rounded Intermediate		Late Intermediate Superficial Intermediate Squamous Intermediate Transitional Intermediate	Cornified Superficials		
Type/Subtype	Parabasal	Low Intermediate	Middle Intermediate	Upper Intermediate	Partly Cornified	Fully Cornified	Squame
Relative Size and Outline	Small, Round	Small Round-Ovoid	Medium Ellipsoid	Large Irregular-Squamous		Large Irregular-Squamous	
Nucleus	Normal	Prominent Nucleus	Prominent Nucleus	Prominent Nucleus	Pyknotic Nucleus	Faint Absent	Absent Nucleus
Cell Diameter Typical (Range)	15μ (9-20μ)	30μ (22-35μ)	45μ (35-60μ)	50μ (40-70μ)		50μ (40-75μ)	
Nuclear Diam. Typical (Range)	10μ (6-16μ)	12μ (8-18μ)		11μ (8-18μ)	6μ (4-8μ)	— (0-8μ)	— —
Nucleus/Cell Ratio Typical (Range)	0.7 (0.6-0.9)	0.4 (0.3-0.5)	0.3 (0.2-0.4)	0.2 (0.2-0.4)	0.1 (.07-.20)	— —	— —
Staining (Diff-Quik) Cytoplasm Nucleus	Med Blue Dk Blue	Med Blue Violet	Lt Blue Violet	Lt Blue Violet	Lt-Med Blue Dk Blue	Lt-Med Blue —	Clear —

ly in Figure 3. The morphological characteristics of the cell types in smears and their stained appearance when using Diff-Quik are summarized in Table 1.

Parabasal Cells

These are the smallest epithelial cells commonly observed in smears; basal cells are only rarely observed. The parabasal cells are round and from 10 to 20 microns in diameter. The diameter of their nucleus is usually greater than 45% of the cell's diameter and it can be as large as 90% of the cell's diameter. The nucleus stains dark blue and the thin ring of cytoplasm is medium to pale blue. Parabasal cells are common in early proestrus, metestrus, and anestrus. They are usually absent from mid-proestrus through the end of estrus.

Small Intermediate Cells

These cells vary considerably in size. They are the growing, transitional cells between the spherical parabasal cells and the larger, more mature, flattened cells into which they develop as they move further away from the basal layers. They thus might be called "early" intermediate cells. The majority of them range in size from 20 to 60 microns in diameter. They vary in shape from nearly round to oval; most are ellipsoid. The cell outline is very regular. As in parabasal cells, the nucleus is large and vesicular, but it is less basophilic. The nuclear diameter is usually 30 to 35% of the cell's maximum diameter. The large cytoplasmic area stains medium to pale blue. The round or oval vesicular nucleus stains orange-violet. The preferential uptake of the orange stain by the nuclei of both small and large intermediate cells is assumed to be related to the extensive metabolic activity of these rapidly enlarging cells, varying from the lower metabolic activity of small parabasal cells in which the nucleus is basophilic. Some nuclei may stain blue, giving the appearance of an oversized parabasal cell.

Small intermediate cells are common in smears at all stages of the estrous cycle except during the period from mid-proestrus through the end of estrus. Small intermediate cells or parabasal cells with a neutrophil in the cytoplasm have been termed metestrous cells because they are not uncommon in vaginal smears collected during metestrus. Though they are not seen in late proestrus or estrus, they are not necessarily characteristic or indicative of metestrus; they may occur during anestrus or early proestrus.[11] Small intermediate cells or large parabasal cells with multiple, clear cytoplasmic vacuoles have been termed foam cells. Although these cells are uncommon, they are seen most often in early metestrus and may be present in smears obtained during anestrus.[11]

Large Intermediate Cells

These cells are characterized by their shape and nuclear appearance rather than their size. They represent a transitional stage between the larger of the regular-shaped, variable-sized, small intermediate cells and the irregular-shaped, squamous, superficial cells. They are squamous in shape with an active, round, normal-sized nucleus.[5,15] They might better be termed late intermediate cells. These cells probably represent the delicate edge between epithelial cell layers with adequate access to nutrients and layers too distant from the basal layers to obtain nutrients sufficient for normal function and nuclear morphology. Due to their unique transitional status, these cells have also been called superficial intermediate cells.[11]

Large intermediate cells are flat, squamous cells that are very irregular in outline. The periphery is folded, angulated, wrinkled, or layered. They contain round, vesicular nuclei similar to the nuclei in small intermediate cells. They range in maximum diameter from 40 to 75 microns. The nuclear diameter is usually less than 35% and may be as little as 15% of the cell's diameter. The cytoplasm stains medium to pale blue; the active nuclei stain orange-violet. Cells that are transitional between large intermediate and partially cornified superficial cells can also be present in smears as large intermediate cells with a slightly shrunken and/or irregularly shaped nucleus that still takes the orange stain.

Large intermediate cells are common during proestrus, rare during estrus, common during early metestrus, and otherwise uncommon.

Superficial Cells

These cells are large and flat. Their nucleus is very faint or pyknotic and dense; it may be absent. The intensity of the cytoplasmic stain can also vary depending on the degree of cornification and/or degeneration. In the category of partially cornified superficial cells we include medium to pale blue cells with distinct, dark pyknotic nuclei or with faint-staining nuclei. In the category of fully cornified superficial cells we include medium or dark blue cells with no nuclei, dark blue cells with an indistinct and condensed nucleus, and the so-called "squames." The last are older keratinized cells that fail to absorb stain and appear nearly transparent and have no nuclear remnants.

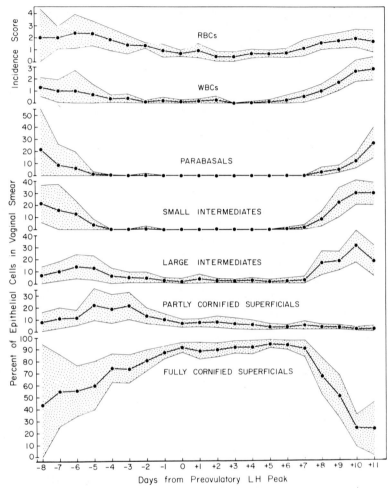

Fig 4. Mean incidence of blood cells (based on relative, subjective scoring) and of epithelial cell types (as actual percentages of epithelial cells present) observed in vaginal smears obtained at known times relative to the day of the preovulatory LH peak in 18 cycles. The shaded areas indicate the 95% confidence intervals for the means shown. Ovulations would occur on day 2, oocyte maturation on day 4-5, and loss of oocyte fertility between day +7 and +9.

Superficial cells are extremely angulated, folded, and irregular in shape. The intensity of their staining is usually increased during estrus and may relate to the degree of cornification. Such a correlation should not be presumed, however, when using the Diff-Quik stain because there is no component in the stain specific for keratin as there is in polychrome stains commonly used for that purpose.[14,15]

Superficial cells range from 40 to 75 microns in diameter. The small pyknotic nuclei, when present, are usually less than 15% of the maximum diameter of the cell.

Superficial cells in various states of disintegration can be seen in small numbers at any stage of the estrous cycle. Normal ones become prominent during proestrus and dominate the smear during late proestrus. They are usually the only epithelial cells present during the fertile period of estrus and rapidly decrease in number immediately thereafter.

Blood Cells

During most of the estrous cycle, erythrocytes and neutrophils present in smears stained with Diff-Quik are similar to their appearance in blood smears. The erythrocytes are round or slightly crenated, semi-transparent, and pale orange or pale blue. Neutrophils have dark blue, multilobular nuclei and a clear cytoplasm with a regular outline. During early and mid-proestrus, as the mucosa through which the leukocytes must migrate thickens and before cell migration is blocked, the leukocytes observed in smears are often degenerate and appear as distorted nuclear remnants without distinct cytoplasmic borders. During estrus, erythrocytes are often not distinct and appear as broken ghosts or cell fragments, suggesting a possible lysis due to changes in the composition of the vaginal mucus.

Changes in Vaginal Cells

The following information is based on studies of vaginal smears obtained daily from colony-housed Beagles throughout proestrus and estrus and subsequently related to the day of the preovulatory LH peak (Fig 4). The considerable variation in cellular content is assumed to be representative of the variation that might be encountered among dogs of any breed. The transition from behavioral proestrus to behavioral estrus is often not synchronous with the preovulatory LH surge. Therefore, for the purposes of this discussion, the terms proestrus and estrus have been used in reference to endocrinologically defined periods, ie the periods immediately before and after the LH peak. A summary of changes in superficial vs nonsuperficial cells related to the day of the LH peak and concurrent changes in the gross appearance of the mucosa is presented in Figure 5.

Anestrus

The epithelial cells in anestrus smears are few to moderate in number. They often are adhering to masses or strands of mucus. The

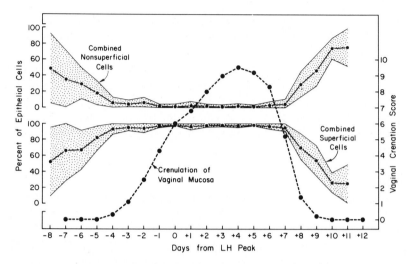

Fig 5. Summary of major changes in the incidence of epithelial cell types in canine vaginal smears considering only the superficial and nonsuperficial cells in relation to the day of the LH peak. Also shown are the mean scores for gross changes in the vaginal surface. The latter are based on a scoring system for extent of crenulation in mucosal folds, including the following: 0-round and edematous; 4-obvious wrinkling and sacculation; 8-obvious, sharp angulation; 10-maximum angulation; 7-thinner, angulated mucosa; 3-very thin, but wrinkled, shedding epithelium; 0-flattened or small rounded folds with patchy coloration.

cells are mostly parabasals and small (early) intermediates (Plate 1a). A few, old, curled superficials and squames from the previous cycle may also be present. Neutrophils are commonly present, but usually are not numerous. The smears are usually unimpressive, except in late anestrus shortly prior to proestrus when there is an increase in the number of epithelial cells, especially small intermediates.

Proestrus

At the onset of proestrus all epithelial cell types are more numerous along with erythrocytes and usually some neutrophils (Plate 1b). During the course of proestrus there is a progressive decrease in the relative number of parabasals and small intermediates, a transient increase in large intermediates, and a progressive increase in superficial cells (Plate 1c,d). During the 7 to 10 days prior to the LH peak, there are typical changes. The parabasal cells decrease from numbers that initially were 5 to 30% of all cells in a smear to less than 5% within 4 to 5 days before the LH peak; they are almost always absent by 2 to 3 days before the peak (Plate 1d). Small intermediate cells disappear in the same pattern. Large intermediate cells initially increase as a percent of the smear's total cells along with superficials until they reach a peak incidence of 5 to 25% by 5 to 6 days before the LH peak; they then decline in number. In most normal estrous cycles, large intermediates are no longer present at the time of the LH peak, having disappeared 1 to 4 days earlier (Plate 1e). In some cycles, however, large intermediates persist into and throughout estrus, apparently due to less than complete cornification of the upper cell layers.

During the week prior to the LH peak, superficial cells increase from a 30 to 60% incidence to comprise 100% of the epithelial cells in the smear by 1 to 5 days before the peak. This is not true when some large intermediates are still present. Neutrophils are rarely present in smears obtained during late proestrus, but in some cycles a few isolated, degenerated neutrophils may persist. Erythrocytes are commonly present throughout proestrus, although their relative abundance may decline. Mucoprotein and cellular debris are common background material in proestrus smears (Plate 1e). Moderate numbers to numerous bacteria may be present as normal flora.

Due to the variation in the time at which vaginal smears contain only superficial cells as well as the retention of large intermediate cells in some cycles, there is no obvious change in cell distribution that is distinctly indicative of the occurrence of the LH peak or of impending ovulation. There are gross changes in the vaginal mucosa viewed endoscopically, however, that can be observed concurrent with the LH peak and ovulation. See normal canine vaginoscopy, page 108.

Estrus

For 6 to 8 days after the LH peak the vaginal smear is dominated entirely by superficial epithelial cells, except in the few cycles in which small numbers of large intermediate cells are retained. Background debris is often absent (Plate 2a). An abrupt clearing of the background is usually indicative of the occurrence of the LH surge. Erythrocytes may be either moderate or abundant or they may be sharply reduced in number despite the presence of a serosanguineous discharge (Plate 1e, Plate 2a, b). Changes in vaginal mucus following the LH surge may promote their lysis. Erythrocytes may also be absent in smears obtained during estrus in some bitches. This may be due to a decrease or cessation in uterine discharge of blood into the vagina in conjunction with any lysis occurring in the vagina. Neutrophils are rare other than isolated, degenerate remnants of the polymorphic nuclei. Parabasals and small intermediate cells are invariably absent in nearly all normal cycles.

There is a progressive increase in the extent of superficial cell cornification during early estrus. The increase is not obvious in Diff-Quik-stained preparations, but has been noticed when tri-chrome stains or hematoxylin and eosin stains are used.[10,14,15] With simple Diff-Quik staining, the distinction between partially and fully cornified cells is not always obvious. In some bitches, however, there is a steady decrease in partially cornified superficial cells containing a distinct pyknotic nucleus from 3 days before to 3 days after the LH peak. Then only anuclear superficials are seen for the last 2 to 4 days of "vaginal" estrus. The borders of superficial cells may become more frayed and indistinct in late estrus, 4 to 6 days after the LH peak. At the same time sheets of epithelium that are several cell-layers thick may become more common, along with an increase in the number of poorly staining squames.

Late Estrus-Early Metestrus
The end of "vaginal" estrus and onset of "vaginal" metestrus occur rapidly over a 1 to 3 day period in which previously absent parabasal cells and intermediate cells reappear in the vaginal smear.[8,9,11] In nearly all normal cycles these cells progress from being entirely absent to being decidedly present. Initially, however, they are only a few cells among all the superficials (Plate 2c,d). Thus the presence of only a few nonsuperficial cells in the smear is usually indicative of the end of estrus and the start of metestrus. This transition is more obvious during the next 1 to 2 days during which nonsuperficial cells become a significant percentage of the total cells present. In rare instances in which a few isolated parabasals or small intermediates are found in a smear obtained during mid-estrus, this end-of-estrus transition may not be clear until these cells increase to represent 1 to 5% of the epithelial cells in the smear (Plate 2d).

Monitoring the time of this appearance of nonsuperficial cells can be extremely useful because it occurs at a rather constant period after the LH peak and can thus be used to predict the expected times of implantation and parturition in bred bitches and to determine retrospectively the times of any breedings or manipulations in relation to the time of ovulation (Table 2). In the majority of cycles the shift occurs 7 to 9 days after the LH peak and involves an increase in small intermediate and parabasal cells. They then comprise 1 to 40% of the epithelial cells after being absent on the previous day. On the following day they increase to comprise 5 to 95% of the epithelial cells while the number of superficial cells declines rapidly. There usually is a simultaneous increase in the number of large (late) intermediate cells, but this is only diagnostic in cycles in which the large intermediates

Table 2. Timing of Reproductive Events in Relation to Reappearance of Nonsuperficial Epithelial Cells in Canine Vaginal Smears During Transition from Late Estrus to Early Metestrus

Parameter	Days From Transition	
	Mean	Range
Preovulatory LH peak	-8	-6 to -10
Onset of behavioral estrus	-7	-2 to -13
Ovulation	-6	-4 to -6
Oocyte maturation	-4	-2 to -4
End of peak fertile period	-3	-1 to -5
Metestrus shift in smear	0	
Latest possible fertilization	2	0 to 4
Early pregnancy palpation	12	9 to 15
Optimal pregnancy palpation	17	14 to 20
Questionable pregnancy palpations	26	22 to 30
Early fetal radiography	39	36 to 42
Prepartum hypothermia	56	53 to 59
Parturition	57	54 to 60

are few or absent throughout most of estrus. Though the transition usually occurs 7 to 9 days after the LH peak, it has been observed occasionally as early as 6 days or as late as 10 days after the LH peak.

In the majority of estrous cycles there is a reappearance of neutrophils in moderate to abundant numbers at the same time as the metestrus shift in epithelial cells (Plate 2c-e). The reappearance of leukocytes in the smear is a less reliable indicator of metestrus, however, because it may occur slowly and may be delayed by several days, or may not involve sufficient numbers to be obvious.[4,11]

References
1. Bell, ET and Christie, DW: Brit Vet J **127** (1971) 113.
2. Bell, ET, Bailey, JB, and Christie, DW: Res Vet Sci **14** (1973) 173.
3. Christie, DW, Bailey, JB, and Bell, ET: Brit Vet J **128** (1972) 301.
4. Concannon, PW: In *Current Veterinary Therapy* VIII, pp 886-901. WB Saunders, Philadelphia, 1983.
5. Dore, MA: J Small Anim Pract **19** (1978) 561.
6. Dore, MA: Irish Vet J (March, 1978) 54.
7. Holst, PA and Phemister, RD: Biol Reprod **5** (1971) 194.
8. Holst, PA and Phemister, RD: Amer J Vet Res **35** (1974) 401.
9. Holst, PA and Phemister, RD: Amer J Vet Res **36** (1975) 705.
10. Linde, C and Karlsson, I: J Small Anim Pract **25** (1984) 77.
11. Olson, PN *et al:* Comp Cont Educ **6** (1984) 288.
12. Olson, PN *et al:* Comp Cont Educ **6** (1984) 385.
13. Phemister, RD *et al:* Biol Reprod **8** (1973) 74.
14. Roszel, JF: Veterinary Scope **19** (1975) 3.
15. Schutte, AP: J Small Anim Pract **8** (1967) 301.
16. Schutte, AP: J Small Anim Pract **8** (1967) 307.
17. Schutte, AP: J Small Anim Pract **8** (1967) 313.

NORMAL CANINE VAGINOSCOPY
BY F.E.F. LINDSAY & P.W. CONCANNON

Introduction
The progressive changes in the vaginal mucosa during the fertile period can be observed directly by endoscopic examination. Serial inspections of the vaginal mucosa will also reveal the dramatic changes during the preovulatory LH surge and ovulation, a period in which there are no obvious changes in vaginal smears. The gross changes in the vaginal mucosa that occur during the decline of estrogen levels at the transition from proestrus to estrus are obvious in genital tracts removed from bitches (Fig 1).

Equipment for Vaginoscopy
Either fiberoptic endoscopes or pediatric proctoscopes less than 12 mm in diameter can be used in most bitches to view changes in the caudal vagina and caudal aspect of the dorsal median fold. A scope with a diameter greater than 8 to 10 mm will rarely pass beyond the caudal tubercle of the dorsal median fold. Instruments 5 to 6 mm in diameter can usually be passed into the cranial vagina to visualize its surface and that of the vaginal cervix and the external cervical os. The close-up views of the entire vagina that are possible with the small-diameter fiberoptic endoscopes have decided advantages for detailed studies. The passage of such instruments, however, through the vagina, recognition of landmark structures, and interpretation of mucosal fold profiles require moderate practice and experience. Pediatric proctoscopes used as canine vaginoscopes have the advantages of easy passage through the vagina and the normal perspective provided by viewing the mucosa from a distance, as well as lower cost, greater durability, and easier maintenance.

Pediatric Proctoscopes
The small pediatric or stricture proctoscope is a light-fitted, double stainless steel tube that is 25 cm long and has an outside diameter of 11 mm (Welch-Allyn #32023). The light housing, which also serves as a handle, attaches to a fiberoptic light port for projection of light down the outer tube. Viewing is done directly through the central tube without magnification. The central tube accommodates a blunt, plastic-tipped obturator, the end of which, when inserted, projects from the end of the scope and facilitates passage of the instrument. After the proctoscope has been inserted and the obturator is withdrawn, viewing is done with the hinged eyepiece fixed in place or

swung aside. The eyepiece serves as an air seal when insufflation is induced with a hand-held air-bulb or an air-pump connected to a valved insufflation port at the base of the scope.

With obturator in place, the proctoscope is passed through the vestibule and into the vagina in an upward direction as described for the insertion of a speculum when collecting vaginal smears (Fig 2). Resistance to passage is common near the cingulum (vestibulovaginal junction) and caudal vagina. Application of moderate, steady pressure must be accompanied by firm thumb-pressure on the obturator handle to utilize the guidance and safety provided by its tip. If natural lubrication is not sufficient, the protruding tip of the obturator and the outer surface of the proctoscope's end can be covered thinly with a medical lubricant. Excess lubricant should be removed to

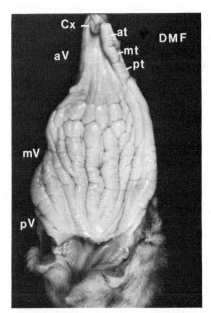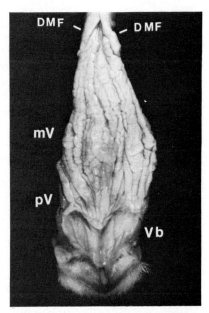

Fig 1. Posterior portions of reproductive tract removed from bitches in late proestrus (A) and early estrus (B), cut open along the dorsal midline and spread open to expose the vaginal mucosa. A. In late proestrus, at the time of peak estrogen secretion and resulting edema, the mucosal folds are thick, round and smooth and produce a gross cobble-stone surface on the mucosa. The dorsal median fold (DMF), with its posterior (pt), middle (mt) and anterior tubercles (at), normally fills and occludes the narrow anterior vagina (aV) and prevents viewing of the cervix (cx), the dorsal surface of which shows here (cx). B. In estrus, when estrogen falls and progesterone increases, fluid retention decreases, and the mucosal folds are sacculated, wrinkled and irregular. In this view the DMF has been sagittally cut through part of its length, with the cervix not exposed and out of view. Also indicated are the levels of the vestibule (Vb), posterior (pV), mid (mV) and anterior (aV) vagina.

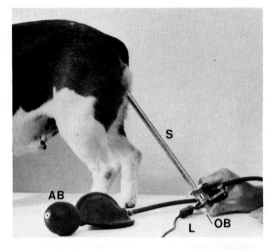

Fig 2. Pediatric proc-
toscopes used for canine
vaginoscopy. Components
include scope (S), obturator
(OB), light-source handle (L)
and air-insufflation bulb
(AB). Initial upward orientation for passage through
vesibule into cingulum,
holding obturator firmly in
place (above), and full insertion followed by removal of
obturator for examination
of mucosal folds (below).

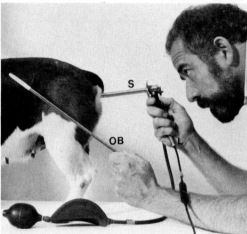

prevent its entering the vaginal lumen. After the scope is in the
vagina and in a horizontal position, it is slowly advanced as far
cranially as possible without undue pressure. This usually brings the
scope into contact with the caudal aspect of the dorsal median fold. In
a medium-sized bitch the insertion will be 12 to 25 cm from the vulval
surface; the average insertion is about 16 cm. Marking rings on the
scope can be used to determine the distance of insertion, as well as the
location of structures or lesions encountered. After the scope is fully
inserted, the obturator is withdrawn and the mucosa is examined for
color, texture, and shape of mucosal folds as the scope is slowly
withdrawn 1 to 4 cm and then slowly advanced to the original posi-

tion. Mild insufflation can then be induced to attempt exposing the vaginal cervix and to facilitate viewing of the vaginal mucosa. Insufflation should only be induced while viewing through the scope so that the extent to which the resulting view is affected by insufflation can be assessed.

Fiberoptic Endoscopes

The construction and application of rigid and flexible fiberoptic scopes used for small animal endoscopy and laparoscopy have been reviewed.[1-4] The equipment described is used by the second author to monitor the periovulatory period in the bitch (Fig 3). Equipment used by the first author to study and photograph the vagina is described elsewhere.[3-5]

The rigid endoscope (Wolf Model #8654.33) is 30 cm long, has an outside diameter of 4 mm, and fits inside a sheath with the same functional length and an outside diameter of 5 mm. The fitting is secured by a breech-mount ring near the eyepiece. The outer sheath serves as an air insufflation channel through a valved port near the breech-lock fitting. Fiberoptic bundles serve the eyepiece and the light-projecting bundles are served by a fiberoptic cable connection port located on the side of the scope near the eyepiece. A larger, standard-sized scope and sheath can be used effectively in most bitches, but scopes with outside diameters over 1.0 cm can prevent close viewing of the cervix.

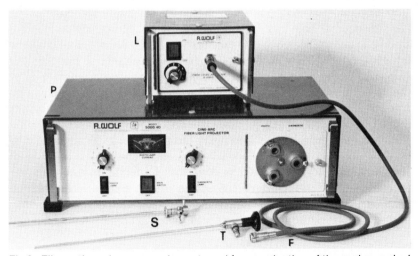

Fig 3. Fiberoptic endoscopy equipment used for examination of the canine vaginal mucosa, including (T) 5 mm x 25 cm telescope, (S) 7 mm sheath with valved insufflation port, (F) fiberoptic light cable, (L) portable diagnostic light source, and (P) high intensity photographic light source.

A diameter greater than 8 mm may not be appropriate for smaller bitches. Offsetting the disadvantage of small viewing area and limited photographic capability with the 4 mm scope and 5 mm sheath, this size of scope can be used in a bitch of any size, it can be passed into the cranial vagina in most bitches, and it can be used to demonstrate the length of the dorsal median fold and location of the cervix in relation to the fold.

The fiberoptic cable is 4 feet long and connects to a dedicated light source or to other light sources via commercially available adaptors. Dedicated light sources include a relatively inexpensive, portable unit containing a variable, low-intensity diagnostic light source (Wolf Model #4008) or a high intensity, blue-light source unit that also incorporates an alternative low-power diagnostic light source into a single cabinet (Wolf Model #5000.40).

In some bitches considerable pressure is placed on the endoscope where it passes over the pelvic brim, and the outer sheath is always used to protect the instrument as well as to provide an insufflation tube. The end of the scope is inserted into the vestibule, spreading the vulval lips manually or with a speculum. Insertion through the cingulum into the caudal vagina is usually done at the same time. The insertion should be viewed through the scope if there is any doubt about its placement or avoidance of the urinary meatus, or when prior digital palpation has revealed the presence of fibrous tags or an imperforate hymen.

Passage of the scope forward along the length of the vagina and all subsequent movements should only be made while viewing through the eyepiece because the pathway may be irregular and the tip of a narrow instrument can perforate or otherwise damage the vagina if undue pressure is exerted against its wall. Obstruction of the view due to moisture, mucus, or debris at the scope's tip can be remedied by withdrawing the scope, rinsing and then reinserting it while holding the sheath in place within the vagina. Slight insufflation induced during observation may aid passage of the scope. Whenever possible, however, the initial passage to the caudal tubercle of the dorsal median fold should be done with minimal or no insufflation to enable an assessment of the shape of the folds of the vaginal mucosa. After initial observations of the vaginal mucosa have been made, a more panoramic view can be obtained by inducing mild to moderate insufflation.

Periovulatory Changes in the Vaginal Mucosa

The vagina's shape has been compared to that of a bottle.[3] The caudal portion is the base of the bottle, the wide, mid-vaginal region is the body of the bottle, and the narrow, cranial portion is the shoulder of the bottle, and the paracervix is the neck. The cervix is placed like a cork into the cul-de-sac or paracervix. The entire mucosal surface is lined by longitudinal (craniocaudal) furrows and inter-furrow folds. The folds are low in anestrus, become large, rounded, edematous, and prominent during proestrus, and become wrinkled and shrunken during estrus (Fig 1). At the end of fertile estrus, the folds become flattened.

The dorsal median fold is a prominent, consistently observed, longitudinal fold on the roof of the cranial vagina and it is a distinct anatomical landmark. The fold is continuous cranially with the dorsal rim of the vaginal cervix (Fig 4). It extends several centimeters along the length of the cranial vagina and is usually divided by 2 or more minor strictures across its length into cranial, middle, and caudal tubercles. The caudal tubercle normally occludes the vaginal lumen. This bulb enlarges during proestrus and it is often mistaken for the cervix. It has been termed the pseudocervix. During estrus the bulb can develop a shape and appearance that is nearly alike to that of the true cervix. The caudal tubercle of the dorsal median fold usually blocks the passage of instruments over 1 cm in diameter, even after extensive insufflation has created a crescent-shaped ventral lumen. After creating a ventral lumen, the scope can be manipulated to view parts of the cervix several centimeters beyond the end of the scope. Instruments less than 6 mm in diameter usually can be easily passed under

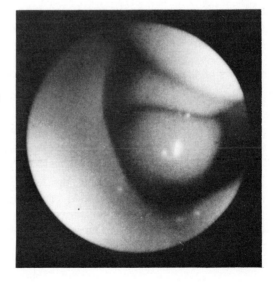

Fig 4. Posterior view of the dorsal surface of the canine cervix, as observed through a fiberoptic endoscope placed under the posterior tubercle of the dorsal median fold (DMF), with the anterior and middle tubercles of the DMF in the foreground.

and along the dorsal medial fold, enabling a close view of the cervix and cul-de-sac.

The cervix usually projects in a ventral, oblique direction with the os faced downward and partially or totally out of view. The surface of the cervix usually observed is actually the dorsal quadrant of the cervical mass and the more dorsal of the furrows that radiate from the os often are only partially visible. Manipulating the cervix through the abdomen will often provide better orientation for viewing. Endoscopic views of the vaginal mucosa at various stages of proestrus and estrus are shown in Figure 5. The extent and time course of grossly visible changes, and their relation to changes in the vaginal smear and to the time of preovulatory LH peak are summarized in Figure 5, page 108.

Anestrus

During anestrus the mucosal folds are very low and due to the thinness of the epithelium and visibility of the underlying microvasculature they are red or pink-red in color. The folds seen in profile are small, round, and flaccid. They often disappear with insufflation (Fig 5a).

Proestrus

During early and mid-proestrus the mucosal folds are enlarged, round, and edematous.[3-5] Transverse furrows develop and produce, in conjunction with longitudinal folds, a smooth, rounded cobble-stone pavement surface (Fig 1a) that appears in the scope as rounded profiles (Fig 5b). The color varies from pink-gray to gray-white to cream-white and finally to paper-white due to progressive thickening and cornification of the epithelium. The texture varies from soft to very firm due to progressive increases in mucosal edema, turgidity, and thickness. The sero-sanguineous uterine discharge appears as red fluid in the furrows of the folds.

Preovulatory Estrus

By late proestrus or early estrus during the fall in serum estrogen levels and the start of the preovulatory LH surge, additional furrows have formed on the surfaces of the mucosal folds. Additional wrinkles or indentations become progressively obvious during the preovulatory LH surge (Fig 5c). Eventually the large, round mucosal folds are subdivided into smaller, rounded crumpled folds and round peaks. Because of the continued withdrawal of estrogen's water-retention effect, there is a progressive increase in mucosal shrinkage, wrinkling, and sharpness of the wrinkled folds viewed in profile (Figs 5c-f). This progressive wrinkling is termed crenulation (Fig 5, p. 108).

Figs 5A-J. Normal canine vaginal endoscopy. (Scores are those used to develop crenulation profile on page 104.)

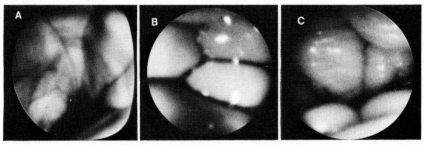

A. Anestrus. Low, flat mucosa. B. Mid-proestrus. Large, round edematous, pink-white folds. Score 0. C. Late proestrus or early estrus, near time of LH peak. Slight wrinkling of thick, round, white folds. Score 2.

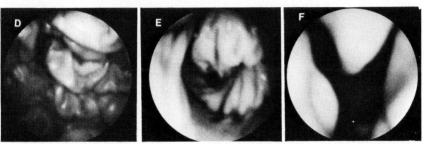

D. Early estrus, around time of ovulation. Crumpled, wrinkled, and shrunken folds with rounded profiles. Score 4-6.
E. Mid-estrus, after ovulation, around the time of oocyte maturation. Angulated folds with sharp peaks on the smaller wrinkles, giving a fluted or concertina appearance. Score 8-10.
F. Close-up view of sharp tip of a mucosal fold during mid-estrus.

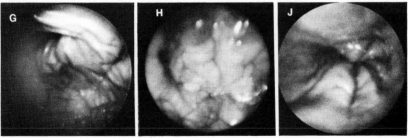

G. Late estrus, 6-7 days after LH peak. Extremely wrinkled, sharply-angulated, but thinner mucosa, giving a crepe-paper appearance. Oocytes have reduced fertility. Score 3 or 7.
H. Early metestrus, 7-9 days after LH peak. Low, soft folds without obvious peaks. Mucosa has both white areas and reddened areas ("patchy hyperemia"). Oocytes unlikely to be fertile after this time. Score 0.
J. Early metestrus. Rosette of low, smooth, flaccid folds formed by spontaneous contraction of vagina in region of posterior tubercle of dorsal median fold. Constricted lumen is at center of rosette. Score 0.

Postovulatory Estrus

The crenulation observed during early estrus reflects moderate angulation, with the previously rounded mounds of mucosa turning into smooth topped peaks (Fig 5d). In mid-estrus, about 3 to 4 days after the LH peak (and thus 1 to 2 days after ovulation), the angulation becomes maximal. The peaks are now sharp-tipped and irregular in appearance (Figs 5e,f). The mucosa also looks drier despite the presence of mucus; a reduction in natural lubrication is often suggested by a tighter fit of the instrument during its passage. During the progression from early to mid-estrus many of the folds on the dorsal aspects of the vaginal lumen, as well as the dorsal median fold, maintain their longitudinal orientation. During the decline of edema they become fluted and the surface then develops long sharp peaks not unlike the pleats of an accordion bellows. In other areas, some shorter folds become pleated and have a concertina-like appearance (Fig 5e). Near the end of the fertile period of estrus (5 to 7 days after the LH peak) the extremely crumpled, wrinkled, sharply angulated mucosal surface is obviously thinner than in mid-estrus (Fig 5g).

Metestrus

The shedding of cornified layers is completed rapidly and within 12 to 36 hours at the end of vaginal estrus the thinner mucosa has a soft, flaccid surface of low, less distinct folds that are round and easily flattened by insufflation (Fig 5h). The resulting color is characteristic of the transition from the end of fertile estrus to the start of vaginal metestrus. The surface becomes variegated, with patches of white mucosa mixed with patches that are thin and red. This change occurs at the same time that nonsuperficial cells are beginning to reappear in the vaginal smear in rapidly increasing numbers. At the same time, intense contraction of the vagina may be noticed in the region of the caudal tubercle of the dorsal fold. The contraction results in closure of the lumen and formation of a rosette of low, soft folds around the closed lumen (Fig 5j).

References

1. Zimmer, JF: In *Current Veterinary Therapy*, VII, pp 954-961. WB Saunders, Philadelphia, 1980.
2. Patterson, JM: In *Current Veterinary Therapy*, VII, pp 969-973. WB Saunders, Philadelphia, 1980.
3. Lindsay, FEF: Pedigree Dig **5** (3, 4) (1980) 8.
4. Lindsay, FEF: J Small Anim Pract **24** (1983) 1.
5. Lindsay, FEF: In *Current Veterinary Therapy*, VIII, pp 912-921. WB Saunders, Philadelphia, 1983.

LAPAROSCOPY
BY DAVID E. WILDT

Introduction

Laparoscopy (observation through an endoscope inserted into the peritoneal cavity) provides the clinician an atraumatic alternative to laparotomy. Its primary advantage is its versatility. The various applications of the technic include inspection of body cavities and inner structures, use in biopsies, administration of drugs, and use for minor surgical procedures. Laparoscopy has become adapted for animals as diverse in size as the mouse and gorilla.[1] The primary use of laparoscopy in most species, including the dog and cat, has been to study reproductive function.

History

A brief discussion of the history of this procedure is pertinent because the development of its application in animals is unique.[2] Unlike most biomedical procedures that were first applied in animals and then in humans, laparoscopy was first used in humans. Various attempts were made throughout the 19th century to view the contents of the human abdominal cavity by using crude transmitters of light. The instruments often consisted of simple cylindrical tubes through which an artificial light was projected. By the end of the 1880's a small light bulb had been attached to the distal end of a cystoscope to view the lumen of the bladder. Though this provided the needed inner illumination, problems arose because of the excessive heat associated with the light source.

A modified cystoscope with optical lenses and distal illumination to view the peritoneal cavity was designed in the early 1900's. During this period the term, laparoscopy, was first used. During the next 30 years, abdominal laparoscopy was refined and used for the diagnosis of many abnormal conditions in human patients. The development of proximal light projection systems in the early 1950's eliminated the dangers of thermal injury and greatly increased the practicality and usefulness of laparoscopy.

A significant development in the 1950's was the use of a quartz rod to transmit light from a proximal light source. In this system the light from an external projector was reflected by an optical prism to the end of a clear rod of fused quartz. Though the procedure provided excellent illumination for the laparoscope, the quartz rods were expensive, fragile, and cumbersome. As a result, the system for transmitting light into the abdominal cavity through flexible fiberoptic

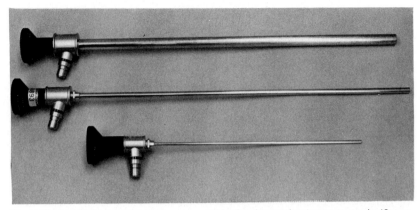

Fig 1. Three 180-degree laparoscopes used in the dog and cat: upper one is 10 mm in diameter; middle one is 5 mm in diameter; lower one is 2.7 mm in diameter (arthroscope).

glass bundles was developed and became extremely popular. In this technic a "cold" light was transferred from an external projector through a flexible fiber cable into the laparoscope and thus into the cavity. The concomitant refinement of optical lenses for the laparoscope resulted in a clear, bright image of the target organ being viewed.

Animal laparoscopy had its beginnings in the 1950's and 1960's, when there was considerable interest in basic reproductive function. A variety of animals was successfully used in laparoscopy studies, including the dog, cat, nonhuman primates, mare, cow, pig, sheep, rabbit, and numerous species of birds, reptiles, and wildlife.[3-11] With the exception of large hoof stock, birds, and reptiles, abdominal laparoscopy was generally similar in most animals in that general anesthesia was induced and then the laparoscope was inserted into the peritoneal cavity through a midventral incision. In cattle, horses, and birds, laparoscopy was often performed with local anesthesia only; a paralumbar incision was made for insertion of the laparoscope.

Laparoscopy was first used in the dog in 1972.[12] Although the technic was not described, the author discussed the potential of laparoscopy in dogs and provided photographs of observations of various liver diseases. The technical details and application of laparoscopy in both dogs and cats were described 5 years later.[13]

Laparoscopy has been found to be a simple and practical procedure for observing the anatomy and function of internal organs and for performing certain diagnostic procedures. It has proved useful in the detection of certain intra-abdominal neoplasms. In animals with known or suspected neoplasms, laparoscopy has been useful in regulating therapy and determining the indications for surgical resection.[14]

Equipment

A wide variety of instruments are suitable for canine or feline laparoscopy. (A list of their manufacturers is provided at the end of this section on laparoscopy.) For a routine diagnostic examination the following instruments are required: laparoscope, trocar-cannula assembly, Verres needle, light projector, and flexible fiberoptic cable. Optional instruments that either facilitate the examination or enable performance of more sophisticated surgical procedures include: an automatic insufflator; auxiliary trocar-cannula and manipulatory or biopsy forceps; heavy-duty light projector; camera and eyepiece adapter.

Laparoscope

The laparoscope is generally identified by its diameter and direction of view; the latter is often expressed in degrees. A 180-degree laparoscope provides a view directly outward from the tip of the instrument and a 130- or 160-degree laparoscope provides a view at an oblique angle.[15] The 180-degree instrument (Richard Wolf Medical Instruments Corp), in particular, enables rapid visual orientation within

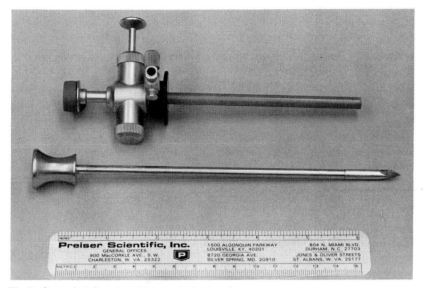

Fig 2. Cannula (above) and trocar (below) unit.

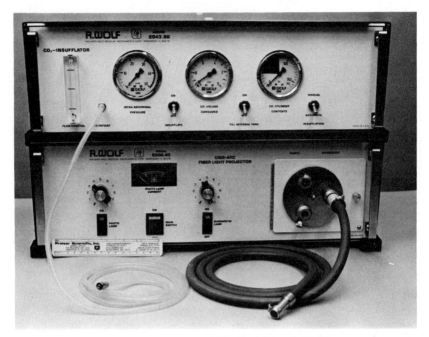

Fig 3. Automatic insufflator (above) and CO_2 hose for establishing a pneumoperitoneum; heavy duty light projector (below) with fiberoptic cable.

the abdominal cavity. The range and size of laparoscope used in the
dog and cat vary from 2.7 to 10 mm in diameter (Fig 1). Although a
10-mm instrument provides a wide field of vision, its use is often
restricted to dogs that weigh more than 10 kg. This size is not recommended for smaller dogs or cats because at least a 2-cm incision is required for insertion of the trocar-cannula. The 5-mm telescope that requires a 1-cm incision is the most versatile instrument for dogs and
cats of any body size. This size of laparoscope is highly recommended
when the instrument's cost is an important consideration. Laparoscopes of comparable size (4 to 7 mm in diameter) are available commercially and are equally suitable for the dog and cat. The 2.7-mm instrument has been useful only for examination of kittens and puppies. The length of incision for its insertion is 0.5 cm or less.

Trocar-Cannula Assembly

The trocar-cannula unit must correspond in size to the type of
laparoscope used (Fig 2). Generally the cannula consists of a channel
with a trumpet or clip valve to prevent loss of pneumoperitoneum

when the trocar is removed. A sleeve and valve for insufflation are on the cannula and are used for additional insufflation during the laparoscopic examination.

Light Projector and Cable

A variety of light sources are suitable for routine examinations or combined diagnostic and photographic use. A small compact unit is relatively inexpensive and provides illumination with a single 150-watt, tungsten-halogen lamp. Although suitable for diagnostic examination, this light source is inadequate for laparoscopic photography. A heavy-duty light projector with alternating lamps (150-watt and a 1000-watt enriched mercury or xenon lamp) is suitable for both diagnostic examination and photography (Fig 3).

The transmission of light from the projector to the laparoscope requires a fiberoptic cable that is available in different sizes. We have routinely used a cable that is 6 mm in diameter (Fig 3).

Verres Needle and Insufflator

The intra-abdominal space must be filled with gas to enable routine examination with a laparoscope. To produce the initial pneumoperitoneum a hollow Verres needle, approximately 120 mm long and equipped with an on-off valve, is used (Fig 4). Gas can be provided by several methods; the most common is the automatic insufflator (Fig 3). This device is connected to a tank of gas. It contains

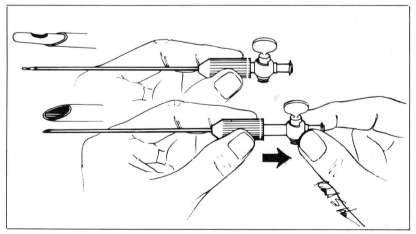

Fig 4. The blunt tip of a Verres needle can be retracted, leaving a sharp point that facilitates penetration of the abdominal wall. From *Animal Laparoscopy,* Williams & Wilkins, 1980.

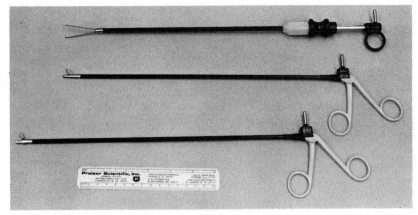

Fig 5. Accessory instruments include a grasping forceps (above), grasping biopsy forceps (middle), and hook scissors (below).

an internal chamber that is filled from the external tank and has a hose attachment that transfers the gas to the Verres needle. The automatic insufflator is convenient and safe because its gauges and flowmeters record the external tank's pressure, internal tank's volume, intra-abdominal pressure, and gas flow rates into the animal. Thus, the problems associated with excessive insufflation are avoided.

A 2nd method of insufflation must be used with caution. It involves use of a commercial gas tank that has a regulatory valve. The gas is transferred through a hose directly to the animal. A step-down regulator valve must be used to permit slow release of gas from the tank to avoid rapid over-insufflation. The abdominal cavity can also be inflated by attaching a sterile syringe (60 ml) directly to the Verres needle and injecting room air. To produce an adequate pneumoperitoneum the syringe must be removed from the needle and refilled with room air several times.

The gases successfully used for insufflation in the dog and cat include carbon dioxide (5% in air or 100%), air, and nitrous oxide.[13,14] Because CO_2 is readily absorbed and is also a product of natural metabolism, it is safest. Because of its combustibility, oxygen is unsuitable. Nitrogen is not used because of its insolubility.

Accessory Instruments

For the dog and cat a manipulatory forceps, biopsy forceps and hook scissors are the most useful accessory instruments (Fig 5). Insertion of these devices into the abdominal cavity is possible after first using an accessory trocar-cannula unit that is either 3 or 6 mm in diameter. Due to its greater rigidity and durability the 6-mm trocar-cannula and corresponding 5-mm auxiliary forceps or scissors are recommended.

Camera and Adapter

Combining laparoscopy and photography is an excellent way of documenting results and obtaining illustrative material. The laparoscope can be adapted to various types of photography, including 35-mm photographs, television videotape, and 8- or 16-mm film. For still photography an SLR camera with a standard 50- or 100-mm lens system is usually used. Most standard SLR cameras can be adapted for laparoscopic photography by using a special ring adapter that screws into the camera lens. This allows the camera to be readily attached and removed from the laparoscope eyepiece (Fig 6). Videotape recording also provides impressive documentation of observations. Portable black and white or color camera units with standard lens systems can also be adapted to attach to the telescope with the same or a similar ring adapter.[11]

Preparation and Anesthesia

Laparoscopy is best performed in a well-equipped surgical suite. This facilitates sterility and ensures access to appropriate equipment

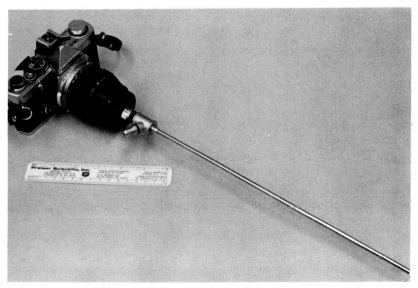

Fig 6. Camera with 100-mm lens and lens adapter fitted to eyepiece of the laparoscope.

needed in emergencies. The instruments are immersed in a germicidal solution of chlorhexidine for 20 minutes prior to use. Autoclavable laparoscopes are available, but they are not recommended because repeated sterilization tends to deteriorate lens seals within the telescope and shortens the useful life of the instrument. In addition, autoclaving is not practical when several animals are to be examined at the same time. Though gas sterilization is effective and safe for laparoscopic equipment, it requires 24 hours of aeration after sterilization before the instruments should be used.

Food is withheld from dogs and cats for 24 and 12 hours respectively, before laparoscopy. Water is usually withheld on the day of examination although an enlarged bladder is rarely a problem.

A surgical plane of anesthesia is induced in dogs with a combination of ketamine hydrochloride (Ketaset) at a dosage of 11.0 mg/kg and xylazine (Rompun) at a dosage of 2.2 mg/kg. Both are administered at the same time in separate IM injections. Anesthesia occurs within 5 minutes or less and a surgical plane of anesthesia is maintained for about 30 minutes. Approximately 20% of small dogs (less than 12 kg) will have a 1-minute tetanic spasm, but no other adverse effects have been observed. The dogs appear to have fully recovered within 1.5 to 2 hours after administration of the drugs.

Ketamine hydrochloride (20.0 mg/kg) and acepromazine (0.18 mg/kg) injected IM at the same time have provided excellent results in the cat. A surgical plane of anesthesia is reached within 5 to 10 minutes and lasts about 30 to 45 minutes. Full recovery occurs within 5 to 7 hours after injection. Occasionally the anesthesia for a dog or cat will require supplementation during a prolonged examination. This can be provided by ketamine administered alone or with an inhalant anesthetic, such as halothane.

The anesthetized animal is placed on its back on a surgical table with tilt capacity and restrained with tie-downs (Fig 7a). After the animal's abdomen has been prepared as for surgery, the table is adjusted so that the patient lies supine at a 30-degree angle. With such positioning the abdominal organs move cranially, thus improving the view of the reproductive organs. In addition, movement of the abdominal organs cranially lessens the danger of injury during insertion of the trocar-cannula unit.

Insertion and Use of the Laparoscope

A pneumoperitoneum is established before inserting the trocar-cannula unit. The Verres needle is inserted through the lower right abdominal wall and into the cavity (Fig 7b). A syringe is attached to the

Plate 1 — CANINE VAGINAL SMEARS

Patrick Concannon

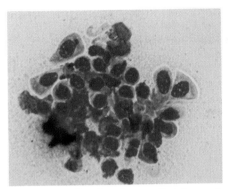

a. Anestrus. Parabasals, small intermediates, and WBCs.

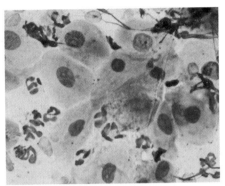

b. Early proestrus. Parabasals, small and large intermediates, RBCs, WBCs. Possible on days -15 to -6 (before LH peak).

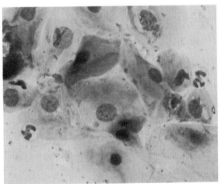

c. Mid-proestrus. Small and large intermediates, superficials, WBCs, RBCs. Possible on days -8 to -4.

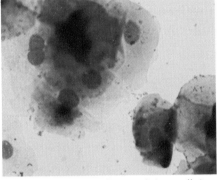

d. Late proestrus. Large intermediates, superficials. Likely on days -6 to +1.

e. Very late proestrus. Superficials, RBCs and considerable debris. Likely on days -4 to +2.

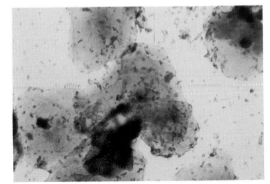

Plate 2 — CANINE VAGINAL SMEARS
Patrick Concannon

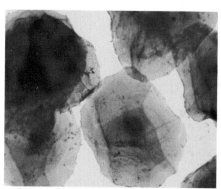

a. Estrus. Fully cornified superficials, no RBCs, few bacteria, clear background. Likely on days +1 to +6 (after LH peak).

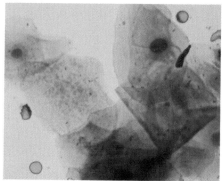

b. Estrus. Full and partially cornified superficials, RBCs. Possible on days -3 to +8.

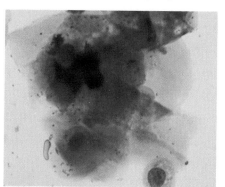

c. End of vaginal estrus. Superficials, RBCs, and parabasals. No WBCs. Possible on days +6 to +9.

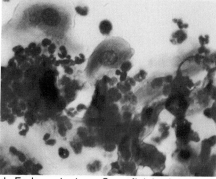

d. Early metestrus. Superficials, intermediates, parabasals, many WBCs. Possible on days +7 to +11.

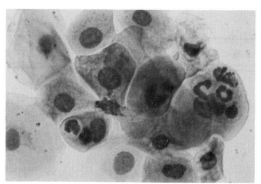

e. Metestrus. Large and small intermediates, superficials, RBC, WBCs, metestrual cells. Possible on days +9 to +15.

Plate 3 — LAPAROSCOPY
David E. Wildt

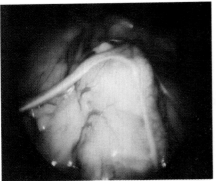

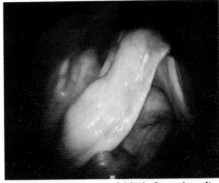

a. Uterine horns of the bitch during anestrus are bright pink, smooth, and narrow. From *Anat Rec* **189** (1977) 443.

b. Left uterine horn of bitch 2 weeks after ovulation. The horn is more pale than in anestrus, swollen, and contains longitudinal ridges.

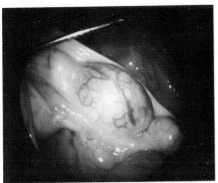

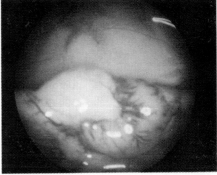

c. Swollen segment (conceptus site) of a highly vascularized gravid uterine horn of a bitch. From *Animal Laparoscopy,* Williams & Wilkins, 1980.

d. Cat ovary covered by the transparent fimbria. From *Current Therapy in Theriogenology,* W. B. Saunders, 1980.

e. Feline ovary with 2 corpora lutea. From *Current Therapy in Theriogenology,* W. B. Saunders, 1980.

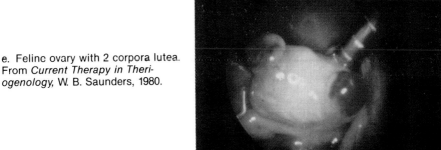

Plate 4 — LAPAROSCOPY
David E. Wildt

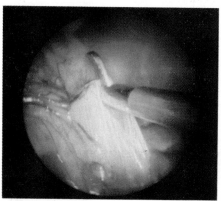

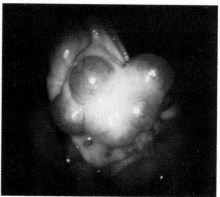

a. Scissors used to extend slit in the ovarian bursa of a bitch. From Anat Rec **189** (1977) 443.

b. Canine ovary during estrus.

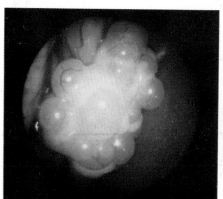

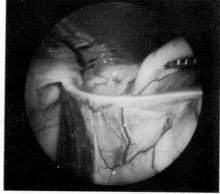

c. Cystic follicles on the ovary of bitch.

d. Left ductus deferens (white tube) in an adult dog is coursing from inguinal canal (left) medially (right). Spermatic artery-vein plexus is located laterally, descending into inguinal canal. From Amer J Vet Res **42** (1981) 1888.

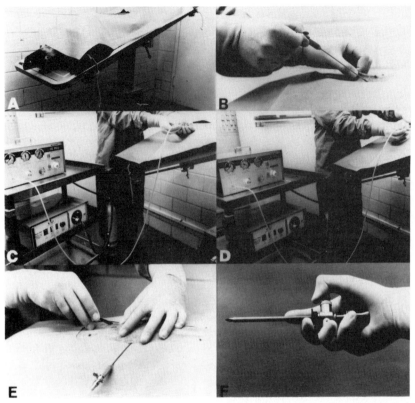

Fig 7. Laparoscopic technic: (A) anesthetized dog in recumbent head-down position; (B) insertion of the Verres needle; (C) attaching the gas hose from insufflator to the Verres needle; (D) monitoring distention of abdominal wall during insufflation; (E) incising skin near umbilicus; (F) grasping the assembled trocar-cannula unit. From *Animal Laparoscopy,* Williams & Wilkins, 1980.

needle and suction is applied to ensure that the needle has not been inadvertently inserted into the bladder. The hose from the insufflator or gas tank is attached to the Verres needle and gas is allowed to flow into the abdominal cavity (Figs 7c,d). The patient's size obviously determines the amount of gas required; the volume needed can vary from less than 0.5 liter for animals weighing less than 2.5 kg to 1 to 2 liters in dogs weighing more than 14 kg. Generally, a sufficient volume of gas has been transferred when the ventral abdominal wall becomes slightly distended. Caution should be exercised to avoid over-insufflation, which can result in respiratory distress. Excessive gas can be removed by detaching the gas hose and opening the valve on the Verres needle.

Following establishment of a pneumoperitoneum, a midline incision (1 to 2 cm depending on the trocar-cannula size) is made in the skin immediately cranial to the umbilicus (Fig 7e). The trocar-cannula unit (Fig 7f) is then inserted at about a 30-degree angle to the longitudinal plane of the animal (Fig 8a). A smooth, twisting motion should be used to insert the unit. An audible "pop" will be heard when the peritoneum is pierced. The trumpet valve of the cannula is then depressed and the trocar is removed and replaced with the laparoscope (Figs 8b,c,e). The hose is removed from the Verres needle and attached to the insufflation sleeve of the cannula (Fig 8d), thus freeing the needle for use as a manipulatory probe. The light cable is then attached to the sleeve of the laparoscopic eyepiece, the lamp projector is switched on, and the examination is initiated (Fig 8f).

During examination, the inserted laparoscope is supported by the midline cannula and not by the telescope itself. The cannula is grasped and elevated slightly ventrally to maintain the intra-abdominal space. When omentum obstructs the view, it can be moved by manipulating the Verres needle. Fogging or soiling of the terminal lens of the laparoscope can often be handled by touching the end of the telescope against internal tissues. Otherwise, the laparoscope can be removed from the cannula and cleaned with sterile gauze.

Laparoscopy can seldom be performed without manipulating internal organs or tissue. The most useful tool for simple manipulations is the Verres needle. In some cases 2 needles inserted at slightly different locations can be used together to manipulate abdominal structures. When it is necessary to perform extensive manipulations or to support heavy organs, insertion of an accessory trocar-cannula is useful. The accessory unit is inserted through a skin incision made 6 to 8 cm lateral to the midline. Insertion is the same as with the midline trocar-cannula unit. After removing the trocar, the 2nd instrument is inserted through the cannula and used to grasp, cut, or move organs (Fig 9). Biopsy forceps can be used to obtain adequate tissue for histopathologic examination and, if necessary, it can be used to obtain multiple samples from the same organ. Most biopsy forceps are serrated on the cutting edge, which minimizes post-biopsy hemorrhage. If bleeding becomes a problem, the biopsy forceps can be attached to an electrosurgical unit to coagulate the bleeding site.

Following examination, the laparoscope and any accessory instruments are removed from their cannulae. Gas is removed from the peritoneal cavity by depressing the trumpet valve of the midline cannula and allowing the gas to escape. The cannula is then removed and a single suture is placed to close the peritoneum, and 2 to 4 sutures are used to close the skin. An antibiotic is usually injected.

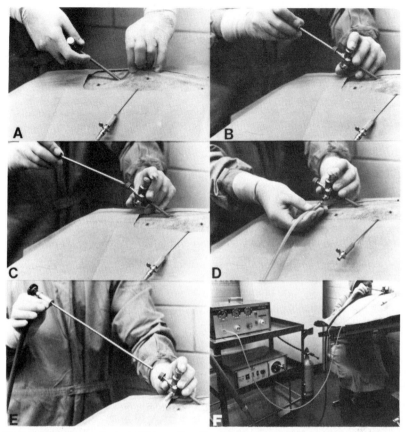

Fig 8. Laparoscopy technic (A) inserting the trocar-cannula unit with a twisting motion; (B) depressing the trumpet valve of the cannula and removing the trocar; (C) releasing the trumpet valve to prevent loss of pneumoperitoneum; (D) attaching the gas hose to the midline cannula sleeve; (E) inserting the laparoscope; (F) inspection through laparoscope. From *Animal Laparoscopy,* Williams & Wilkins, 1980.

Results and Contraindications

The lens system of the laparoscope provides a superior visual field and a panoramic view that encompasses large areas of the abdominal cavity. The varying degree of magnification that is available often provides a better view than can be obtained by laparotomy. Unlike laparotomy, laparoscopy is rarely accompanied by bleeding that obscures the visual field.

The major advantage of laparoscopy is the opportunity it provides to examine the abdominal cavity directly either once or repeatedly with only minor surgical intervention. This has been especially important in reproductive research that may require serial examina-

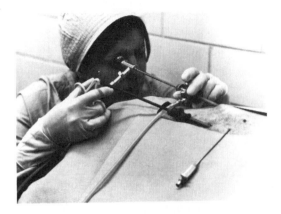

Fig 9. Laparoscopic ex-
amination with the acces-
sory instrument inserted
through an auxiliary can-
nula. From *Animal Lapa-
roscopy*, Williams & Wilkins,
1980.

tions of ovarian activity in individual animals. Some bitches and queens have been subjected to more than 100 laparoscopic examinations. A healthy dog or cat can usually tolerate anesthesia and laparoscopic examinations performed every 48 hours for 7 to 12 days. Daily laparoscopy has been performed in dogs and cats for 3 to 5 days without causing a problem or interfering with the reproductive cycle. In addition, adhesions do not result in animals subjected to considerable manipulation or repeated examinations.

Laparoscopy is contraindicated in animals with peritonitis or coagulopathies. It also is not recommended for animals suspected to have bowel-peritoneal adhesions because there is an increased risk of visceral perforation during insertion of the trocar-cannula. Animals with cardiovascular or respiratory impairment may be compromised by insufflation with gas and the head-down position. Subcutaneous emphysema has occurred during improper insufflation with gas. Obesity causes problems in visualization that generally can be overcome by repositioning the animal or moving fat deposits with the accessory probe.

Laparoscopy in Reproduction

Laparoscopy has been used most extensively in studies of reproduction. Although the procedure has considerable clinical application in the diagnosis of infertility in dogs and cats, there have been few reports on the subject because laparoscopy is still a new procedure in clinical veterinary medicine.

Uterine Disease and Reproductive Function

Uterine disease in animals has been readily detected by laparoscopy. Early changes associated with pyometra, metritis, or cystic glandular hyperplasia in cats have been apparent through alternations in uterine morphology. Both open and closed forms of pyometra have been diagnosed in queens by performing laparoscopy.

The current reproductive status of a bitch or queen can be determined in part by the appearance of the uterus viewed laparoscopically. This is associated with the fact that uterine morphology is partially dependent on the concentrations of circulating hormones,which vary with the stage of the reproductive cycle. When reproductive hormones are at basal levels, as in anestrus, the uterine horns are small in diameter, very smooth and flaccid, and generally pink (Plate 3a). During active periods, such as estrus and metestrus, the ovaries produce larger quantities of hormones that markedly alter the uterine appearance. At these times the uterine horns swell, coil slightly, and appear to contain sequentially enlarged segmentations and longitudinal ridges (Plate 3b). The horns also have more tone, are avascular, and often grayish. Because these uterine changes do not occur in the anovulatory bitch or queen, this laparoscopic observation can be used to predict with reasonable accuracy if ovulation has occurred.

Laparoscopy is especially helpful in cases in which a bitch exhibits estrous and mating behavior but fails to conceive. In such cases, laparoscopic examination of the ovary is difficult because the canine ovary is normally encapsulated in a bursa. It still would be possible to predict whether or not ovulation had occurred by inspecting the uterus. If the uterine horns are similar in appearance to those of a normal post-ovulatory bitch, it could be presumed that ovulation has occurred and that infertility was a result of some other factor(s).

Diagnosis of Pregnancy

Changes in the gross appearance of the uterine horns enable the early diagnosis of pregnancy. In the gravid bitch and queen, conceptus sites (observed as sequential swellings) are detected as early as the 21st to 25th day of gestation. Individual conceptus sites are very distinct by the 4th week of pregnancy and are usually characterized by marked vascularization (Plate 3c).

Laparoscopic examinations between the 3rd and 4th weeks of gestation by the previously described procedures have not caused problems. Abortions have not occurred and animals examined in this manner have had normal parturitions and litters. Both the bitch and queen appear to tolerate repeated laparoscopic examinations during pregnancy. In one bitch the laparoscopic examinations were initiated 2 weeks post-ovulation and continued at 5- to 7-day intervals through the 6th week of gestation. Her parturition and litter size were normal.

More recently, 11 queens subjected to routine laparoscopy on days 33, 38, and 40 of gestation (day of mating = day 1) had normal gestation periods and litters.[16]

Potential litter size can be estimated during laparoscopic examination by counting the number of sequential swellings in each uterine horn. Because accumulation of fluid within a uterine horn makes manipulation of the horn difficult, it is best to make the count before the 40th day of pregnancy. Though determination of the number of embryos developing *in utero* by laparoscopy is an accurate estimate of potential litter size, 100% accuracy cannot be expected when the count is made early in pregnancy. Normal embryonic attrition occurs in both the dog and cat, and thus affects litter size.

Laparoscopic examination of the uterus may also have application in diagnosing retained or mummified fetuses in an unhealthy, postparturient bitch.

Uterine Infusion, Flushing, and Insemination

This technic in which foreign agents are placed in the uterus probably has more research than clinical relevance. It could be useful, however, when a clinician desires to administer medicinal agents directly into the uterus.

Laparoscopic methods have been used in other species for direct uterine or oviductal deposition of spermatozoa and embryos and to flush and collect embryos.[17-20] In experiments in dogs designed to determine whether or not spermatozoa require vaginal exposure to achieve capacitation, sperm have been deposited directly into the uterus. Numerous other reproductive studies in animals will conceivably involve laparoscopic technics. They are exemplified by a procedure that involves immobilizing a uterine horn to facilitate intrauterine penetration with a needle (Fig 10).[21]

Evaluating Ovarian Activity

Laparoscopy affords a rapid and simple means of assessing ovarian activity in the cat. The queen's ovaries are found by locating the uterine horns and tracing each one cranially and laterally to its terminus. A fimbria or pocket of peritoneum normally covers each ovary and it can easily be removed by manipulation with an accessory probe (Plate 3d). All aspects of the ovary can then be inspected (Plate 3e).

Laparoscopy has facilitated studies in our laboratories concerning the relationship of ovarian morphology to numerous other factors in reproduction. Laparoscopy was performed initially to observe normal sequential changes in the ovarian follicle and corpus luteum (CL)

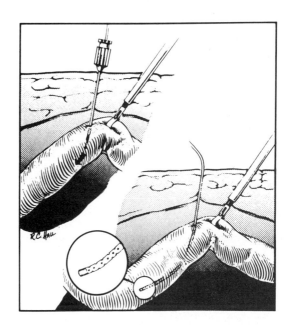

Fig 10. Segment of uterine horn is grasped with accessory forceps. A 16-gauge needle is inserted into the horn and cannulated with polyethylene tubing. The needle can then be withdrawn, leaving the tubing within the uterine horn. From J Reprod Fertil **44** (1975) 301.

throughout the reproductive cycle (Plate 3e).[22] The information obtained was used to study the effects of exogenous gonadotropins on ovarian activity, the relationship of ovarian morphology to sexual behavior, and endocrine changes during estrus, the luteal phase, and pregnancy through postpartum estrus.[23-29] The laparoscopic examinations in cats had no detectable effect on the estrous cycle or endocrine functions.

Similar studies of reproduction have been performed in the bitch. In the dog a bursa composed of fat and smooth muscle conceals most of the ovarian surface. The bursal pouch has a slitlike opening (1 to 2 cm long) and in less than a fifth of the dogs examined one or both slits were long enough to enable manipulation of the ovary through it for inspection.

The ovary can also be exposed in an anesthetized dog by using a cautery scissors. Under laparoscopic observation the scissors is used to lengthen the bursal slit by cutting the tissue nearest to the cranial terminus of the uterine horn (Plate 4a). If hemorrhage can be controlled by electrocoagulation, formation of adhesions can be avoided and the bursa can be removed to enable an unobstructed view of the ovary (Plate 4b). This has facilitated detailed studies of the changes associated with ovulation and the relationship of ovarian morphology to sexual behavior and reproductive hormone concentration.[30-33]

Though laparoscopy is useful for diagnosing ovarian disorders in the queen, the reproductive anatomy of the bitch precludes similar application of the technic. In the latter species there is some indecision about identifying through laparoscopy such abnormalities as infantile ovaries or cystic follicles (Plate 4c). The oviduct of the bitch courses through the bursa from the lateral to medial ovarian pole. Because it is difficult to identify, an oviduct could be damaged or severed when cutting a bursa to expose the ovary. The possibility of inadvertently affecting a bitch's fertility by performing certain laparoscopic procedures should probably contraindicate their use to diagnose suspected ovarian disease. This may not apply if the owner or breeder has decided that there is "nothing to lose." In such cases a single ovary could be surgically exposed and evaluated by the laparoscopist. By not disturbing the other ovary or its bursa the animal's reproductive potential is thus maintained.

Diagnosis and Treatment of Ovarian or Parovarian Cysts

Ovarian cysts in the cat appear as enlarged, fluid-filled follicles on the surface. Though they usually do not affect the animal's general health, these cysts can cause prolonged estrus. The cause of follicular cysts in the cat has not been extensively studied, but gonadotropic hyperpituitarism or suppression of normal release of pituitary gonadotropin due to insufficient gonadal production of steroids may be implicated. Attempts to ovulate or luteinize these aberrant follicles with exogenous hormones (human chorionic gonadotropin) are generally unsuccessful.

Ovarian cysts can best be treated by laparoscopic aspiration (Fig 11). This involves inserting a 20-gauge, 4-cm needle through the abdominal wall and using the laparoscope to direct it to the ovarian surface. The needle is then inserted near the apex of the follicular dome, a syringe is attached to the needle's hub, and suction is applied. To prevent recurrence of a cyst, it may be necessary to cauterize the site.

Parovarian cysts are occasionally found in both the bitch and queen. Neither the cause nor significance of these structures is known. Parovarian cysts are filled with fluid that can be aspirated.

Ovarian-Uterine Horn Biopsy

Although not reported in the dog or cat, ovarian biopsy has been performed routinely by laparoscopy in other species, including women.[34,35] A standard biopsy forceps is used to grasp and obtain tissue at the target site on the ovary. Hemorrhage is reportedly negligible and it can be controlled by electrocoagulation. An ovarian neoplasm could conceivably be diagnosed in this manner, especially in the cat.

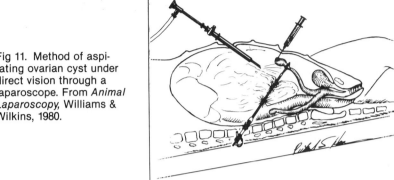

Fig 11. Method of aspirating ovarian cyst under direct vision through a laparoscope. From *Animal Laparoscopy*, Williams & Wilkins, 1980.

Obtaining a sample of common neoplasms of the female genital tracts of animals would probably require an initial incision with an accessory scissors and then removal of tissue with a grasping forceps. Because the uterus is a highly vascularized organ, control of hemorrhage would be required by using electrocoagulation.

Laparoscopy in the Male Dog and Cat

In the male dog and cat each vas deferens is easily located and observed from its opening in the urethra to its descent through the abdominal inguinal ring (Plate 4d).[36] Also clearly visible are the spermatic artery and vein coursing along the dorsal lateral abdominal wall. The prostate gland is difficult and often impossible to distinguish due to its location, which varies with the position and volume of the bladder.

Laparoscopy may be useful in diagnosing such anomalies as incomplete differentiation of the reproductive tract, spermatocelic lesions of the vas deferens, and retained testes.

Sterilization of Males

Laparoscopy has recently been used to develop and test new procedures for sterilizing adult and prepubertal male dogs and adult male cats.[36] After inserting a laparoscope into the anesthetized animal's abdominal cavity, the vasa deferentia were identified. Sterilization was achieved by occluding 1 to 2 cm of the vasa deferentia by using an ancillary bipolar forceps and electrocoagulation (Fig 12). Adult cats have been sterilized similarly by severing the vasa deferentia with an accessory scissors.

Within 48 hours after occluding the vasa deferentia of dogs, the sperm counts were zero. Live sperm were detected in the ejaculates of

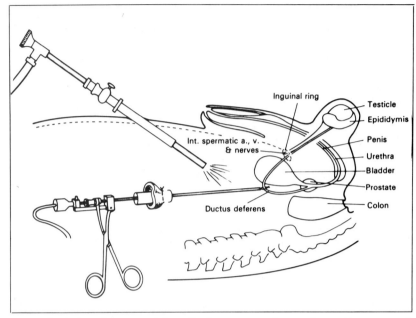

Fig 12. Occlusion of the vasa deferentia. An accessory forceps is used to grasp and cauterize each vas deferens. From Amer J Vet Res **42** (1981) 1888.

some cats as long as 120 hours after surgery. Sterilization of the prepubertal dogs (16 weeks old) resulted in chronic azoospermia without influencing their body weight or testicular development. Sterilization by laparoscopy also had no effect on the animal's libido or copulatory ability. Prepubertal dogs with bilaterally occluded vasa deferentia were able to have penile erections and azoospermic ejaculations at ages comparable to sham-sterilized dogs.

Compared with scrotal vasectomy technics the intra-abdominal procedure requires less time. In addition, the laparoscopic incisions are made at relatively avascular sites that are difficult for the animal to lick or bite during postoperative healing. The greatest potential for laparoscopic sterilization of male dogs and cats is when mass sterilizations are being performed, such as in pet population control programs.

Sterilization of Females

Laparoscopy is used extensively to control fertility in women and its use for sterilizing female dogs and cats should be investigated further. Preliminary studies have involved altering the uterine horn of the bitch or queen by electrocoagulation and/or cutting. Ligation or coagulation of the oviduct as performed in women is both difficult and time-consuming in the bitch and queen. In experimental studies, uterine horn ligation by laparoscopy has proved safe and effective when the horns were cauterized near the ovarian bursae. Additional research is required to further develop this procedure and to devise methods of eliminating ovarian function. Because the cat's ovaries are quite accessible, future studies involving ovarian cautery, intraovarian injection of sclerosing agents, and electrocoagulation of the ovarian blood supply are warranted.

Manufacturers of Laparoscopic Equipment

Richard Wolf Medical Instruments Corp
7046 Lyndon Avenue, Rosemont, IL 60018

American J. Mueller
110 Technology Park, Norcross, GA 30092

Dyonics, Inc
71 Pine Street, Woburn, MA 01801

Eder Instrument Company, Inc
5115 North Ravenwood Avenue, Chicago, IL 60640

Karl Storz Endoscopy-America, Inc
658 South San Vicente Boulevard, Los Angeles, CA 90048

Acknowledgment: The author thanks Drs W. Richard Dukelow, Richard M. Harrison and Mitch Bush for their contributions to this chapter; Ms Jane Koeser for manuscript preparation; and Mr Paul Guthrie for photographing laparoscopy procedures. Some of this work was conducted in the Institute of Comparative Medicine, Baylor College of Medicine, with the partial financial support of the Ralston Purina Company.

References

1. Harrison, RM and Wildt, DE: In *Animal Laparoscopy.* Williams & Wilkins, Baltimore, 1980.
2. Harrison, RM: In *Animal Laparoscopy,* pp 1-14. Williams & Wilkins, Baltimore, 1980.
3. Wildt, DE: In *Animal Laparoscopy,* pp 31-72. Williams & Wilkins, Baltimore, 1980.
4. Harrison, RM: In *Animal Laparoscopy,* pp 73-94. Williams & Wilkins, Baltimore, 1980.
5. Witherspoon, DM *et al:* In *Animal Laparoscopy,* pp 157-168. Williams & Wilkins, Baltimore, 1980.
6. Maxwell, DP and Kraemer, DC: In *Animal Laparoscopy,* pp 135-156. Williams & Wilkins, Baltimore, 1980.
7. Wildt, DE: In *Animal Laparoscopy,* pp 121-132. Williams & Wilkins, Baltimore, 1980.
8. Seeger, KH and Klatt, PR: In *Animal Laparoscopy,* pp 107-120. Williams & Wilkins, Baltimore, 1980.
9. Dukelow, WR: In *Animal Laparoscopy,* pp 95-106. Williams & Wilkins, Baltimore, 1980.
10. Bush, M: In *Animal Laparoscopy,* pp 183-198. Williams & Wilkins, Baltimore, 1980.
11. Bush, M *et al:* In *Animal Laparoscopy,* pp 169-182. Williams & Wilkins, Baltimore, 1980.
12. Lettow, E: Vet Med Rev **2** (1972) 159.
13. Wildt, DE *et al:* Amer J Vet Res **38** (1977) 1429.
14. Johnson, GF and Twedt, DC: Vet Clin No Amer **7** (1977) 77.

15. Prescott, R: In *Animal Laparoscopy*, pp 15-30. Williams & Wilkins, Baltimore, 1980.
16. Chan, SWY *et al:* J Reprod Fertil **65** (1982) 395.
17. Morcom, CB and Dukelow, WR: Lab Anim Sci **30** (1980) 1030.
18. Meredith, S *et al:* Proc Amer Soc Anim Sci Abst 91 (1979) 117.
19. Ariga, S. and Dukelow, WR: Primates **18** (1977) 453.
20. Ariga, S. and Dukelow, WR: Fertil Steril **28** (1977) 577.
21. Wildt, DE *et al:* J Reprod Fertil **44** (1975) 301.
22. Wildt, DE and Seager, SWJ: In *Current Therapy in Theriogenology*, pp 828-832. WB Saunders Co, Philadelphia, 1980.
23. Wildt, DE *et al:* Lab Anim Sci **28** (1978) 301.
24. Wildt, DE and Seager, SW: Horm Res **9** (1978) 130.
25. Chakraborty, PK *et al:* Lab Anim Sci **29** (1979) 338.
26. Wildt, DE *et al:* Horm Behav **10** (1978) 251.
27. Wildt, DE *et al:* Endocrinol **107** (1980) 1212.
28. Wildt, DE *et al:* Biol Reprod **25** (1981) 15.
29. Schmidt, PM *et al:* Biol Reprod **28** (1983) 657.
30. Wildt, DE *et al:* Anat Rec **189** (1977) 443.
31. Wildt, DE *et al:* Biol Reprod **18** (1978) 561.
32. Wildt, DE *et al:* Biol Reprod **20** (1979) 648.
33. Wildt, DE *et al:* J Anim Sci **53** (1981) 182.
34. Bush, M *et al:* JAVMA **173** (1978) 1081.
35. Kleppinger, RK: In *Endoscopy in Gynecology*, pp 80-84. Amer Assn Gynec Laparoscopists, 1978.
36. Wildt, DE *et al:* Amer J Vet Res **42** (1981) 1888.

TESTICULAR BIOPSY
BY THOMAS J. BURKE

Introduction

Testicular biopsy has been performed extensively in the diagnosis of infertility in man.[1,7] Its application in dogs and cats is relatively recent. The role of testicular biopsy has changed in human medicine with the advent of non-invasive diagnostic technics, such as cytogenetic procedures and gonadotropin assays by radioimmunoassay.[7] Many of these newer procedures are either not widely available or have yet to be fully developed for clinical use in the dog and cat. Therefore, veterinary practitioners may have to rely on biopsy of the testis more than physicians.

Indications

Testicular biopsy should be performed only after a thorough examination assures that the patient is infertile and that the cause of the infertility cannot be established by any other means. Biopsy should always be correlated with one or more analyses of semen.

According to one author, the indications for testicular biopsy include acquired azoospermia, palpable degeneration of the testes, and suspicion of neoplasia.[8] Reports vary concerning the value of a biopsy in identifying oligospermic men. Partial obstruction of the excurrent duct system has caused oligospermia and reduced sperm motility in men.[9] Congenital bilateral aplasia of the excurrent duct system has been reported in dogs.[2,10] I would include acquired or apparently congenital oligospermia as an indication for biospy as well as apparently congenital azoospermia.

Contraindications

Other than a patient's inability to withstand general anesthesia, there are no specific contraindications for testicular biopsy. Postsurgical atrophy of a testis is usually the result of poor technic that results in excessive hemorrhage or infection.[4] Transient lowering of sperm counts and motility following biopsy have been reported in man, dog, and other species.[5,6,9] In a study of 100 normal men subjected to bilateral testicular biopsy, the sperm counts decreased in 39, rose in 4, and were unchanged in 57.[9] The average decrease was 42%. The men that had decreases fell into 2 groups: one with a maximal decrease by the 2nd week after biopsy and return to normal by the 10th week and a group with a maximal decrease between the 2nd and 4th weeks after biopsy and a recovery that did not begin until week 10 and was complete by week 18. Decreased sperm counts were more likely to occur in patients with higher pre-biopsy counts.

In a study of 24 normal Beagles subjected to testicular biopsy, the post-biopsy sperm counts were 110% of the presurgical count during the first 4 weeks, but after 2 subsequent biopsies of the same testis at 4-week intervals the counts fell to 88% and 82% of the original count.[5] By 7 weeks after the 3rd biopsy, the sperm counts were near normal. Sperm motility was unaffected. In an unpublished study of 4 dogs that were biopsied twice with a 2-week interval there was decreased sperm motility in 3 of the 4 dogs and decreased sperm output in all 4 animals.[6] The latter was not severe, however. Long-term changes were not assessed. The cause of this drop in semen quality has been theorized to be related to local inflammation, surgical trauma, or an immune reaction.[4,6] It has been observed in dogs, however, that biopsy alone did not induce sperm-agglutinating antibodies.[6]

The owner should be made aware of the possible complications associated with testicular biopsy. I prefer a situation in which there is "everything to be gained and nothing to lose." As a consequence, most of my biopsy patients have been either severely oligospermic or azoospermic. The remainder have had abnormal testicular masses.

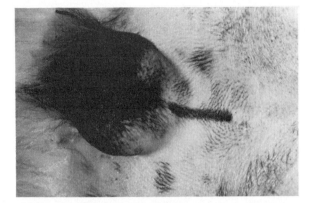

Fig 1. Site of incision
for testicular biopsy
is marked with a
black line cranial to
the scrotum.

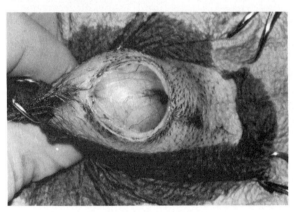

Fig 2. Positioning of
a testis for biopsy.
The pressure exerted
digitally should be
steady and gentle.

Operative Procedures

Aspiration and punch biopsy technics have been described.[4] Their
value is limited, however, because they have been associated with
serious artifacts and the chance for formation of sperm granulomas is
increased with punch biopsy.[8] The method of choice for obtaining
testicular tissue for histologic examination is incisional.[3,7,8] It requires
general anesthesia and aseptic technic. Because nearly all patients
presented for testicular biopsy are in good condition and are seldom
aged, these requirements are seldom a problem.

The preoperative examinations should include an assessment of
clotting function because postoperative hemorrhage can be a serious
complication. Assessment of activated clotting time and inspection
of the platelets in a peripheral blood smear are usually adequate.

In man the usual site of incision is through the scrotum directly
over the site to be biopsied.[1,9] This approach has also been recommended for the dog.[3] I have observed wound dehiscences however,

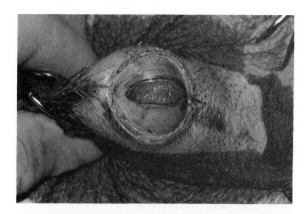

Fig 3. Testicular parenchyma is bulging through the incised tunica albuginea.

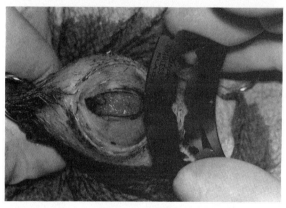

Fig 4. A razor blade is used to obtain the biopsy specimen. It is bowed slightly as the cut is started at the cranial end of the testis.

caused by patients when this technic was used. For this reason, I prefer a midline antescrotal incision as for routine castration (Fig 1). After preparing the site for surgery, an incision is made through the skin and subcutaneous tissue. The testis to be biopsied is then brought to the incision by gentle manipulation (Fig 2). Care must be taken to ensure that the ventral surface of the testis is presented to avoid incising the epididymis. This may be difficult if the testis is severely atrophied. The tunica vaginalis is incised and any fatty tissue is removed. Then with pressure being applied gently to the sides of the testis, a 1.5- to 3-cm incision is made through the tunica albuginea with a scalpel. The testicular parenchyma will then bulge through the incision (Fig 3). A gas-sterilized, double-edged razor blade is used to obtain the biopsy specimen. It is held between a thumb and middle finger and bowed slightly (Fig 4). Starting at the cranial end of the testis with the razor blade resting on its surface the tissue is incised using a slight side-to-side motion while pushing the

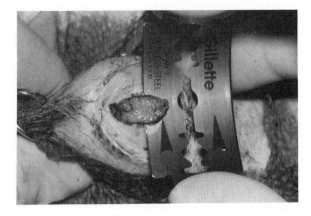

Fig 5. The blade is moved slightly side-to-side as the testicular parenchyma is severed.

blade caudally (Fig 5). If the tissue sample does not separate freely at the caudal end of the incision, it should be snipped free with a sharp scissors. The sample should not be grasped with a forceps. The specimen is then dropped into a jar containing Bouin's fixative (Fig 6).[3,9] Formalin should not be used as a fixative because it may produce artifacts.[7] The blade is removed from the jar with a forceps and the jar is filled to overflowing with the fixative solution and capped (Fig 7). This prevents wave action in the jar, which could damage a specimen being transported.

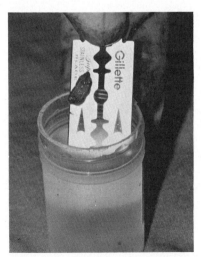

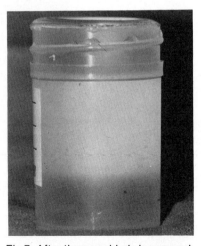

Fig 6. Transfer of the testicular sample and razor blade into a fixative solution. The fixative container is made of rigid plastic.

Fig 7. After the razor blade is removed from the fixative container, the jar is filled to overflowing with the fixative to prevent wave damage to the specimen while being transported.

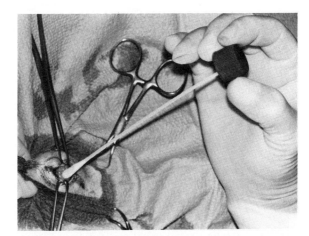

Fig 8. Sample of testicular parenchyma is taken for culturing.

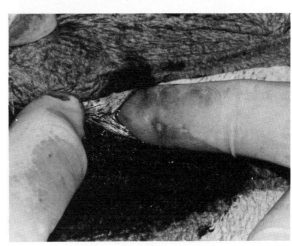

Fig 9. Repositioning the testicle into the scrotum.

The testicular parenchyma can be cultured by touching a swab to the incised area (Fig 8). The edges of the tunica albuginea are then grasped with an Allis forceps to stabilize the incision during closure. Simple interrupted sutures with an absorbable material are used to close the tunica albuginea. The testis is then replaced in the scrotum (Fig 9). The tunica vaginalis and subcutaneous dead space and then the skin are closed with absorbable sutures. Self-mutilation of these surgical wounds has not been a problem. If both testes are to be sampled, only one skin incision is required.

Hemorrhage is minimal. The larger vessels can usually be identified and ligated prior to severing them. Bleeding from smaller vessels is usually controlled with hemostats and, if necessary, by liga-

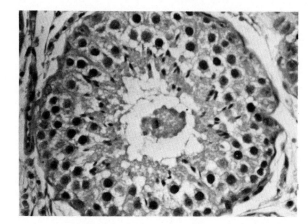

Fig 10. Histologic appearance of testicular tissue.

tion. They should not be cauterized because this may result in artifacts in the tissue to be examined.

This method of testicular biopsy will produce tissue with the fewest artifacts (Fig 10). Though the histopathologic examination does not always enable identification of the exact cause of an abnormality, it usually enables an accurate prognosis and serves as a guide for therapy.

Animals that have undergone a testicular biopsy examination are kept in the hospital overnight so that they can be observed for evidence of hemorrhage or wound damage. Antibiotics are not prescribed routinely after surgery.

References

1. Colgan, TJ *et al:* Fertil Steril **33** (1980) 56.
2. Copland, MD and MacLachlan, NJ: J Small Anim Pract **17** (1976) 443.
3. Fanning, ML: In *Current Veterinary Therapy V.* WB Saunders Co, Philadelphia, 1974.
4. Finco, DR: Vet Clin No Amer **4** (1974) 377.
5. Hunt, WL *et al:* J Anim Sci **24** (1965) 921.
6. Larsen, RE: Unpublished data.
7. Levin, HS: Hum Path **10** (1979) 569.
8. Schille, VM: In *Current Therapy in Theriogenology.* WB Saunders Co, Philadelphia, 1980.
9. Silber, SJ and Rodriguez-Rigau, LJ: Fertil Steril **36** (1981) 480.
10. Majeed, ZZ: J Small Anim Pract **15** (1974) 263.

PROSTATE BIOPSY
BY THOMAS R. CHRISTIE

Introduction

Obtaining a sample of representative tissue is often required in the diagnosis of prostatic disease. A good sample often provides information that aids differentiation of prostatic neoplasia, hypertrophy, and infection. Because of the difficulties associated with major surgery of the prostate, a biopsy should be considered in most cases.

Prior to performing a biopsy of the prostate, the gland should be examined carefully. The examination should include palpation (both rectal and abdominal) of the prostate, radiographs (including positive-contrast urethrography), a CBC, and a urinalysis. Fluid from the prostate should be examined microscopically and cultured.

The technics used most commonly are the percutaneous perineal needle biopsy, the percutaneous transabdominal needle biopsy, and the wedge biopsy by direct visualization.[1] Obtaining prostate tissue after laparoscopy may have distinct advantages and this procedure is slowly gaining favor among veterinary clinicians.

Because prostatic disease is often multifocal, it may be difficult to obtain a representative sample of the diseased tissue without direct visualization of the gland.[2] Infections and abscesses often result in accumulation of fluid and pockets of pus within the prostate's parenchyma and dissemination is almost certain if one of these pockets is punctured by a biopsy needle. For these reasons it is preferable to perform a laparoscopy and obtain a wedge of tissue that is being visualized. Anesthetic risk, time, and cost must also be considered in selecting the biopsy technic for each case.

Percutaneous Perineal Technic

Percutaneous perineal biopsy of the prostate should be attempted only when the entire gland can be palpated rectally. This procedure is also favored when the gland is easily immobilized.

This technic requires a bit more expertise than other methods. The surgeon should be familiar with the anatomy of the area and the technic should be practiced before it is attempted on a live animal.

An area on one side of the anus is clipped and prepared as for surgery. Selection of the side to be penetrated depends on the surgeon's judgment after rectal palpation. If there is no preference on this basis, the operative site is selected to facilitate immobilization of the

CHAPTER 2

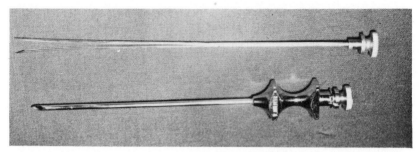

Fig 1a. A Franklin-modified Vim-Silverman needle consists of a needle with stylet and cutting prongs.

gland with the finger of one hand and advancement of the needle with the other. Thus for a right-handed surgeon the right side is preferred.

Sedation with acepromazine (0.2 mg/lb given IM) and induction of local anesthesia with 2% Xylocaine are usually sufficient for this biopsy procedure. The patient is then positioned in lateral recumbency on the side opposite to the perianal area prepared for surgery. Alternately, the animal may be held in a standing position by an abdominal sling. Pressure over the abdomen is applied by an assistant to force the abdominal viscera and prostate caudally.

A Franklin-modified Vim-Silverman biopsy needle is suitable for this procedure (Fig 1a). The tip of this needle obtains the biopsy specimen with minimal damage to prostate parenchyma (Fig 1b). The use of this needle has been adequately described in other sources.[3,4]

The prostate is retracted and immobilized as far caudally as possible from within the rectum and transabdominally. A stab incision is then made 1 to 2 cm in the prepared site beside the anus while being careful not to incise the anal sac or rectum. The biopsy needle with

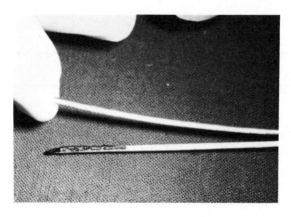

Fig 1b. A biopsy specimen has been obtained in the tip of the cutting prongs.

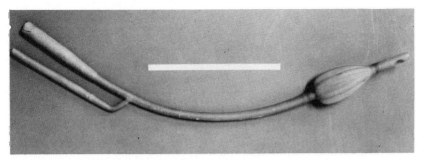

Fig 2a. Foley-Bardex catheter with inflatable bulb.

stylet is inserted just through the capsule of the diseased gland. The stylet is then removed and the cutting prongs are advanced into the prostatic tissue. The needle should be directed parallel to the median plane of the gland so that the urethra is not likely to be punctured. The outer cannula is then advanced over the cutting prongs and the instrument with tissue specimen is removed. Digital pressure should be applied to the prostate for several minutes after the needle is withdrawn. One or 2 sutures are then placed to close the small skin incision.

Potential complications of this technic are infection, hemorrhage, and puncture of the bladder, urethra, colon, or other perineal structures.[5] A urethral fistula may form subsequently. Evidence of blood loss, fever, shock, or abdominal pain within the first 24 hours after surgery are signs of complications. If urethral puncture is suspected, a positive-contrast urethrogram should be obtained to disclose its size and location.

Most urethral tears made with a modified Vim-Silverman needle can be repaired with a urethral stent. This involves passing the largest catheter possible through the urethra beyond the tear and into the urinary bladder. When a urethral tear is extensive, a temporary

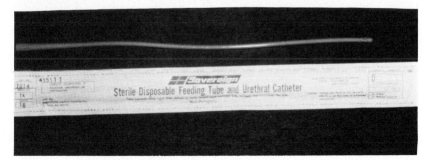

Fig 2b. Brunswick feeding tube.

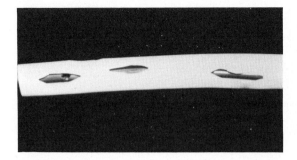

Fig 3a. A fenestrated
Penrose drain has been
placed over a fenes-
trated Brunswick drain.

perineal urethrotomy should be considered to facilitate passage of a
catheter. A Foley-type catheter with an inflatable balloon or a soft
Brunswick catheter is suitable for this purpose while the urethra is
healing (Figs 2a,b). The catheter is attached with sutures and left in
place for 5 days. A broad-spectrum antibiotic should be administered
during this period.

If a significant amount of urine collects in the abdominal or pelvic
cavity after a urethral tear, it should be drained. A fenestrated
Penrose drain and a fenestrated Brunswick-type catheter should be
used to provide continued drainage of urine. The catheters should be
sutured together with the Penrose drain over the Brunswick-type
(Fig 3a). The Penrose drain is then sutured to the skin (Fig 3b).

Percutaneous Transabdominal Technic

This prostate biopsy is performed when, because of the animal's
conformation or the size of the prostate, it is possible to immobilize
the gland against the abdominal wall either by rectal or transab-

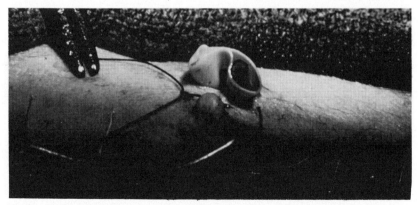

Fig 3b. The combined Penrose and Brunswick drains are sutured to the skin.

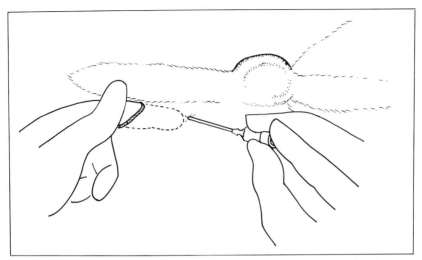

Fig 4. The surgeon's index finger is inserted through a skin incision to immobilize the prostate and to guide the biopsy needle.

dominal manipulation. The danger of damaging abdominal viscera is less with this technic because of the anatomy involved as well as the decreased distance the needle must be passed to enter the prostate.

For this procedure the patient is placed in either dorsal or lateral recumbency and a 5 x 5-cm area lateral to the preputial orifice is prepared for surgery. A combination of a sedative and local anesthetic usually is adequate for restraint of the patient.

The prostate is pressed tightly over the prepared surgical site with a finger in the rectum and a hand over the abdomen. A stab incision is then made and a modified Vim-Silverman needle is used to obtain the sample of prostate tissue.

In an excellent modification of the technic just described a keyhole incision is made into the abdominal cavity at the prepared site. The surgeon then inserts an index finger through this incision to guide the biopsy needle to the immobilized prostate and thus help to ensure selection of a suitable sample of tissue (Fig 4).

Wedge Biopsy Under Direct Visualization
Though this method of obtaining prostate tissue requires more time and surgical manipulation than the others described, it is not necessarily the procedure with greatest risk. Being able to see the gland gives the surgeon the optimum control in selection of the biopsy site and thus reduces the possibility of iatrogenic damage and increases the probability of obtaining a representative sample.[6]

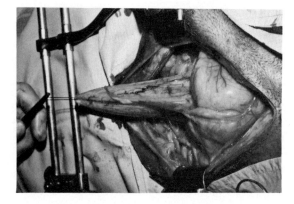

Fig 5. Cranial traction
on the bladder has
moved the prostate to
the abdominal incision.

The ventrocaudal abdomen is prepared for surgery prior to induction of general anesthesia, if possible. The abdominal incision is made along the ventral midline from a point 2 to 4 cm caudal to the umbilicus to a point 1 cm cranial to the prepuce. The incision is then curved gently around the prepuce and extended caudally to the level of the inguinal nipples. If possible, the parapreputial portion of the incision should be made medial to the nipples to avoid the caudal superficial epigastric vessels. The preputial artery and vein are then double-ligated and transected near the cranial preputial orifice.[7] The prepuce and penis are reflected laterally by dissection along the plane of the external rectus muscle sheath. The abdominal cavity is entered through the linea alba and the urinary bladder is drawn exteriorly by gentle cranial traction (Fig 5). The prostate is then exposed by dissecting the paraprostatic fat from the ventral prostatic raphe that separates the gland into 2 lobes (Fig 6). After dissecting the fat from the gland and reflecting it laterally, the prostatic vessels can be seen

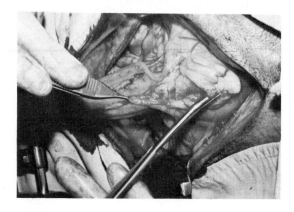

Fig 6. Removal of para-
prostatic fat to expose
the gland's capsule.

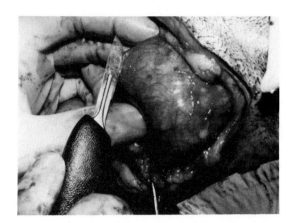

Fig 7. The elliptical-shaped wedge of tissue is made transversely if possible.

branching from the urogenital vessels in the inguinal area. Care should be taken to avoid these vessels when selecting a site for obtaining a wedge of tissue.

An elliptical specimen is excised from the diseased prostate by incising a wedge from the gland's surface (Fig 7). A wedge that is 5 to 8 mm long and 5 mm deep is usually large enough to provide the needed information and leave a defect that is small enough to manage. It is preferable to make the wedge transversely, if the size of the prostate allows, to minimize the severing of smaller prostatic vessels. Because of its vascularity, cut surfaces of the prostate bleed profusely.

Either 3-0 or 4-0 gut sutures are placed to close the wedge defect. The sutures should include the prostatic capsule and parenchyma in a simple interrupted pattern. Digital compression of the wedge defect over the capsular closure for several minutes usually provides adequate hemostasis. Gelfoam or Surgicel may be used if hemorrhage from the cut surface persists. The biopsy site should then be liberally flushed with sterile Ringer's solution. A drain need not be installed unless the surgical site has been contaminated.

The patient's ventral midline is closed with simple interrupted sutures of chromic gut or polyglycolic material. The preputial reflection is closed with a subcutaneous suture pattern using 3-0 or 4-0 chromic gut. Simple interrupted sutures are used to close the skin.

References
1. Leeds, EB and Leav, I: JAVMA **154** (1969) 925.
2. Christie, TR: In *Pathophysiology in Small Animal Surgery.* Lea & Febiger, Philadelphia, 1981.

3. Finco, D: Vet Clin No Amer **4** (1974) 367.
4. Christie, TR: In *Current Techniques in Small Animal Surgery,* 2nd ed. Lea & Febiger, Philadelphia, 1983.
5. Barsanti, JA *et al:* JAVMA **177** (1980) 160.
6. Morrow, DA: *Current Therapy in Theriogenology.* WB Saunders Co, Philadelphia, 1980.
7. Annis, JR and Allen, AR: *An Atlas of Canine Surgery.* Lea & Febiger, Philadelphia, 1967.

CULTURE TECHNICS
BY THOMAS J. BURKE

Introduction

The results of any laboratory test can be no more accurate than the quality of the sample submitted. This is especially true for bacterial cultures. The primary objective is to obtain representative material that is not unduly contaminated. The sample must then be transported to the laboratory in such a manner as to preclude additional contamination or loss of organisms.

All equipment used to collect a sample for culturing, including lubricants, should be sterile. The specula used should be heat- or gas-sterilized because contact of the swab with chemically sterilized instruments may destroy organisms. If the sample cannot be put on culture media immediately after its collection, a "transport" medium should be used. The sample should be refrigerated until and during transportation to the laboratory.

The laboratory personnel should be instructed to attempt to culture both aerobic and anaerobic organisms. Many potential pathogens of the reproductive tract are anaerobic or microaerophilic.[1,2] The author also requests that an estimate of the degree of growth (light, moderate, or heavy) of each isolate be made and reported. This facilitates interpretation. Cultures for particular organisms, such as Brucella or Mycoplasma, should be prearranged with the laboratory so that special media, etc., can be prepared.

Vaginal Cultures

Culture of material from the vestibule and vagina caudal to the urethral orifice has little value because this area is usually heavily

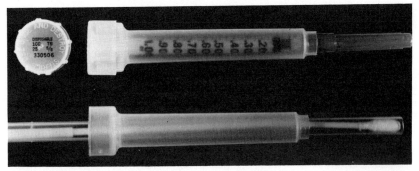

Fig 1. A disposable syringe case can be used as a speculum to obtain vaginal contents for culture.

contaminated with normal flora, including a variety of gram-negative rods and gram-positive cocci.[16] An exception would be the culturing of material from an abscess or pustule.

In cases of suspected bacterial vaginitis the material to be cultured is obtained with a standard-length sterile swab after the vulva has been washed with a povidone-iodine solution, rinsed, and dried. A speculum is inserted into the vagina to protect the swab from contacting the caudal vagina and vestibule. Ideally the material for culture should be obtained from an area ventral to the mid-

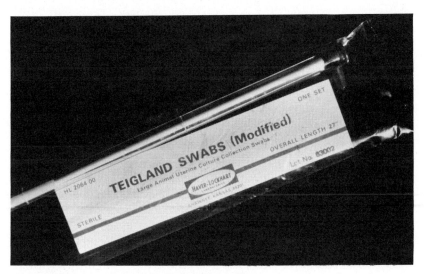

Fig 2. Modified Teigland swab. Notice its length.

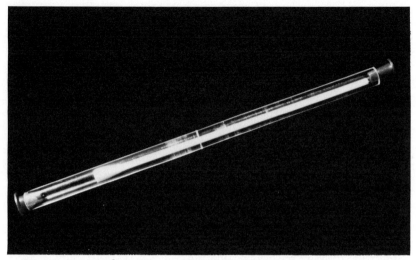

Fig 3. After obtaining a sample, the Teigland swab can be broken to a size more convenient to handle and mail.

sacrum. Plastic guides for insertion of human tampons have been used instead of a speculum,[5] as have disposable tuberculin syringe cases (Fig 1).

Culture material from the cranial vagina can be obtained with a longer swab. I prefer to use a modified Teigland swab that is 27 inches (68 cm) long (Fig 2). To use this swab a speculum is inserted until the pseudocervix is encountered, and then the Teigland swab guard is advanced until resistance is encountered. The tip of the swab is then advanced a centimeter or so and the swab is rotated. This instrument has a sterile outer guard that helps to ensure minimal contamination during passage of the swab through the caudal and middle vagina. After the sample is obtained, the swab and guard can be broken to a size more convenient for transportation to the laboratory (Fig 3).

Swabs with wooden shafts should not be used, especially to obtain material from the cranial vagina because they may break and be difficult to retrieve.

Uterine Cultures
Material cannot be obtained from the uterus for culture without penetrating the abdomen. The uterus can be exposed by a laparotomy

and entered through an incision or a sample of uterine contents can be obtained by infusing and then withdrawing sterile saline solution with a syringe and needle. It is also possible to excise a small piece of uterus for culture.

When the cervix is open (proestrus and estrus), culture of pericervical material will usually reveal the organisms present in the uterus as well as those that have migrated from the anterior vagina.[1] Culture of a pericervical swab may, however, reveal only organisms considered to constitute the normal vaginal flora. These organisms are usually present in low numbers and mixed cultures are very common.[2,5]

I regard the recovery of a single organism in high numbers (heavy to moderate growth), if associated with a history of infertility, to be suggestive of bacterial endometritis and will institute treatment on this basis. The therapy is based on bacterial sensitivity tests and is continued for 3 to 4 weeks. The results in reference to a change in fertility have been encouraging.

Culture of Samples from Male Genitalia

Obtaining samples of prostatic fluid is described in another section of this chapter. Semen may be cultured by collecting the 2nd fraction only of the ejaculate in a sterile tube. This is difficult and the sample usually contains some prostatic fluid. A testicular sample for culture may be obtained by excision or needle aspiration. Both technics require general anesthesia.

The vas deferens' contents may be sampled by infusion and aspiration of sterile saline solution with a syringe and 25- to 27-gauge needle. The ducts must be exposed surgically.

Culturing material from the glans penis is usually an exercise in futility because the preputial sheath is inhabited by numerous organisms similar to the bacteria normally found in the caudal vagina.[3,4] Culture of a single organism in large numbers, however, can be significant in the treatment of severe balanitis or balanoposthitis.

References

1. Baba, E et al: Amer J Vet Res **44** (1983) 606.
2. Hirsh, DC and Wiger, N: J Small Anim Pract **18** (1977) 25.
3. Allen, WE and Dagnall, GJR: J Small Anim Pract **23** (1982) 325.
4. Ling, GV and Ruby, AL: Amer J Vet Res **39** (1978) 695.
5. Olson, PNS and Mather, EC: JAVMA **172** (1978) 708.
6. Platt, AM and Simpson, RB: Southwestern Vet **27** (1974) 76.

RADIOLOGIC EXAMINATION
BY STEPHEN K. KNELLER

The use of radiography to evaluate the genital system varies depending on the organ, interests, and experience of the examiner, severity of the clinical signs, and the equipment available. Some structures, such as the male cat's accessory sex glands, cannot be evaluated radiographically. Other structures, such as the oviducts, can be evaluated only by tedious and time-consuming procedures. To examine some structures, however, radiography is one of the best procedures. This assumes that the radiographs are top quality, and for this purpose excellent reference sources are available.[1-4]

Radiographs are obtained and inspected from 2 different perspectives. One is for the purpose of studying a particular structure. The other is to discover unanticipated abnormalities. In the following discussion both perspectives are considered.

Radiography of the Uterus

Generally, the uterus of the queen and bitch is not visible on a survey radiograph unless the organ is enlarged. An exception may occur when there is an excessive amount of fat in the caudal abdomen, the intestine is empty, and the contrast and definition of the

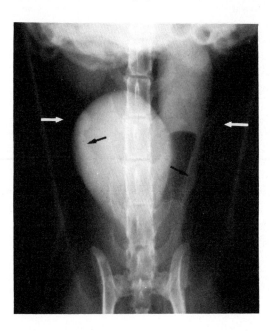

Fig 1. Ventrodorsal view of normal, 4-year-old queen made with a horizontal beam as cat is suspended head down after injection of CO_2 into peritoneal cavity. Ovaries (white arrows) and uterine horns (black arrows) are visible. Gas-filled small intestines are at top of radiograph. Urinary bladder and gas-filled colon are visible in center of film.

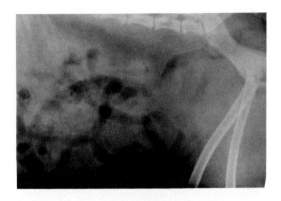

Fig 2a. Radiograph of 9-year-old Poodle with vaginal discharge and palpable abdominal mass. This lateral view is difficult to interpret because of feces in colon.

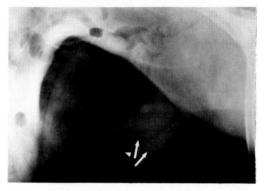

Fig 2b. Lateral view of dog in Fig 2a was obtained as caudoventral abdomen was compressed with a wooden spoon. Small intestine (arrowhead) and larger uterus (arrows) are visible. Palpable mass was enlarged uterus.

radiograph are optimal. In such cases it should not be assumed that the uterus is enlarged just because it is visible. To evaluate the size of the uterus in a radiograph it can be estimated that the diameter of a normal, nongravid uterus in anestrus is approximately half of the diameter of a loop of small intestine (Fig 1). Because there usually is better contrast in radiographs of the cat's abdomen, the uterus is occasionally visible in a nongravid queen.

Uterine Enlargement
    Because the uterus is of soft tissue density, it will usually be indistinguishable unless grossly enlarged. By emptying the colon and urinary bladder, it is possible to remove interfering densities and allow the uterus to be in a more natural position. Overlying skin folds and muscle masses of the hindlimbs can cause confusing shadows and to diminish their effect the limbs should be pulled caudally. The abdomen should not be stretched, however, because this will compress the caudal abdominal shadows and reduce definition of intra-abdominal structures.

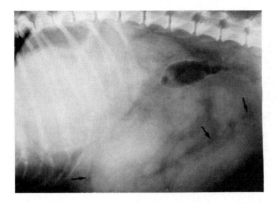

Fig 3. Lateral view of 11-year-old Australian Shepherd with history of apathy and weakness. She also had a distended abdomen. Large, tubular soft-tissue density (arrows) is in caudoventral abdomen, displacing other organs cranially.

A compression device can be used to separate the abdominal structures (Fig 2).[5,6] Such devices include paddles, wooden spoons, and other low-density objects. When applying compression, care must be taken not to injure fragile organs. In fact, compression should not be applied unless interpretation of survey radiographs is difficult and it is necessary for organ evaluation. With compression, the exposure can usually be decreased because of the change in tissue thickness. Reduction of exposure to 50% is usually sufficient.

Another simple technic that may enhance visualization involves elevation of the animal's rear quarters and gentle ballottement of the abdomen prior to radiography. This causes other abdominal organs to move forward and thus decreases the number of obscuring structures. Though the uterus is seen best on a recumbent lateral view, the ventrodorsal view can also provide valuable information and it should not be omitted.

The uterus may appear slightly enlarged with soft-tissue density during the first 2 trimesters of gestation and during the first 3 to 4 days after parturition. If pregnancy can be ruled out and parturition has not recently occurred, an enlarged uterus should be considered abnormal.

To distinguish an enlarged uterus from intestine the following differences are helpful:

1. A minimally enlarged uterus will usually not contain gas as the small intestine commonly does.

2. The uterus will not have a peristaltic configuration and will usually be uniform in diameter. Segmentation may be seen in a minimally enlarged gravid uterus; a larger uterus will become more uniform in appearance. Although a filled, nongravid uterus may be sacculated, it is nearly always tubular in shape (Fig 3). Its convoluted structure may cause it to appear

Fig 4. Lateral view of a 15-year-old German Shepherd that had vaginal discharge for 18 hours. Dog was alert, had been in estrus 8 weeks before. Tubular mass was palpable in caudoventral abdomen. Abdominal compression was applied as this film was made. Both horns and body of uterus (black arrow) are visible between colon and bladder. Wooden spoon (white arrow) used for compression is also visible.

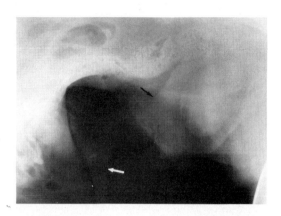

saccular, but the tubular shape can usually be traced. Although rare, uterine neoplasia may result in localized enlargement.

3. By the time that a uterine abnormality is clinically evident, the uterus is usually larger than normal small intestine. Therefore, tubular soft-tissue densities that are larger than small intestine in the caudal abdomen are usually an enlarged uterus or colon.

4. By careful scrutiny of a radiograph an enlarged uterus can often be traced to the pelvic brim between the colon and neck of the bladder (Fig 4).

Normal Gravid Uterus

Because of known and theoretical effects of x-radiation on developing fetuses, radiography is not recommended during pregnancy unless it is considered necessary. When pregnancy is discovered, however, in an animal with no history of having been bred, the staging of gestation by radiographs can be useful. Although there is some variation, information is available to help predict fetal age and expected parturition date from the evidence provided by radiographs (Fig 5.)

Table 1. Radiographic Assessment of Fetal Age

Structure Recognized	Days Before Expected Parturition	
	Queen	Bitch
Maternal uterine enlargement	44-46	30-35
First fetal skeleton	25-27	18-22
Scapula, humerus, and femur	20-22	12-15
Metacarpal-metatarsal bones and radius, ulna and tibia	13-15	10-12
Phalanges, caudal vertebrae, and sternum	10-12	5-10
Molar teeth	5-7	3-8

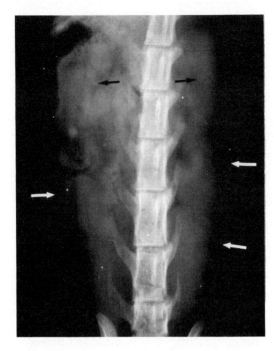

Fig 5a. VD radiograph of 3-year-old pregnant queen reveals rounded uterine enlargements (white arrows) typical of pregnancy about 3 weeks prior to fetal mineralization. Black arrows = kidneys. Though cystic endometritis may appear similar, in normal animals the fetuses will continue to develop and mineralize.

Breeding dates used in the past to calculate fetal age have been shown to be less reliable than expected because of the variation in time of ovulation related to breeding.[7] In Table 1 radiographic evidence is used to assess the age of canine and feline fetuses.[8,9] Even with good-quality radiographs, however, the size, shape, and content of the dam's abdomen will cause variation in the appearance of these structures. In larger, more rounded abdomens they are more difficult to recognize. The lateral view is usually more informative.

Dystocia

Radiographs are often useful in the diagnosis and assessment of dystocia. Although much information can be obtained by palpation, radiographs provide more definite data about the number, size, and, within limits, the viability of the retained fetuses. When many fetuses are present, however, the number is more difficult to determine. The dam's entire abdomen should be included on the radiograph because some fetuses may be located near the liver. Both the fetal vertebrae and skulls should be counted because it may be difficult to see other body structures. For example, the spinal columns and skulls can be counted as a total that is divided by 2. The dam's pelvis should be examined for evidence of prior fractures that

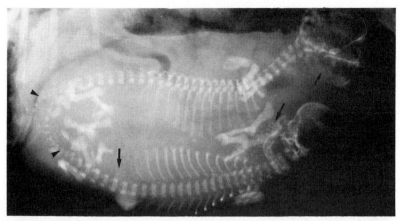

Fig 5b. Lateral radiograph of an 18-month-old Pekingese reveals 2 mature fetuses. Caudal vertebrae (arrowheads), metatarsal bones (large arrows), and teeth (small arrow) are visible. Phalanges were visible on the original radiograph, but not on this photograph.

could decrease the diameter of the pelvic canal. This assessment can also be made by digital palpation.

Pelvimetry as used in human medicine has little application in predicting dystocia in domestic animals. Geometric distortion of the pelvis results in erroneous assessment of birth canal size and the variation in size and shape of the pelvises and fetuses among animals makes it nearly impossible to calculate normal ratios. This is further complicated by such factors as molding of the fetal body and expansion of the pelvic canal during parturition.

Except for brachycephalic breeds, the skull of the dog and cat is small in relation to the rest of the body; therefore skull size has little relationship to dystocia. A very large fetus will occasionally be unable to pass through the birth canal of a bitch or queen. When dystocia occurs, radiographs can be obtained to determine if dystocia is due to fetal malposition (Fig 6).

Abnormal Pregnancy and Fetal Death

Early in pregnancy radiographs have little use in determining whether or not fetuses have died. During this stage of pregnancy, a normal uterus should continue to enlarge gradually. Gas in the uterus during pregnancy reflects breakdown of tissues. In late pregnancy when fetal structures are visible, there is more evidence that can be used to diagnose fetal death. For example, malalignment of cranial bones is commonly accepted as evidence of fetal death, especially when the bones overlap. It should be noted, however, that some mal-

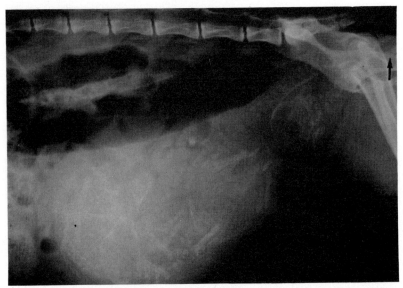

Fig 6. Dystocia in a 4-year-old queen. Forelimbs of fetus (arrows) are visible at vulva. Fetal head is turned backwards, obstructing birth canal. Such observations should be confirmed with lateral and VD radiographs.

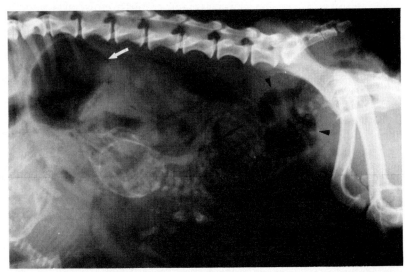

Fig 7a. Dystocia in 2-year-old Dachshund. Rear quarters of 1 of 2 fetuses are in pelvic canal. Gas in fetus's gastrointestinal tract (arrowheads), major vessels (small, black arrows), and around the diaphragm (large, black arrows) indicates fetal death. Large pocket of gas (white arrow) is likely in the uterus. Two dead fetuses were delivered after injection of oxytocin.

Fig 7b. Two-year-old Doberman reportedly bred 1 month previously. Bitch was depressed and had a thin, bloody discharge at the vulva. Three fetal skeletons can be seen. The radius, ulna, and tibia of 1 fetus can be seen (small arrows), indicating parturition is less than 2 weeks away. One fetus (white arrow) is hard to recognize because it is macerated. It is surrounded by a large pocket of gas that appears in contrast to the placenta (large, black arrow).

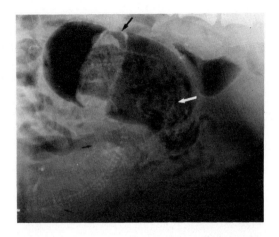

alignment can occur in the live fetus during labor if the fetal skull is within the pelvic canal.[10] The presence of gas in the heart, vessels, and subcutaneous tissues of the fetus and in the fetal membranes and uterus is more diagnostic of fetal death. Care must be taken, however, not to mistake gas in the gastrointestinal tract of the dam for gas in or around the fetus (Figs 7, 8).

Fig 8a. VD radiograph of 1-year-old queen bred 50 days previously. Sudden onset of vomiting and diarrhea preceded signs of shock. Five fetal skeletons can be seen and "uncomfortable" positions of some suggest that they have died. Gas pocket (arrow) caudal to stomach may be in uterus or transverse colon. (See 8b, lateral view.)

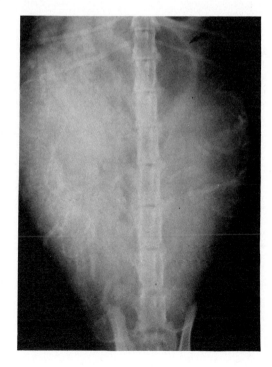

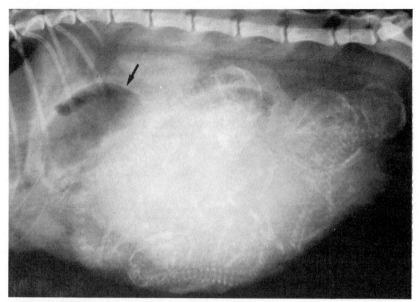

Fig 8b. Lateral view of animal in 8a. Gas pocket (arrow) caudal to stomach may be in uterus or transverse colon.)

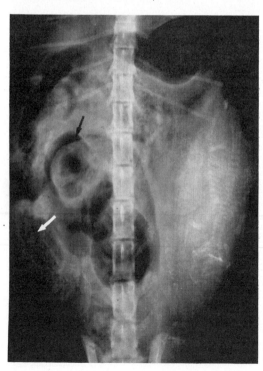

Fig 8c. Same cat as in Figs 8a,b taken after 3 days of supportive therapy. Gas in uterus (black arrow) surrounds fetus. Gas is in heart and vessels of a fetus (white arrow).

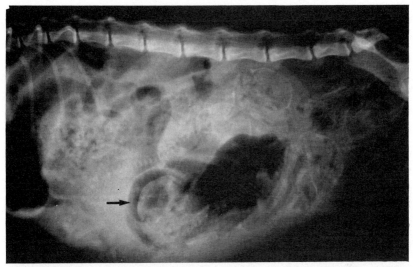

Fig 8d. Same cat as in Figs 8a-c, taken at same time as view 8c. Gas in uterus surrounds fetus. Radiographs of queen's thorax also revealed signs of pneumonia not present 3 days earlier.

An earlier though less reliable sign of fetal death is an abnormal posture of the fetus. Because of normal movement, viable fetuses will lie in a "comfortable" position. When muscle tone of a fetus is lost, it may assume an "uncomfortable" position and often be located in the ventral abdomen (Figs 9, 10). This has been referred to as fetal hyperflexion and the C-sign.[10,11] It may include hyperextension and other positional abnormalities of a fetus. Although positional abnormalities may be seen earlier than other signs, they can be interpreted incorrectly. Other procedures, such as ultrasonography, should be performed to obtain additional evidence.

Occasionally 1 or 2 fetal skeletons may be considerably less mineralized than the remainder of the litter. This may be an indication of fetal death if it is known that there was only one breeding (Fig 11).

Abnormal Nongravid Uterus

Pyometra and other conditions that cause enlargement of the uterus appear similar in radiographs. For this reason, the condition will be referred to as an enlarged uterus; this assumes that pregnancy has been ruled out. Identification of an enlarged uterus on survey radiographs has been discussed earlier. A greatly enlarged uterus may displace other organs from the caudal ventral abdomen.

All normal causes for uterine enlargement are linked with reproductive processes. If the patient's status in this regard is clear, one

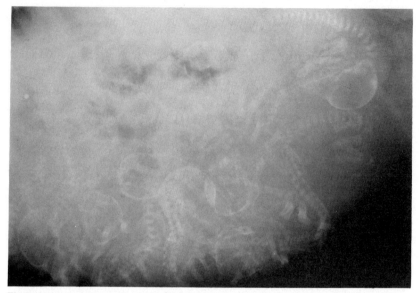

Fig 9. Lateral radiograph of a 7-year-old Setter with chronic renal disease. She was 1 week overdue, according to estimate, and had a thick discharge at the vulva. Eight full-term fetal skeletons are visible, gathered together in the ventral abdomen. A cesarean section was performed and 8 dead fetuses were found.

can assume that an enlarged uterus is abnormal. Enlargement of the uterus without distinct segmentation 25 to 30 days following estrus is most likely due to pyometra.[12]

Special Radiographic Procedures: When a survey radiograph reveals questionable density in the caudal abdomen, uterine enlarge-

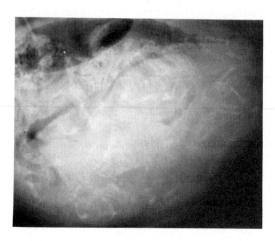

Fig 10. Lateral radiograph of a 3-year-old Persian queen that had started to labor 2 days previously and passed amniotic fluid. She was presented because of marked lethargy for 2 hours. Five fetal skeletons are gathered in the mid-ventral abdomen, suggesting that they are dead.

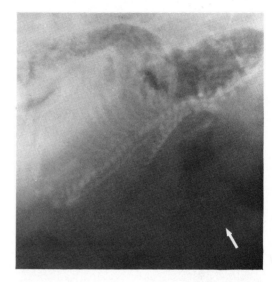

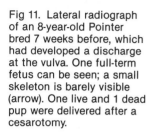

Fig 11. Lateral radiograph of an 8-year-old Pointer bred 7 weeks before, which had developed a discharge at the vulva. One full-term fetus can be seen; a small skeleton is barely visible (arrow). One live and 1 dead pup were delivered after a cesarotomy.

ment should be considered as a cause. When uterine or ovarian enlargement is suspected, the visibility of the abdominal organs can be enhanced by injecting gas into the abdomen.[13] Although air is used most commonly, either nitrous oxide or carbon dioxide is preferred because they are absorbed more readily. The technic for performing pneumoperitoneography has been described in detail.[3,13] The procedure involves aseptic injection of the gas just caudal and to the right of the umbilicus and distributing the gas by turning the animal. Dosages of 65 to 110 ml/kg have been recommended.[13] The abdomen should not be overfilled because respiration and circulation may be compromised. Smaller volumes of gas can be given if the animal's rear quarters are elevated to move the gas to the caudal abdomen, especially when the radiographs are obtained with a horizontal x-ray beam. In this position, all organs move cranially except the uterus, urinary bladder, and colon. Small lesions, including abnormalities of the uterine stump, may be identified with this technic (Fig 12).

When the technic just described is used in an obese animal, fat in the prepubic area will appear as soft tissue in contrast to the gas. This can lead to an erroneous diagnosis. Care must be taken to not restrict breathing for extended periods by keeping the animal in the inverted position. The exposure must be decreased by reducing either the milliamperage or exposure time by half.

If a uterine rupture is suspected, this lesion can be confirmed by injecting an organic iodide, such as sodium diatrizoate, into the uterus through a catheter. The dosage of contrast medium varies de-

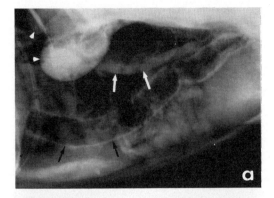

Fig 12a. Lateral pneumo-peritoneogram of a 1-year-old Poodle spayed 3 months previously. A puru-lent discharge persisted at the vulva for 2 months despite treatment. Kidneys (white arrowheads), colon (black arrows), and tubular soft-tissue structure (white arrows) are outlined by gas. Pelvic inlet is obscured.

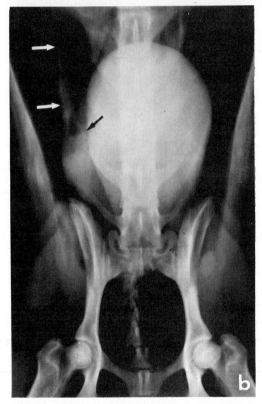

Fig 12b. VD radiograph of Poodle in 12a, obtained with her rear quarters ele-vated, and using a horizon-tal beam. A rounded, soft-tissue mass (black arrow) is on right side of bladder; it is continuous with a tubu-lar, soft-tissue structure (white arrows). Laparotomy revealed an abscess at the uterine stump and metritis of the right uterine horn, which had not been re-moved during original surgery.

pending on the size of the uterus; it is usually 3 to 15 ml. The presence of a rupture is disclosed if contrast medium is seen in the abdominal cavity.

If there is no radiographic evidence of a uterine abnormality and the uterus is not palpably enlarged when clinical signs indicate

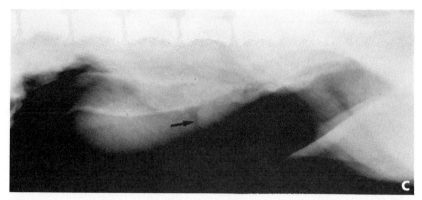

Fig 12c. Lateral view of same Poodle, also obtained with rear quarters elevated, and using a horizontal beam. Gas has concentrated in caudal abdomen, and small bowels are displaced cranially. Black arrow indicates soft-tissue mass referred to in Fig 12b.

uterine disease, a less frequently used diagnostic procedure (hystero-salpingography) can be performed. Abnormalities of the endometri-um, retained placenta, and uterine tube abnormalities have been diagnosed by performing this procedure. It involves injecting a small amount of organic iodide through the cervix into the uterine horns. Because the procedure is performed infrequently and produces vari-able results, more detailed descriptions of it should be studied before attempting this technic.[11,14,15]

Radiography of the Uterine Tubes, Ovaries, and Vagina

The uterine tubes and ovaries are not readily accessible for radio-graphic examination. Lesions located caudoventral to the kidney may be ovarian abscesses or neoplasms. Excretory urography may be per-formed to outline the kidneys when dealing with lesions suspected of being in an ovary.

Because the vagina can easily be palpated and examined endo-scopically, there is little need for radiographic evaluation of this struc-ture. Vaginography can be useful, however, when more direct methods of examination are limited due to the patient's size or the nature of the disease. The dosage of a contrast medium (air or an iodinated material) varies considerably because of the range in vaginal capacity. Enough medium (2 to 20 ml) should be used to dis-tend the vagina slightly. The vaginal infusion may be made by gravi-ty rather than syringe injection to reduce the risk of rupturing the

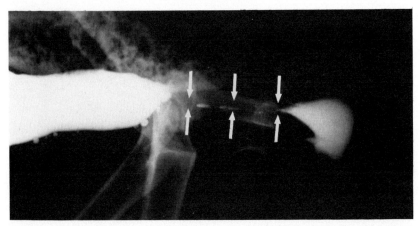

Fig 13. Lateral vaginogram of a 1-year-old bitch spayed 2 months earlier because of a vulvar discharge. Discharge persisted after surgery. Vaginoscopy revealed a soft-tissue mass obscuring entire vault. Oil-base contrast medium (20 ml) was injected through a fistula that joined the vagina. Filling defect (arrows) indicates that the mass is not amenable to surgery.

vagina. The vaginal injection should be made slowly and not forcibly. Likewise, if a balloon catheter is used, care should be taken to not overdistend the vagina. Following the injection of a contrast medium, radiographs are obtained to assist detection of vaginal fistulae, developmental anomalies, and masses (Fig 13).

Radiography of Male Reproductive Organs
Radiography has little application for evaluation of genital disease in male cats. Urethrography has been recommended, however, prior to performing surgery to relieve urinary obstructions. In the dog the prostate gland and urethra can be studied radiographically. They are seen best on lateral views, but a ventrodorsal view may add significant information. If material of mineral density is not present in the urethra, this structure will not be visible on survey radiographs. Use of a contrast medium will then be required to disclose the urethra.

Retained testes may appear on radiographs as abdominal masses if they become enlarged or neoplastic (Fig 14). The iliac lymph nodes and adjacent vertebrae and pelvis may become affected by neoplasms or infections of the male genitalia (Fig 15). When bony structures are involved secondarily, it has been my experience that neoplasia is the cause (Fig 16). Spinal lesions that are suggestive of discospondylitis should prompt an examination for *Brucella canis.*[11]

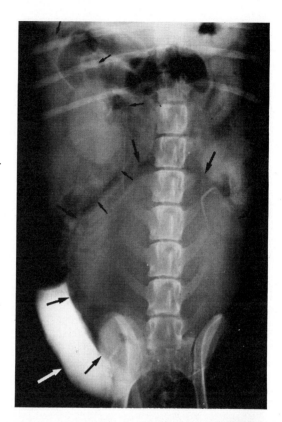

Figs 14a,b. VD and lateral excretory urograms of a 7-year-old Schnauzer presented for abdominal tenseness. Physical examination revealed a mass in the caudal abdomen and only 1 scrotal testis. Bladder (white arrow) is filled with contrast medium and displaced ventrally and to the right by large prostatic cyst (large black arrows). Slightly smaller mass (Sertoli-cell tumor) is in right cranial abdomen (small black arrows).

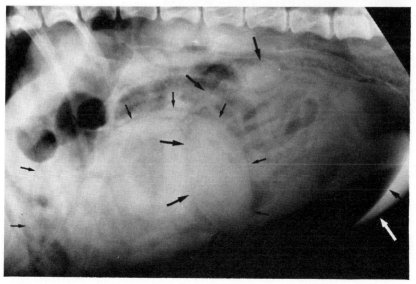

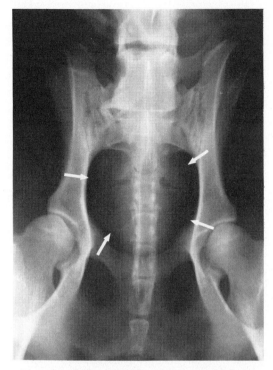

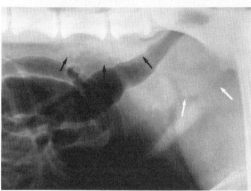

Figs 15a,b. VD and lateral radiographs of a 9-year-old Doberman with abdominal pain and enlarged prostate gland. Prostate (white arrows) is displacing bladder cranially. A soft-tissue density (black arrows) beneath 6th and 7th lumbar vertebrae contrasts with the fat around it.

Prostate Gland

The prostate gland of normal male dogs (up to 4 to 5 years old) is rarely visible on radiographs. It may be seen at the brim of the pubis when the bladder is full and appears as a small, rounded, soft-tissue mass that is partially hidden by the ilium. Minimal enlargement of the prostate gland has been attributed to normal aging, benign hy-

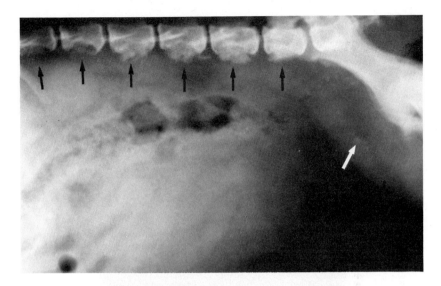

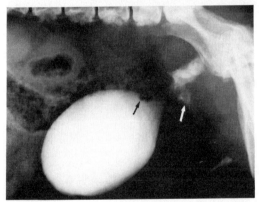

Figs 16a,b. Plain radiograph and urethrocystogram of Beagle with dysuria for 3 weeks and recent edema of prepuce and hindlimbs. On plain film, small mineral densities (white arrow) are present and bony irregularities are seen on the ventral surfaces of lumbar vertebrae (black arrows). Urethrocystogram reveals filling defect in bladder (black arrow) and contrast medium ventral to urethra, indicating extravasation of medium into cystic areas of prostate gland (white arrow). At necropsy a prostatic adenocarcinoma was found, that had metastasized widely.

pertrophy, and low-grade prostatitis.[11] Normal prostate glands of Scottish Terriers may be slightly larger than the prostate of most other dogs. If a smooth prostate is visible radiographically but is smaller than the widest diameter of the ilial wing, it should not be considered abnormal unless it is painful or otherwise abnormal.

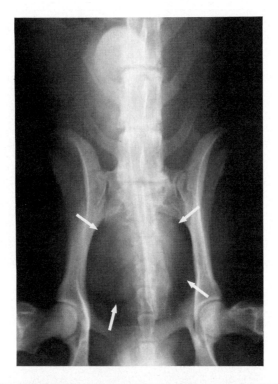

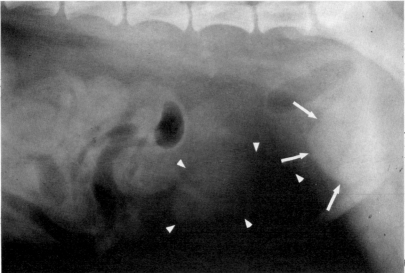

Figs 17a,b. VD and lateral radiographs of 6-year-old Sheltie with hematuria for 10 days. Prostate gland (arrows) is enlarged, smooth, and rounded, suggesting benign hypertrophy or hyperplasia. Bladder is displaced cranially (arrowheads).

Figs 18a,b. Plain radiograph and urethrocystogram of 6-year-old Pointer with abdominal pain and palpable mass in caudal abdomen. On plain film, 2 masses (arrows) with smooth rounded borders are seen in caudal abdomen. One of these is presumably the bladder. Small metallic densities are gunshot. On urethrocystogram, bladder (arrow) is displaced cranially. Urethra is shown passing through enlarged prostate gland, later found to be cystic and hyperplastic.

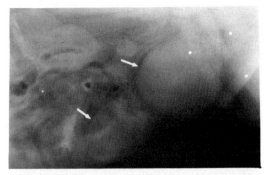

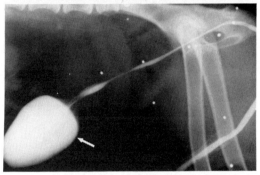

Prostatic enlargement may be due to hypertrophy, hyperplasia, inflammation, abscessation, or neoplasia. On survey radiographs, prostates that are hypertrophic and hyperplastic will usually be smooth, rounded, and symmetrical with relatively well-defined borders (Fig 17). Cystic hyperplasia, abscessation, and neoplasia may result in larger asymmetrical masses with well-defined borders (Fig 18). Inflammation and neoplasia may result in smooth, symmetrical enlargement with ill-defined borders due to the reaction of surround-

Fig 19. Radiograph of 11-year-old Pointer with dysuria and painful prostate gland. Prostate is within normal size range at pelvic brim (large arrow). Rectum (small arrows) is elevated by a mass beneath it, subsequently found to be inflamed prostate tissue.

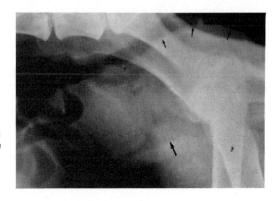

ing tissues (Fig 19). The tissue of a neoplastic prostate gland may blend into the density of the urinary bladder. An irregular periosteal reaction on the caudal lumbar vertebrae or pelvis is also characteristic of prostate neoplasia (Fig 16). Cysts also develop occasionally in neoplastic prostates.

Cystic hyperplasia or abscessation of the prostate gland may result in masses larger than a full bladder. Neoplastic prostates without cysts, however, will rarely become as large as a normal full bladder without causing urinary obstruction. It has also been reported that prostatic cysts and neoplasms result in larger masses than hypertrophy or inflammation of the prostate gland.[17]

Urethra

Urethral abnormalities that are visible on survey radiographs are limited to calculi and mineralization of the urethral wall. A fracture or osteomyelitis of the os penis is also apparent.

Contrast Radiography

Cystograms, prostatograms, and urethrograms involve the use of contrast medium to outline the cavities of the urinary bladder, prostate gland, and urethra. Because these procedures entail catheterization of a single orifice, they can be performed in combination. The order of their investigation varies depending on the area of major interest. If it can be assumed that the entire urethra is patent, some clinicians prefer to pass a catheter into the bladder and empty it. The bladder is then filled with contrast medium. This is followed by injection of the contrast medium into the prostatic urethra and then into the distal urethra. Other clinicians prefer to fill the distal urethra first and then to inject the medium into the prostatic urethra and finally the bladder. The most logical procedure may be to examine the area of primary interest first.

When performing a prostatogram, some clinicians prefer to have the bladder distended with liquid at the time that the contrast medium is injected. Though more contrast medium is likely to be forced into the prostatic orifices when the bladder is filled, the small amount of prostatic reflux is often insignificant.

If the urethra is obstructed, the injection should be made just distal to the obstruction. Because of the urethra's tendency to become spastic when exposed to foreign material, sites of narrowing, especially at the ischial arch, may erroneously be interpreted as obstructive lesions. For this reason, some clinicians inject a local anesthetic into the urethra before passing a catheter and injecting a contrast medium.

Cystography

A cystogram can be used to identify the extent of a prostatic enlargement and the shape of the prostate's cranial border as well as the extent of invasiveness of a prostatic mass. This procedure is useful in evaluating the size of the prostate gland when it is poorly visualized on survey radiographs and difficult to palpate, and when a mass is apparent but difficult to characterize. With larger masses of the prostate gland, the patency of the ureters should be evaluated by urography. Because the prostate gland is located in the retroperitoneal space, pneumoperitoneography is of limited value in examining it.

Encroachment of the prostate gland on the bladder can be identified by filling defects and irregularities in the caudal portion of the bladder wall (Fig 16). The bladder normally tapers to the prostatic urethra with no indentation.

To evaluate the condition of the prostate gland, a positive contrast medium, such as diluted organic iodide, is preferred to air. Any organic iodide medium that is used for IV urography will be satisfactory. To prevent obliteration of small defects as well as to decrease the possibility of subsequent inflammation, the contrast medium should be diluted to make a 5 to 10% concentration of iodine.[19] A soft, flexible catheter should be passed into the bladder. If desired, the tip of the catheter can be passed to the prostatic urethra to obtain a prostatogram at the same time. Better radiographs are obtained by making 2 separate injections because the exposure should be made during injection for the prostatogram and after the bladder is filled for the cystogram. The catheter should be large enough to nearly occlude the urethral lumen or have an inflatable cuff to prevent backflow of the contrast medium.

Prostatography

In this procedure, radiographs are obtained during injection of contrast medium into the prostatic urethra under pressure. The purpose is to disclose patent cavities or ducts connected to the urethra and to evaluate the size and shape of the prostatic urethra. Gross abnormalities, such as cysts and abscesses, are also revealed (Fig 20).

Opacification or filling of prostatic ducts has been reported as both normal and abnormal.[18,20,21] Because of the variations (amount of pressure and volume) in technic, the presence or absence of contrast medium in prostatic ducts and cysts alone has little significance. For example, cysts may be present but not revealed by the contrast

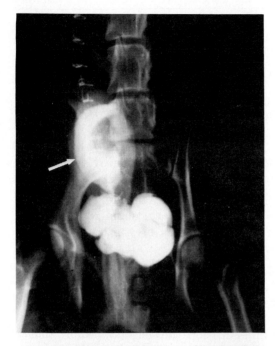

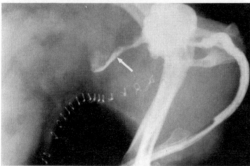

Figs 20a,b. VD and lateral urethrograms of 8-year-old Pekingese with dysuria and enlarged prostate gland. Metal sutures are from previous abdominal surgery. Contrast medium is filling cystic areas within prostate; bladder (arrow) is only partially filled with medium.

medium. When cysts are filled with contrast medium, their presence and patency are obvious (Fig 21).

The prostatic urethra is usually slightly wider than the remaining proximal urethra. It may have striated filling defects if not completely distended during the injection of contrast medium.[18] As narrowing of the prostatic urethra may reflect spasticity, stenosis should not be diagnosed until the narrowing has been demonstrated several times by repeated injections (Fig 22). Unusually large prostatic urethras are not indicative of disease. The prostatic urethra of older dogs tends to be larger than that of younger dogs. Neoplastic, cystic, and inflam-

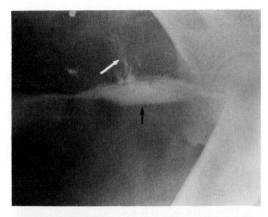

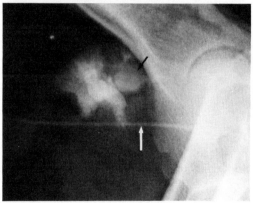

Figs 21a,b. Urethrogram of 6-year-old Doberman with chronic bloody discharge from urethra, and enlarged prostate gland. In Fig 21a the prostatic urethra (black arrow) and small prostatic ducts (white arrow) are filled with the medium. In Fig 21b contrast medium fills cystic area (black arrow) in prostate dorsal to catheter (white arrow).

matory lesions may occasionally cause narrowing of the prostatic urethra.

Urethrography

Urethrography is performed primarily to evaluate urinary disorders, especially following trauma and with dysuria. From the standpoint of reproduction, there are few conditions that warrant urethrography which do not also cause dysuria. Urethrography is an effective method for revealing urethral rupture or stricture.

The technic involves obtaining radiographs after injection of contrast medium into the distal urethra near the middle of the os penis. If a lesion is suspected but not confirmed, the catheter should be advanced to a point just distal to the suspected site and the injection repeated. The urethra may normally be narrower at the ischial arch or wider just caudal to the prostatic gland.

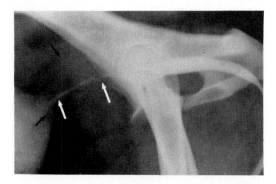

Fig 22. Urethrogram of 10-year-old Sheltie with dysuria, urine retention, and dribbling of urine. Urethra is filled with contrast medium, but prostatic urethra is narrowed (white arrows). Repeated urethrograms revealed urethral irregularity due to compression by an enlarged prostate gland (black arrows).

It is difficult to fill the urethra with contrast medium without having the medium leak from the urethral orifice. To control such leakage, the catheter used should be as large as possible. In addition, the penis and sheath can be compressed by tying gauze strips or umbilical tape around them or by carefully clamping them with tongue forceps. A more frequently used technic is to insert a cuffed catheter.[22] These catheters are very effective in preventing backflow of contrast medium, but they must be used carefully. If a urethral

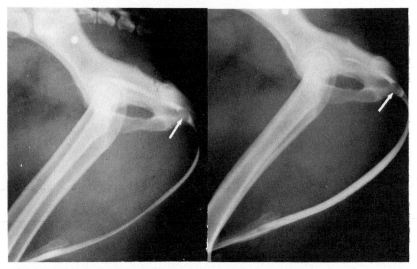

Figs 23a,b. Urethrograms of 5-year-old Dalmatian with history of urinary calculi. Dog was presented for severe dysuria. Catheter could be passed only to ischial arch. Filling defect in urethra is present at the ischial arch (arrow). Variation in urethral filling in the 2 films is due to differences in time and rate of contrast medium injection. Following use of local anesthetic and gentle pressure, a calculus was repelled into the bladder and then removed surgically.

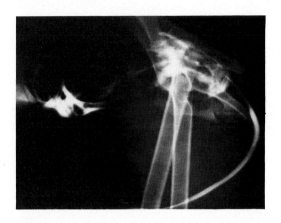

Fig 24. Urethrogram of 3-year-old mongrel recently hit by a car. Pelvic fractures were palpable, but the bladder was not. Contrast medium extravasated from pelvic urethra into surrounding tissues and abdominal cavity, revealing that the urethra was ruptured.

stricture or blockage does exist, an injection of fluid under pressure can result in rupture of the urethra.

Another potential hazard associated with use of a cuffed catheter in the urethra is damage to the urethral mucosa. Such damage can be caused by over-inflating the cuff or by leaving it inflated for an extended period. Despite the hazards associated with use of cuffed catheters in the urethra, they are useful and can be used to advantage if proper care is taken.

Sedation or general anesthesia of the patient is recommended when performing urethrography. Without sufficient sedation the animal may attempt to urinate when the contrast medium is injected. The subsequent urethral contractions can result in radiographic signs that are misinterpreted. To minimize urethrospasm, a topical anesthetic (2% lidocaine) may be injected into the urethra before injecting the contrast medium. The urethral catheter is filled with the anesthetic agent before catheterization and the remainder of the anesthetic is then injected into the urethra after inserting the catheter.[18] In this way, air is removed from the catheter and the presence of air bubbles in the radiographs is avoided.

To obtain a radiograph with the urethra dilated, the exposure is made as the last portion of medium is being injected. It is advisable to use slightly more contrast medium than is expected to fill the urethra (5 to 20 ml) because the urethra is open to the bladder.

As with other radiographic studies, repeating the procedure to confirm an observation is worthwhile (Fig 23). In some cases, however, the diagnosis is unmistakable and its confirmation is unnecessary (Fig 24). Although not widely used, lubricant gel (may contain an anesthetic) may be mixed with an equal amount of an organic iodide.[22]

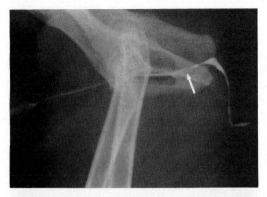

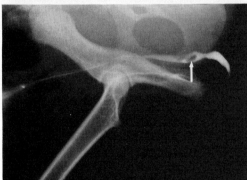

Figs 25a,b. Urethrograms of castrated male cat with urinary obstruction. Lateral view (25a) reveals slight irregularity in pelvic urethra (arrow). Oblique view (25b) reveals filling defect at that site (arrow).

When this is done, the contrast medium tends to remain in the urethra after injection and thus enables the radiographs to be obtained without the pressure of injection. Besides providing a more natural image of the urethra, the backflow around the catheter is decreased due to the viscosity of the mixture. Care is needed to remove air bubbles from the mixture of contrast medium and gel.

Prior to obtaining urethrograms, the patient should be placed in lateral recumbency with the hindlimbs pulled forward to obtain a survey radiograph. A urethral catheter is then inserted and the animal is put in the same position for urethrography. The injection of contrast medium should be made rather rapidly (within 3 seconds) but not forcibly. The x-ray exposure is made near the end of injection. If additional radiographs are to be obtained, the injection of contrast medium must be repeated except when using the mixture of gel-contrast medium.

Oblique ventrodorsal radiographs may be required to fully evaluate the urethra (Fig 25). Oblique views are useful for viewing the dorsal and ventral portions of the urethra separately because they are superimposed on ventrodorsal views.

References

1. O'Brien, T: In *Radiographic Diagnosis of Abdominal Disorders in the Dog and Cat,* pp 1-7. Covell Park Veterinary Company, Davis, CA, 1978.
2. Morgan, J: In *Techniques of Veterinary Radiology.* 3rd ed. Veterinary Radiology Associates, Davis, CA, 1982.
3. Ticer, J: In *Radiographic Technique in Small Animal Practice. pp 3-70.* WB Saunders, Philadelphia, 1975.
4. Kleine, L: In *Small Animal Radiography.* CV Mosby, St. Louis, 1983.
5. Carrig, C: JAVRS **17** (1976) 178.
6. Farrow, C: JAAHA **14** (1978) 337.
7. Concannon, P: JAVR **44:8** (1983) 1506.
8. Boyd, J: J Small Anim Pract **12** (1971) 501.
9. Rendano, V: In *Current Veterinary Therapy VIII,* pp 947-948. WB Saunders Co, Philadelphia, 1983.
10. Farrow, C: JAVRS **17** (1976) 11.
11. Bartels, J: In *Radiographic Diagnosis of Abdominal Disorders in the Dog and Cat. pp 615-660.* Covell Park Veterinary Co, Davis, CA, 1978.
12. Ackerman, N: In *Radiology of Urogenital Diseases in Dogs and Cats,* p 22. Venture Press, Davis, CA, 1983.
13. O'Brien, T: In *Radiographic Diagnosis of Abdominal Disorders in the Dog and Cat,* p 74. Covell Park Veterinary Company, Davis, CA, 1978.
14. Cobb, L: Vet Rec **71** (1959) 66.
15. Reid, J: JAAHA **9** (1973) 367.
16. Adams, W: JAVRS **19** (1978) 80.
17. Stone, E: JAAHA **14** (1978) 115.
18. Ticer, J: Vet Rad **21** (1980) 2.
19. Park, R: In *Radiographic Diagnosis of Abdominal Disorders in the Dog and Cat,* p 563. Covell Park Veterinary Company, Davis, CA, 1978.
20. Root, C: In *Radiographic Techniques in Small Animal Practice,* p 413. WB Saunders Co, Philadelphia, 1975.
21. Kealy, K: In *Diagnostic Radiology of the Dog and Cat,* p 125. WB Saunders, Philadelphia, 1979.
22. Johnson, G: In *Current Veterinary Therapy VI,* p 1189. WB Saunders, Philadelphia, 1977.

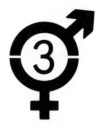

Artificial Control
of Reproduction

OVULATION INDUCTION IN CATS
BY EMERSON D. COLBY

Introduction

The induction of ovulation in the domestic cat is at best a refined experimental procedure. It should not be undertaken until the queen's complete breeding history is known. Ovulation has been induced by various methods in queens to arrest estrus for short periods and thus control fertility.

The cat is an induced ovulator and ovulates approximately 24 hours following coitus. The mediation under natural conditions is considered to be neurohumoral and is stimulated by vaginal and/or cervical stimulation. The spines of the male penis are not essential to the process, but they undoubtedly add significantly to the vaginal stimulation. The results of experimental denervation of both the vagina and cervix have supported the theory that only stimulation to the vaginal area will result in ovulation.

Ovulation Induction

Artificial induction of ovulation in the cat has been practiced for many years in studies of the effects of ovarian follicle maturation and of pseudopregnancy. A variety of methods can be used to stimulate the release of luteinizing hormone (LH) in addition to the use of hormones or hormone-releasing agents. Manipulating the vagina with a glass rod will induce LH release as will use of a medicine dropper to obtain material for a vaginal smear. Considerable attention has been given recently to the use of hormones to initiate ovulation. This interest has undoubtedly been prompted by the advent of the radioimmunoassay technic, which reliably measures the blood levels of hormones.

187

Use of Follicle-Stimulating Hormone (FSH)

Follicle-stimulating hormone has been used successfully to induce estrus in the domestic cat. Both FSH-P and PMSG can induce ovulation when given in sufficient dosages. FSH-P is made from porcine pituitary glands and it contains some LH. PMSG is made from the serum of pregnant mares and it contains more LH than FSH-P. The PMSG product used most commonly to induce estrus is marketed as an experimental compound known as Gestyl. It has a half-life of 26 hours and is found in the blood of pregnant mares between the 40th and 140th days of gestation.

Human chorionic gonadotropin (HCG) is secreted by the human placenta and is found in urine soon after conception. It is obtained from the urine of pregnant women. HCG is commonly used to induce ovulation in cats and is given prior to or immediately after mating. When used to induce ovulation following treatment with FSH-P, from 250 to 500 IU of HCG have been given IM. This has been reported to cause the ovulation of over 90% of mature follicles. The most commonly used product is called Pregnyl. I prefer to give this product at a dosage of 250 IU for 2 consecutive days.

Gonadotropin-releasing hormone (GnRH) is secreted in the hypothalamus and is currently available under the commercial name, Cystorelin (CEVA). Its most singular advantage is that it is not a foreign protein as are the other hormonal preparations and it causes the release of the endogenous pituitary LH. It is given IM in doses of $25\mu g$.[1]

Luteinizing hormone-releasing hormone (LHRH) has been used to stimulate the release of LH by queens in estrus. A dosage of $25\mu g$ given IM causes the release of enough endogenous LH to cause ovulation. It has been postulated that not only the level of serum LH but also its duration above baseline levels is a factor in the ovulation of domestic cats in estrus.[2]

Recent studies of ovulation in cats have revealed that a single mating may be insufficient to induce ovulation. This indicates that only occasionally does a queen have a single mating, ovulate, and carry a litter to term. When the serum levels of LH were monitored independently in 2 groups of queens, it was found that there is a direct relationship between the number of copulations and levels of LH, and subsequently the number of ovulated follicles.[3,4] The data indicate that 3 or more matings per day is the optimum for stimulating adequate release of LH and that repeated matings over a 4-hour period do not deplete pituitary LH. Peak levels of serum LH occurred 1 to 4 hours following uninhibited matings over a 4-hour period. LH is released in a surge and may persist at high levels for up to 12 hours. When there is no repeated breeding stimulation, LH returns rapidly to baseline values. Increased levels of LH produced by the administration of exogenous hormones last a much shorter time.[5]

For most efficient breeding in cats it appears that a minimum of 3 matings should be allowed daily until the queen refuses the male. This schedule should result in optimal release of LH and thus cause ovulation of all mature follicles.

In the absence of ovulation, subsequent estrous periods will occur approximately every 16 days with a mean duration of about 7 days. There is an interestrual interval of about 9 days.[6] The formation of the corpus luteum follows ovulation immediately and the CL reaches its maximum growth between 17 and 21 days. The normal size of a feline CL is approximately 0.3 cm.

References

1. Chakraborty, PK *et al:* Vet Clinics No Amer **12:1** (1981) 85.
2. Chakraborty, PK *et al:* Lab Anim Sci **29** (1979) 338.
3. Wildt, DE *et al:* Endocrin **107** (1980) 1212.
4. Concannon, P *et al:* Biol Reprod **23** (1980) 111.
5. Shille, VM and Stabenfeldt, GH: Adv Vet Sci Comp Med **24** (1980) 211.
6. Shille, VM *et al:* Biol Reprod **21** (1979) 953.

INDUCTION OF ESTRUS
BY P.K. CHAKRABORTY & S.W.J. SEAGER

Introduction
The development of systems for measuring blood hormone concentrations (radioimmunoassay) and of technics to observe ovarian activity sequentially (laparoscopy) have enabled a better understanding of factors influencing female reproduction. Such knowledge is an important prerequisite to development of methods to stimulate ovarian activity and reproductive behavior.

The female cat (queen) is an induced or reflex ovulator, meaning that ovulation occurs only after mating or a comparable stimulus.[1,2] The queen is polyestrous and her behavioral estrus occurs at 14- to 21-day intervals, but she may have periods of anestrus depending on the geographical location.[3-5] More recent observations indicate that the cat does not always ovulate following a single copulation and that the frequency of mating is important in regulating the release of luteinizing hormone (LH) and thus initiating the ovulatory process.[6,7]

The domestic bitch in contrast to the queen is a spontaneous ovulator. She usually attains sexual maturity between 6 and 12 months of age, and can show estrous activity during any season of the year.[4-8] Recent reports have documented the changes in blood hormone concentrations and the ovarian activity during the proestrous-estrous period. They attest to the critical role played by LH at the end of the proestrous period in initiating the ovulatory process.[9-11]

There is a great need by breeders and veterinarians to develop effective and predictable drug treatments to induce estrus and ovulation in dogs and cats. Methods for inducing estrus and ovulation are especially important when valuable bitches or queens fail to conceive following ovulation and have prolonged periods of sexual inactivity. These frustrating delays demonstrate the need for medical intervention.

There currently is no hormonal treatment that is always effective in inducing sexual behavior and ovulation in the cat and dog. There are a number of reasons for failure of gonadotropin treatments, but the primary ones are impure gonadotropins and variable endocrine function in the females at the time exogenous hormones are given. For example, pregnant mare serum gonadotropin (PMSG) has both follicle-stimulating hormone (FSH) and luteinizing hormone (LH) activity. Although both hormones are necessary for development of mature follicles, a PMSG preparation rather high in LH-like activity can cause early luteinization of follicles prior to demonstration of behavioral estrus. In addition, an animal may unknowingly receive repeated doses of an FSH-like preparation during the early follicular phase and become "hyperstimulated," often resulting in cystic follicles and prolonged estrous behavior.

Hormonal Preparations

The objective of giving hormones to induce reproductive function includes stimulation of both mating behavior and ovulation. Though administration of estrogens or related compounds can produce intense estrual activity, these hormones can inhibit ovarian function, including ovulation. For this reason, continued treatment with estrogens (except intermittent low doses as described subsequently for the bitch) is discouraged.

The ovulatory process in all mammalian species has 2 distinct components, the development and maturation of ovarian follicles and subsequent ovulation and formation of corpora lutea (CL). Formation and development of ovarian follicles are primarily under the stimulus of FSH released from the pituitary gland. The pituitary also regulates the ovulatory process by releasing LH during the late preovulatory stage of the estrous cycle. Estrous behavior and sexual receptivity are a direct consequence of increased follicular estrogens in the queen and a combined effect of estrogens and increasing levels of progesterone in the bitch.

Several hormonal preparations that are currently available can mimic the activities of endogenous FSH and LH and they have been utilized extensively for this purpose in many mammalian species. These hormonal compounds include porcine FSH (FSH-P), pregnant mare serum gonadotropin (PMSG), human chorionic gonadotropin (HCG), and gonadotropin-releasing hormone (GnRH).

Although any FSH preparation can be used, the major considerations in selecting a particular preparation are availability and quality. Currently the preparation that is widely available is a partially purified FSH fraction obtained from porcine pituitary glands (FSH-P, Burns Biotec, Oakland, California). Though most of the LH activity would have been eliminated from this product during its purification, we have observed that FSH-P can at times exert LH-like activity in both the cat and dog.

The very potent compound (PMSG) obtained from serum of pregnant mares has been used widely to successfully stimulate follicular activity in many species of animals. The most commonly available product is Gestyl (Organon, West Orange, New Jersey). The major problem associated with use of PMSG appears to be the considerable variation in potency from one commercial lot to another. PMSG is also a large molecule and has been suspected to cause an immunologic or refractory response to repeated injections. In addition, PMSG has an inherent LH-like activity and if given carelessly it can hyperstimulate the ovaries.

HCG isolated from the urine of pregnant women has been used routinely to induce ovulation, most often in combination with PMSG. When a suitable dose was used, this preparation has been very effective and safe. The major commercial compound is Pregnyl (Organon, West Orange, New Jersey).

Since its discovery, synthesis, and characterization, GnRH and several of its more potent synthetic analogs have proved to be highly effective in inducing ovulation in a variety of mammalian and non-mammalian species. This compound is currently available as Cystorelin (CEVA Laboratories, Overland Park, Kansas) GnRH has certain advantages over HCG in that it is not a foreign protein and thus is incapable of causing antibody production when used repeatedly. This compound acts primarily on the pituitary gland and induces ovulation through discharge of LH by the animal's own pituitary gland. It is also useful in identifying cases of pituitary dysfunction.

The results of some recent studies indicate that pulsatile infusion of anestrous bitches with 10 to 25 micrograms of GnRH every 2 to 4 hours for 7 days can induce a fertile estrous cycle. This can be accomplished by subcutaneous implantation of a small osmotic pump identified as Alzet (Alza Corporation, Palo Alto, California) that can be removed later.

Estrus and Ovulation Induction in the Cat

There are a few reports concerning the successful induction of estrus and ovulation in the queen. PMSG has been given in single and multiple injections and is quite effective in inducing estrus.[12,13] The feline ovary appears to be very sensitive to this hormone, however, and its use has been associated with formation of follicular cysts or premature luteinization of follicles. Routine use of PMSG is thus not recommended in the queen.

FSH-P is highly effective in stimulating follicle development and sexual behavior in the queen. Multiple injections are necessary. The most effective dosage has been 2 mg given daily IM until signs of estrus were observed. Because of the hyperstimulatory effects observed with prolonged use of this compound, it should not be given longer than 5 days, even in the absence of overt estrous behavior. If the queen does not display estrual activity within 7 days after the last FSH-P injection, the treatment can be repeated in 5 to 6 weeks.

Both HCG and GnRH will cause rupture of vesicular follicles that develop after natural estrus or FSH-P treatment. Neither compound is indicated when a queen in estrus is to be mated naturally. To ensure that ovulation occurs with natural mating, it is recommended that the queen be mated 2 to 3 times daily on 2 or 3 successive days beginning with the first day of behavioral estrus. When artificial insemination is the breeding method, ovulation must be induced by administering exogenous gonadotropin. The number of follicles ovulating has been shown to increase with the dose of HCG. At dosages of either 240 IU or 500 IU, HCG has caused ovulation of over 90% of all mature follicles. A dose of 250 IU of HCG given IM is recommended on the first 2 days of estrus. Although a single injection of 5 to 25 μg of GnRH increased serum LH levels in estrous queens, only the 25-μg dosage consistently caused ovulation.[14] Giving single or multiple injections of GnRH has not resulted in development of cystic follicles.

The 5-day administration of FSH-P followed by 2 days of HCG has resulted in viable ova. Pregnancies and viable offspring have occurred in queens stimulated by gonadotropin and naturally mated or artificially inseminated with fresh or frozen semen.[15]

Estrus and Ovulation Induction in the Bitch

Even when the bitch is not pregnant, the functional lifespan of her corpora lutea may sometimes last more than 3 months. Some bitches may not show any estrual activity for prolonged periods (10 months or longer), or they may fail to show signs of estrus following a pseudo-pregnancy. In certain breeds, estrus may occur only once a year.

It has been observed that a single injection of combined PMSG and HCG induced estrus in anestrous bitches within 2 to 6 days following the treatment.[16] Subsequent studies have either not confirmed the efficacy of this treatment or observed highly variable results. In more recent studies a variety of treatment regimens have utilized estrogens in low doses in addition to FSH-P, PMSG, and HCG.

Intramuscular injections of 250 to 500 IU of PMSG/daily for 10 days or 20 IU of PMSG/kg/day for 10 days combined with 500 IU of HCG on the 10th day induced estrous behavior and ovulation in 14 of 25 bitches.[17] None of these animals appeared to have any functional corpora lutea prior to initiation of the hormone treatment and the duration of proestrus appeared to be shorter than the length observed in natural cycles. In a more recent study, approximately 60% of a group of bitches ovulated (8/15) following either IM or SC injection of 44 IU of PMSG/kg/day for 9 days followed by injection of 500 IU of HCG on the 10th day.[18] The responding animals exhibited signs of estrus within 10 to 15 days after initiation of treatment, but only 50% of the ovulating animals displayed signs of estrual behavior. As in the previous study, none of the animals appeared to have functional corpora lutea prior to treatment and ovulation was confirmed by the collection of ova and determination of progesterone concentration.

Pretreatment with estrogens, either estrone or estradiol, has appeared to be helpful in inducing estrus, especially in bitches with elevated progesterone levels lasting longer than 60 to 90 days following the last estrous activity. Pretreatment with 100 to 300 mg of estrone per day for 5 to 6 days was effective in inducing vaginal bleeding in 100% of a small group of anestrous bitches. When treated subsequently with a combination of 200 to 400 IU of PMSG and 100 IU of HCG given IM once on the day that bleeding stopped and again on the day that estrus started, 86% of the animals (6/7) conceived and delivered an average litter of 4.2 pups following natural or artificial breeding.[19]

We have used various combinations of FSH-P, PMSG, HCG, and GnRH following pretreatment with either progesterone or estradiol. Our results indicate that, although progesterone pretreatment was

Table 1. Schedule for Induction of Estrus and Ovulation in the Dog and Cat

Species	Estrus induction	Ovulation induction	Schedule
Dog	PMSG; 20-50 iu/kg/day or 500-1000 iu PMSG/day, 2 treatments 6 days apart	1. HCG, 500-1000 iu/day on 1st and 2nd day of estrus. 2. GnRH, 2 treatments of 50 μg each, 6 hr apart on 1st day of estrus.	PMSG treatment given on kg/day basis, inject up to 9 days in succession
Cat	FSH-P, 2 mg/day until induction of estrous behavior	1. Mating 3-4 times. 2. HCG, 250 iu/day on 1st & 2nd day of estrus. 3. GnRH, 25 μg on 2nd day.	FSH-P treatment not to exceed 5 days

ineffective, administration of estradiol (200 mg/day given every other day for 3 doses) consistently induced a proestrous-like vaginal discharge 4 to 7 days later and persisted as long as 7 days. Estradiol pretreatment was especially effective in bitches that had greater than basal progesterone levels, indicating some degree of persisting luteal function. Daily injection (IM) of 5 mg of FSH-P did not appear to induce follicular development when monitored by periodic laparoscopic examinations. PMSG was more effective in inducing estrus, follicular development, and ovulation in the bitch. When 500 to 1000 IU of PMSG and 500 to 1000 IU of HCG were given IM simultaneously on the first day that vaginal bleeding stopped and again 6 days later, 80% of all treated animals displayed estrous behavior that lasted 5 to 9 days. Ovulation was confirmed in 60% of these animals either by a rise in serum progesterone concentration or pregnancy following artificial insemination. Both HCG and GnRH were equally effective in inducing ovulation of developed follicles.

Many dog breeders have been frustrated by breeding bitches that appear to cycle normally. Though examinations reveal nothing that would prevent them from getting pregnant, these animals remain barren after multiple breedings. Such bitches display signs of estrus at regular intervals, and mate naturally, but they do not conceive. A large proportion of these bitches may be exhibiting a disassociated estrus-ovulation syndrome. Normally, about 80% of bitches will start to ovulate within 1 to 2 days after behavioral estrus (standing heat). Some of them, however, can ovulate 2 or more days prior to the 1st day of standing heat, and therefore they may breed naturally but not conceive. These bitches can be identified by analyses of their reproductive hormones, especially LH and progesterone. Based on such analyses, the time for ovulation can be accurately estimated and the animals can be bred by artificial insemination with either fresh or frozen semen. Thus the sexual activity in these particular animals may not be a limiting factor in their reproductivity.

Various treatment regimens and schedule of treatments for inducing estrus and ovulation in the cat and dog have been summarized in Table 1.

Based on various available reports and our experience, several factors appear to be important in inducing estrus and ovulation in the anestrous bitch:

1. Presence or absence of functional corpora lutea. If a high progesterone level persists beyond 3 months following the last estrus, pretreatment with either estrone or estradiol is recommended.
2. Although based on preliminary data, giving gonadotropin IM appears to be more effective than its SC injection.
3. Use of PMSG is more effective than FSH-P. Depending on the size of the animals, giving 2 split doses of 500 to 1000 IU each of PMSG 6 days apart or 20 to 50 IU of PMSG/kg/day for 9 days appears to be equally effective in inducing follicular development and estrous behavior.
4. HCG (500 to 1000 IU/day given on 2 successive days) and GnRH (2 injections of 50 μg each given 6 hours apart) appear to be equally effective in causing ovulation.
5. The incidence of pregnancy is increased when bitches are either mated naturally or bred artificially once every other day up to 3 matings starting on the 1st day that the male is accepted.
6. Induction of fertile estrous cycle is more likely when natural breeding or artificial insemination occurs approximately 4 months or more following the last estrous cycle.

References

1. Greulich, WW: Anat Rec **58** (1934) 217.
2. Dawson, AB and Friedgood, HB: Anat Rec **76** (1940) 411.
3. Scott, PP: In *Reproduction and Breeding Techniques for Laboratory Animals.* p 206. Lea & Febiger, Philadelphia, 1970.
4. McDonald, LE: *Veterinary Endocrinology and Reproduction,* p 421. Lea & Febiger, Philadelphia, 1975.
5. Wildt, DE, Charman Guthrie, S, and Seager, SWJ: Horm Behav **10** (1978) 251.
6. Concannon, P, Hodgson, B, and Lein, D: Biol Reprod **23** (1980) 111.
7. Wildt, DE, Seager, SWJ and Chakraborty, PK: Endocrinol **107** (1980) 1212.
8. Stabenfeldt, GH and Shille, VM: In *Reproduction in Domestic Animals,* p 499. Academic Press, New York, 1977.

Dr. Paul Minnick

209 - 745 - 9688

Elk Grove

Source of PMSG

9. Concannon, PW, Hansel, W and Visek, WJ: Biol Reprod **13** (1975) 112.
10. Wildt, DE *et al:* Biol Reprod **20** (1979) 648.
11. Chakraborty, PK *et al:* Biol Reprod **22** (1980) 227.
12. Colby, ED: Lab Anim Care **20** (1970) 1075.
13. Wildt, DE *et al:* Lab Anim Sci **28** (1978) 301.
14. Chakraborty, PK *et al:* Lab Anim Sci **29** (1979) 338.
15. Platz, CC *et al:* J Reprod Fert **52** (1978) 279.
16. Scorgie, NJ: Vet Rec **51** (1939) 265.
17. Thun, R *et al:* Amer J Vet Res **38** (1977) 483.
18. Archbald, LF *et al:* VM/SAC, p 228, 1980.
19. Takeishi, M *et al:*Jap J Anim Reprod **22** (1976) 71.

USE OF PROGESTINS
BY JOHN D. RHOADES & GRANT H. TURNWALD

Progesterone is a steroid that has a core molecular structure similar to other steroid hormones, such as estrogens, testosterone, and corticosteroids.[1] The main source of progesterone in the dog and cat is the ovary, irrespective of pregnancy.[2,3] A large number of progestogenic hormones has been synthesized and progesterone is the most important one.[4]

Progestogens act on the estrogen-primed uterus of the bitch to stimulate endometrial growth and secretion, thus preparing the uterus for implantation of the fertilized ovum. This effect on the uterus can also be induced by administration of progestogens to the nonpregnant bitch.[5] The progestogens also suppress myometrial activity, decrease uterine contractility, and thus help to maintain pregnancy.[2] They also suppress pituitary secretion of gonadotrophins, and in turn delay estrus and prevent ovulation. This results in suppression of early signs of proestrus in the bitch. There is also a local anti-estrogenic effect independent of pituitary or hypothalamic function.[5]

Use of progesterone to delay or suppress estrus in the bitch was first reported in 1952.[6] Prior to this time its use was limited because of the short duration of action. A repositol preparation of the hormone became available at that time for use as an estrus-delaying agent. The use of progesterone to delay estrus in the bitch then became a common practice during the 1950's and 1960's.[7,8] Among the numerous progestogens used to suppress or delay estrus in the bitch and queen, the most frequently used by veterinarians in this country have been progesterone in oil, hydroxyprogesterone acetate, and medroxyprogesterone acetate.[4,5,9,10]

If progestogens are used improperly, they can cause serious side effects in the bitch and queen. Their long-term usage in oral or parenteral forms has predisposed animals to the endometrial hyperplasia-pyometra complex, mammary neoplasia, and other organic dysfunctions including diabetes mellitus.[4,10,12] Both short-term and long-term administration of progestogens may cause transient side effects, including increased appetite and weight gain, decrease in activity, mammary enlargement, and changes in temperament (generally less aggressive).[10] The effects of progesterone in the bitch are cumulative.[4]

Megestrol acetate (Ovaban) is the only progestogen currently approved in the US for suppression of estrus in the bitch. Megestrol has been used by European veterinarians for suppression of estrus since the mid-1960's. It has been available for use in the US since 1975.[11] It is a potent synthetic progestogen that is excreted mainly through the liver in the dog. It has a half-life of about 8 days.[11] Megestrol is currently recommended to interrupt the estrous cycle in proestrus and postpone the onset of proestrus.

To prevent estrus, megestrol should be given during the first 3 days of proestrus when vulvar swelling and sanguineous discharge occur.[10] It should be administered for 8 days at a rate of 2.2 mg/kg (1 mg/lb) of body weight (Fig 1). If treatment is started too early, there may be an early return of post-treatment estrus. If treatment is delayed beyond the 3rd day of proestrus, there is a marked decrease in its efficacy. Vulvar swelling and vaginal discharge will decrease by the 3rd or 4th day after treatment is started. If mating occurs during the first 3 days of treatment, administration of megestrol should be discontinued and a decision made in regard to treatment for mismating.[10,11] If mating occurs after 3 days of megestrol administration, the bitch will not conceive.[13] The regular course of treatment should be completed.[10] Onset of estrus varies (2 to 9 months) following administration of megestrol acetate during proestrus, but it usually occurs 4 to 6 weeks earlier than anticipated.[14,15] It has also been recommended that commencing on the first 3 days of proestrus, megestrol be administered at a dosage of 2.2 mg/kg for 4 days and then at a dosage of 0.55 mg/kg for 16 days.[15]

To postpone estrus, megestrol acetate should be given during late anestrus. Its administration should be started at least one week prior to onset of proestrus. The dosage to postpone estrus is 0.55 mg/kg (0.25 mg/lb) daily for 32 days.[10] For longer postponement of estrus after the 32 days of treatment it has been recommended that megestrol be given at a dosage of 0.1 to 0.2 mg/kg twice weekly for as long as 4 months. If this treatment is given, the bitch should be allowed to have a normal estrous cycle before further treatment with megestrol.[16] If the approximate date of the next estrus is unknown, vaginal cytology can be performed to predict its occurrence. When erythrocytes are seen in an atraumatically obtained vaginal smear, estrus is likely imminent and an attempt to postpone it would probably be ineffective. If therapy to postpone estrus is begun in late anestrus, the next estrus should occur within 5 to 6 months. When megestrol is given in early to mid-anestrus, it usually will not delay the next estrus.[16]

No problems in fertility, litter size, or sex ratios have been reported when megestrol has been used to suppress or postpone estrus in the bitch.[11,17] Because of its relatively short half-life and the short duration of treatment needed to produce its desired effects, megestrol acetate has proved to be safe for suppression or postponement of estrus in the bitch. It should not, however, be used in bitches with evidence of uterine disease or any other reproductive disorder.[13] Megestrol should not be used in bitches during their 1st estrus nor in bitches with mammary neoplasms.[13] It is likewise contraindicated for pregnant bitches and diabetic dogs. Megestrol should not be used to postpone estrus indefinitely and its use for more than 2 consecutive treatments should be avoided.[13,14]

Accurate assessment of the stage of the estrous cycle is especially important when megestrol acetate is being considered for administration during proestrus. An owner may not detect proestrus until 3 to 4 days after it has started. It may also be difficult for a veterinarian to assess the stage of proestrus by cytology.

Megestrol is not used widely in the US to control reproduction in dogs. It is used, however, to suppress estrus in hunting dogs and in dogs appearing in shows.[14]

Though megestrol is used to control estrus in the cat by European veterinarians, it is not currently approved for such use in the US. To postpone estrus in the queen, megestrol is given at a dosage of 2.5 mg per cat daily for as long as 18 months if the queen is in anestrus.[15] If the queen is in diestrus (between cycles within a breeding season), megestrol can be administered at a dosage of 2.5 mg per cat daily for as long as 60 days (Fig 1).[15] With either dosage schedule it is recommended that cats be allowed to have a normal estrus before further therapy is given.[15] More recent studies indicate that signs of estrus in queens can be controlled by giving 5 mg of megestrol daily for 3 days.[18] Following the initial 3 days, from 2.5 mg to 5 mg have been given to queens once weekly for 10 weeks to maintain anestrus. With this treatment the signs of estrus, such as vocalization, rolling, and seeking of males disappeared in 41% of the queens after the 3rd day.

Fig 1. Megestrol Acetate for Control of Reproduction in the Dog and Cat

Species	Indication	Commencement of Therapy	Daily Dose	Duration of Therapy	Contraindications
Canine	Estrus prevention	1st 3 days of proestrus	2.2 mg/kg	8 days	Reproductive disorders First estrus Mammary neoplasia Pregnancy >2 successive treatments Diabetes mellitus
	Estrus postponement	Anestrus >1 week prior to onset of estrus	0.55 mg/kg	32 days	As above
Feline*	Estrus postponement	Anestrus (between breeding seasons)	2.5 mg/cat	Up to 18 months	As above
		Diestrus (between cycles)	2.5 mg/cat	Up to 60 days	

*Megestrol acetate is not currently approved for the cat in the US.

After 7 days of treatment, there was no evidence of estrus in 92% of the queens.

The most common side effect of megestrol in queens has been increased weight.[10,18] Other side effects that occur less frequently include diarrhea, listlessness, change in urine odor, temperament change, mammary enlargement, change in hair color, and pyometra.[18] Mammary neoplasia and diabetes mellitus have also been associated with administration of megestrol in queens.[19,20] Return to normal estrous cycle by queens that have been treated with megestrol varies depending on the time of year and such factors as the number of daylight hours present when the drug is discontinued.[10] In one study, most of the queens remained in anestrus from 1 to 3 months.[18]

As in the dog, megestrol acetate should not be given to cats with mammary neoplasia, evidence of uterine disease or any other reproductive disorder, or diabetes mellitus.

References

1. Guyton, AC: *Textbook of Medical Physiology,* p 1005, 6th ed. WB Saunders Co, Philadelphia, 1981.
2. McDonald, LE: *Veterinary Endocrinology and Reproduction,* p 274, 3rd ed. Lea & Febiger, Philadelphia, 1980.
3. Stabenfeldt, GH and Shille, VM: *Reproduction in Domestic animals,* p 499, 3rd ed. Academic Press, NY, 1977.
4. Stabenfeldt, GH: JAVMA **164** (1974) 311.
5. Cox, JE: J Small Anim Pract **11** (1970) 759.
6. Murray, GH and Eden, EL: Vet Med **47** (1952) 467.
7. Borst, LM: Allied Vet **29** (1958) 27.
8. Burch, GR: Small Anim Clin **1** (1961) 149.
9. Sokolowski, JH *et al:* JAVMA **153** (1968) 425.
10. Burke, TJ: In *Current Veterinary Therapy VII,* p 1237. WB Saunders Co, Philadelphia, 1980.
11. Burke, TJ and Reynolds, HA: JAVMA **166** (1975) 285.
12. Weikel, JH *et al:* Toxic Appl Pharm **33** (1975) 414.
13. Q & A guide to use of Ovaban. Anim Heal Div, Schering Corp, Kenilworth, NJ, 1974.
14. Wildt, DE *et al:* JAAHA **13** (1977) 223.
15. Cited by Burke, TJ: Vet Clin No Amer **12** (1982) 79.
16. Burke, TJ: *Current Therapy in Theriogenology,* p 674. WB Saunders Co, Philadelphia, 1980.
17. Wildt, DE and Seager, SWJ: Vet Clin No Amer **7** (1977) 775.
18. Houdeshell, JW and Hennessey, PW: VM/SAC **72** (1977) 1013.
19. Oen, EO: Nord Vet Med **29** (1977) 287.
20. Hutchinson, JA: Canad Vet J **19** (1978) 324.

ANDROGENS FOR CONTROL OF REPRODUCTION
BY JAMES H. SOKOLOWSKI & THOMAS J. BURKE

Introduction

Many compounds have been tested for their antiestrual effects in the dog and cat (Table 1).[1,2] Safety evaluations of medroxyprogesterone acetate, melengestrol acetate,[3,4] and megestrol acetate[5] have been reported.

When drugs are considered for control of reproduction in pets, it should be remembered that they usually are used to suit the owner's convenience. Veterinarians should discuss the various methods of birth control that are available and help to select a method that meets the client's needs and causes the fewest undesirable side effects in the pet.

Effects of Androgens

Of the compounds used to alter reproductive function in the dog and cat, the androgenic steroids apparently have the fewest life-endangering effects.[6] Testosterone and some of its analogs alter anatomic development of genetic females and prevent estrous activity in the dog. Additional effects that have been reported include hypercalcemia, masculinization of female fetuses, sodium retention,

Table 1. Drugs Used to Control Reproduction in the Dog & Cat

Progestogens	Miscellaneous
Progesterone	Ethamoxytriphetol
Repository progesterone	Malucidin
Hydroxyprogesterone acetate	
Medroxyprogesterone acetate	
Megestrol acetate	
Melengestrol acetate	**Estrogens**
Delmadinone	Diethylstilbestrol
Chlormadinone	Ethynylestradiol
Norethisterone acetate	Estradiolcypionate
Methylestrenolone	
Prostaglandins	**Androgens**
$F_1\alpha$	Testosterone
$F_2\alpha$	Testosterone propionate
E_1	Stanozolol
E_2	Mibolerone

gynecomastia, liver dysfunction, priapism, decreased ejaculation volume, and gonadotropin inhibition. Though testosterone has been used frequently for this purpose, especially in racing Greyhounds, failure to return to normal estrous cyclicity and to regain fertility after cessation of therapy is common.

Of the androgenic steroids, only mibolerone has been studied in any detail in the dog.[6] Only a limited amount of information is available for the cat.[6,11]

Mibolerone Studies

Early studies of mibolerone in dogs and rodents revealed that this compound had androgenic, anabolic, and antigonadotropic activity, but had no progestational or estrogenic activity.[7] Compared to methyltestosterone in rats, mibolerone was 41 times more potent as an anabolic agent and 16 times more potent as an androgen.[7] Studies of mibolerone's safety revealed that the oral LD50 dose was greater than 1,600,000 mcg/kg in the mouse. The oral LD50 dose in dogs apparently exceeded 30,000 mcg/kg.[6]

When mibolerone was administered orally to adult male and female Beagles at dosages as high as 10,000 times the projected daily dose for 28 days, there was a reduction of stainable lipid in the adrenal cortices, enlargement of the clitoris, thickening of the myometrium, and inhibition of spermatogenesis. All of the treated dogs had periodic episodes of excessive lacrimation. There also appeared to be a drug-related increase in renal, uterine, and prostatic weights and a decrease in ovarian, testicular, and thymic weights.[6]

In another study of mibolerone, male and female Beagles were used to evaluate the influence of the host's maturity, duration of treatment, sex and dosage.[8] The immature animals in this study were 6 to 7 months old and had not been in estrus; the mature animals had had an estrus (maximum of 2 primiparous or multiparous bitches per group). The immature males were 6 months of age at the start of the study, and the mature males were more than 10 months old. During the 2 years of this study the animals were monitored periodically by physical examinations, blood cell counts, blood chemical evaluations, bone marrow biopsies, urinalyses, and direct inspection of tissues after laparotomy. Semen was collected on the last day of treatment. The time needed to ejaculate, and the percentage of live sperm were assessed.

In the study referred to above, mibolerone blocked tertiary but not primary and secondary development of follicles. It caused an enlargement of the clitoris and maintenance of prepuberal ovarian and uterine-cervix weights in the immature animals. Weight of the kidneys was increased slightly, but there was no evidence of altered morphology or function. Prostatic weights were decreased in immature males given the highest dose. Protein-bound iodine levels were decreased without morphologic or functional changes of the thyroid. There was also a significant decrease (not dose-related) in serum cholesterol levels in both immature and mature females and males.

In the same study described above, the treated animals had a slight increase in mean SGOT levels. The SGPT levels were statistically (P <.05) higher in mature females receiving the highest daily dose, but there was no histologic evidence of hepatic necrosis. It was postulated that the mibolerone caused a change in the permeability of the hepatocellular membrane that enabled release of the enzymes into plasma. Peculiar eosinophilic, crystalline, intranuclear inclusions were observed in the hepatocytes.[9] These bodies appeared to be protein in nature, as determined by electron microscopy. They did not disrupt the hepatocytes.[9]

Histologic examination of testicular and epididymal tissues along with microscopic examination of semen revealed that spermatogenesis was not affected by the mibolerone. Fertility was not evaluated. Following cessation of mibolerone administration, estrous cycles recurred rapidly. The average period from the last treatment to recurrence of estrus was 70 to 90 days. Reduced reproductivity was subsequently observed to occur primarily in the immature bitches given mibolerone.

In another study, adult bitches were treated with mibolerone starting 1, 3, or 6 days after the first of 2 breedings.[10] They were treated daily until their puppies were weaned (42 days old). Conception and implantation were not prevented in these bitches. The length of gestation for all 3 groups was within the limits (59 to 67 days) observed for all bitches in the colony. Similar numbers of puppies were delivered in the 3 groups, except for the bitches that were given 60 mcg mibolerone daily starting on the first day after breeding. Though this group of bitches weaned the fewest puppies, the differences were not statistically significant.

Masculinization has been observed in female puppies whelped by dams treated with mibolerone starting shortly after breeding. Gross masculinization in female pups was reflected by an increase in anogenital distance. Examination of the reproductive tract revealed marked anatomical alterations. No gross effects were observed in male progeny.

Bitches from 13 breeds (German Shepherd, Basset Hound, Boston Terrier, Cocker Spaniel, Pekingese, Miniature Poodle, Toy Poodle, Collie, Dachshund, Brittany Spaniel, Labrador Retriever, Scottish Terrier, and Beagle) were used in a long-term study of mibolerone's efficacy and safety.[5] Drug-related effects that were observed over a period of 6 years included enlargement of the clitoris (not objectionable in over 98% of the bitches), slight vaginal discharge, a statistically significant decrease in cholesterol levels, and a statistically significant increase in SGPT (alanine transaminase) level. The gross side effects in this study were similar to those reported previously. Statistical evaluation of serum chemistry results revealed that the only consistent effect was a decrease in the cholesterol level.

Implications of Side Effects

Because cholesterol biosynthesis and catabolism is a primary hepatic function and secondary in other organs, the mibolerone-induced hypocholesterolemia is of special interest. Possible causes of this statistically significant (P <.05) decrease in serum cholesterol include hyperthyroidism, extensive damage of hepatic parenchyma, and acute hepatic cirrhosis. It seems most likely that the persistent hypocholesterolemia in mibolerone-treated bitches is due to a direct androgenic-anabolic effect of mibolerone on liver metabolism rather than alterations in thyroid or hepatic function. This opinion is supported by previous studies in which decreases in protein-bound iodine were not accompanied by hypercholesterolemia as would have been expected if the bitches had clinical hypothyroidism.[6]

It was observed that SGPT levels increased significantly (P <.05) in all breeds studied at some time periods. Because elevations of this enzyme are generally considered to reflect hepatic necrosis primarily, the necrosis should have been detectable histologically and it should have resulted in alterations in other hepatic functions. It was concluded that elevations of SGPT are due to slight alterations in the permeability of the hepatocellular membrane. Another anabolic steroid, 19-nortestosterone homofarnesate, did not induce morphologic changes in the kidneys and liver.

Though alterations in blood cell counts have been associated with the use of steroids, consistent hematologic changes have not been observed in bitches receiving mibolerone.

Changes in body weight associated with administration of androgens have been attributed to either a positive increase in nitrogen retention or an increased retention of fluids. Increase in body weight was not observed, however, among the bitches in the studies of mibolerone. This suggests that estrus-preventive doses of mibolerone are either not anabolic or that these effects are not observed in the dog.

It is evident from the tests reported that mibolerone is biologically active and is effective in preventing estrous activity in dogs at very low doses. The apparent effects of mibolerone on bitches are consistent with the effects of other androgens in this species.

References
1. Sokolowski, JH: Friskies Research Dog, Summer, pp 1-3, 13-15, 1974.
2. Sokolowski, JH and Zimbelman, RG: AJVR **37** (1976) 939.
3. Zimbelman, RG: Symposium on Cheque, 1978.
4. Sokolowski, JH and Van Ravenswaay, F: Canine Practice **5** (1978) 53.
5. Burke, TJ and Reynolds, HA Jr: JAVMA **167** (1975) 285
6. Sokolowski, JH: Symposium on Cheque, 1978.
7. Lyster, SC and Duncan, GW: Acta Endocrinol **43** (1963) 399.
8. Sokolowski, JH and Geng, S: AJVR **38** (1977) 1371.
9. Johnston, RL and Goyings, LS: Symposium on Cheque, 1978.
10. Sokolowski, JH and Kasson, CW: AJVR **39** (1978) 837.
11. Burke, TJ, Reynolds, HA Jr, and Sokolowski, JH: AJVR **38** (1977) 469.

ARTIFICIAL INSEMINATION IN CATS
BY NICKOLAS J. SOJKA

The materials and methodology for artificial insemination (AI) of cats have changed little since the technic was first reported in 1970.[1] Either frozen extended semen, whole semen, or saline-extended fresh semen (0.1 to 0.2 ml) is deposited in the cranial vagina or caudal cervix with a 0.25-ml syringe and a 20-gauge needle with silver solder or polyethylene tubing at the tip (Fig 1). Impregnation has been achieved with fresh, whole, and extended semen that contained from 5 x 10^6 to 3 x 10^8 spermatozoa/dose. Concentrations of 50 to 100 x 10^6 motile spermatozoa/dose are recommended for previously frozen semen. Queens to be inseminated artificially may be immobilized with 6 mg/kg of ketamine hydrochloride if care is taken to keep the queen's hindquarters elevated for 20 minutes following deposition of semen to allow it to pool at the cervical os.[2]

Artificial insemination of queens has rarely been as successful as natural breeding in conception rate or litter size. This difference may

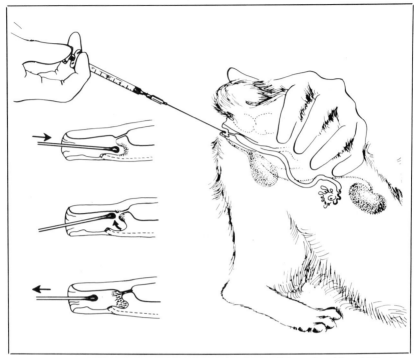

Fig 1. Semen is deposited in the cranial vagina or caudal cervix with a 0.25-ml syringe and a 20-gauge needle with silver solder or polyethylene tubing at the tip.
Closeup shows direction of movement of the needle.

be due, however, to the fact that virgin queens were used in the
original research of AI and their capacity for reproduction is less than
that of multiparous queens.

The breeding behavior of cats and the associated hormonal
physiology are described in Chapter 1, but some repetition is indicated relevant to the use of AI in cats. As with natural breeding, AI
should be performed only when the queen is exhibiting all the signs of
estrus. Selecting the specific day for insemination during estrus is
less important than the extent of sexual stimulation. Because multiple breedings have been demonstrated to be more successful than single breedings, it is reasonable that 2 inseminations be made. Each insemination should be followed by cervical stimulation with either a
smooth glass rod or the insemination needle or tube. This is done to
elicit the necessary reflex of the vagina and accompanying ovulation.
In lieu of stimulation, ovulation is generally ensured by IV or IM injection of 50 IU human chorionic gonadotropin (HCG). The induction
of ovulation in the cat appears to be an all-or-none phenomenon and

requires sufficient vaginal stimulation to cause a large sustained release of luteinizing hormone (LH) from the pituitary to assure the required effect on the ovary.[3,4]

If facilities for hormonal quantitation are available, changes in serum LH levels from pre-insemination concentrations to post-insemination (up to 8 hours after initial AI) should be measured. An increase of 20- to 200-fold should result in pregnancy between fertile animals or pseudopregnancy if either the queen or tom is infertile.[3] Failure of at least pseudopregnancy after a significant rise in serum LH levels would indicate an ovarian or uterine cause of the infertility.

Technics for increasing the probability of ovulation by using exogenous hormones are described in Chapter 1. Their effects on the future reproductive capacity of a queen are unknown. It may be advisable, however, to restrict their use to occasions in which other methods to induce ovulation have failed.

References

1. Sojka, NJ et al: Lab Anim Sci **20** (1970) 198.
2. Platz, CC et al: J Reprod Fert **52** (1978) 279.
3. Concannon, P et al: Biol Reprod **23** (1980) 111.
4. Wildt, DE et al: Endocrinol **107** (1980) 1212.

ARTIFICIAL INSEMINATION IN DOGS
BY STEPHEN W.J. SEAGAR

Introduction

With the increase of purebred dog breeding and the increased sophistication of dog breeders, reproductive failure in both the male and female dog has become a focus of attention. Veterinarians are routinely asked to collect semen for fertility evaluation, and for artificial insemination (AI). Semen is evaluated for AKC certification of the fertility of male dogs over 12 years of age, fertility assessment prior to a stud dog's sale, or to diagnose suspected infertility. During the past 15 years, we have collected and evaluated more than 11,000 ejaculates from more than 100 species of purebred dogs, and many crossbred varieties. In the majority of cases the semen was either artificially inseminated directly or frozen and maintained in liquid nitrogen for subsequent insemination.

To collect and evaluate semen and to perform AI successfully, veterinary practitioners should have the required equipment, become experienced with the procedures, and allot sufficient time for performing the procedures.

Equipment and Procedure

The equipment needed for semen collection and evaluation includes an artificial vagina (latex rubber cone), plastic graduated centrifuge tubes, a small temperature-controlled incubator and/or slide warmer (preferably both), disposable laboratory supplies (pipettes, microscope slides, cover slips, examination gloves) a binocular microscope with a mechanical stage (preferably with phase contrast) with low and high power and oil immersion lenses, a hemacytometer, spectrophotometer, or cell counter, suitable stains and reagents to examine sperm morphology.

A specific appointment should be made for collection and evaluation of semen. The dog should not be used for breeding for at least 4 days prior to examination. If the dog has not been used regularly as a stud, as many as 3 collections and examinations may be required for a reliable assessment of the semen.

A veterinary hospital is usually a strange and even hostile environment for a male dog, and this may affect the quality of his semen. When collection of semen is especially difficult, the veterinarian may decide to perform the procedure at the breeder's home. In such case the required equipment for immediate examination of the collected semen is also transported. Only one collection in the dog's usual environment may be needed to gain his confidence. Semen can be collected satisfactorily from most dogs at the veterinary hospital. It is impossible, however, to collect an adequate semen sample without the dog's cooperation. Therefore, time spent in making the animal feel relaxed and familiar with the veterinarian is time well-spent.

Preliminary Examination

When a dog is presented for semen evaluation, his exterior genitalia should first be examined. After examination gloves are put on, the dog is approached and reassured by voice and gestures. He should be restrained on a leash by the owner or an assistant. After patting and stroking the animal, the testes are palpated gently and assessed for smoothness, mobility, size, and firmness. The owner should be asked whether there has been any noticeable decrease or thickening of the dog's scrotal skin or any other change in the appearance of the scrotum.

After the testes have been examined, the penis should be felt within the sheath and a note made concerning the amount of exudate at the preputial orifice. The dog's penis is then gently slid from the sheath and inspected for color, adhesions, injuries, scars, or spotting on the surface. The owner should be asked about the dog's urination habits and whether or not they have changed recently.

Semen Collection

Prior to attempting collection of semen, the veterinarian should make certain that all needed equipment is at hand. This includes checking the microscope and accessory equipment used for the initial examination. The examiner should also have established measures to prevent any interruption of the examination. When collecting semen for evaluation, the dog's owner is asked to also bring, if possible, a bitch that is in heat. This greatly facilitates semen collection. Though it is not necessary to have a bitch of the same breed, one of similar size is preferred.

If it is not possible to have a bitch in heat present, the veterinarian should have a supply of Q-tip teasers. These are made by inserting a cotton-tipped applicator that has previously been moistened in saline solution into the vagina of a bitch in estrus. The cotton tip is rolled gently against the vaginal wall and removed. The Q-tip is then wrapped in Saran Wrap and stored in a plastic container kept in a freezer. The teasers are thawed for 15 minutes prior to use. Bitches used for their preparation should have a negative test for *Brucella canis*.

Many examination rooms in veterinary hospitals are relatively slippery and it is important in semen collection that both the dog and bitch have secure footing. Most studs will not have adequate pelvic thrusts unless they have secure footing. This is especially true for older dogs. To provide secure footing, we use a rubber-bottom mat that is about 6 feet long. Such a mat can also be used to facilitate natural breeding.

After the mat is rolled out, the bitch is led to it and restrained by the handler. The handler should stand on the bitch's right side and if there is any indication that the bitch may bite, she should be muzzled. The handler should restrain the bitch's head and while kneeling insert his hand under the bitch's chest to keep her standing. The handler's supporting arm should not be at right angles to the bitch, but at a more longitudinal angle. Otherwise, the male may hit the handler's arm as he mounts and cause him to dismount.

The male dog is then brought into the room on a short leash. He should not be allowed to urinate after he enters the room because this will usually result in the presence of urine in the ejaculate. If the dog does urinate after entering the room, his urethra should be stripped of urine. If the bitch being used as a teaser is not in estrus, a thawed Q-tip "teaser" is placed in front of the male's nose as he is led toward the bitch. The teaser is discarded after the dog's penis becomes erect and pelvic thrusts are being made.

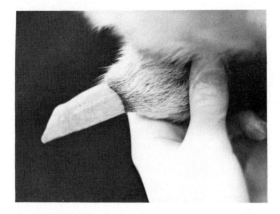

Fig 1. The dog's penis is stimulated through the preputial sheath with digital manipulation and massage.

The artificial vagina is kept in the examiner's pocket prior to its use to keep it near body temperature. The dog's penis is massaged digitally through the preputial sheath (Fig 1) and when the penis is approximately 40 to 50% erect, the preputial sheath is slipped behind the bulbus glandis. If the dog's penis is allowed to enlarge more than this, it will be difficult to slip the preputial sheath behind the bulbus glandis. If this should happen, the dog should be taken away from the bitch for a few minutes until his penis is less swollen. The stud is then returned to the bitch and his preputial sheath is pushed back over the bulbus glandis before the penis is more than 50% erect. This procedure is especially important in a young dog that can become excited quickly and have a preputial sheath orifice that has not reached its maximum size.

After the dog's erect penis is exposed, the artificial vagina is slipped on and up over the bulbus glandis (Fig 2). The examiner should

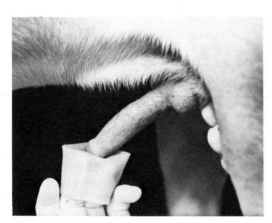

Fig 2. Once the erect penis has been exteriorized, the artificial vagina is slipped on and up over the bulbus glandis.

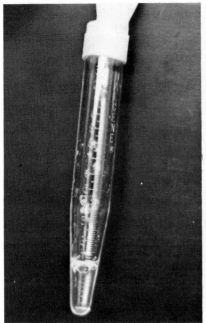 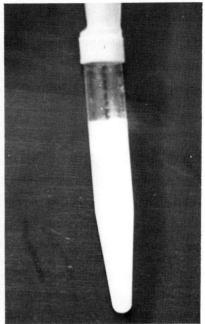

Fig 3. The first ejaculate fraction should be clear, 1-2 mls in a medium-sized dog.

Fig 4. The second ejaculate fraction appears milky, indicating the presence of sperm.

prevent the presence of hair between the dog's penis and the artificial vagina. A hand is then placed between the dog's hindlimbs and the bulbus glandis is encircled through the artificial vagina. A "tie" is then simulated by exerting gentle but firm downward pressure with the encircling fingers. The examiner's other hand is used to hold the centrifuge tube for semen collection. The semen should be inspected as it is ejaculated. The 1st portion (1 to 2 ml in a 25 to 30 lb dog) should be clear (Fig 3). The 2nd portion (1 to 3 ml) is rich in spermatozoa (Fig 4) and the 3rd portion is 2 to 4 ml. The dog's ejaculatory pattern should be noted because it should be consistent in the future.

After 1 to 2 ml of the 3rd portion of an ejaculate have been collected, the artificial vagina is removed gently from the dog's penis. At this time the dog's penis is greatly enlarged and its superficial vessels can easily be damaged, resulting in pain, infection, and subsequent lack of libido.

Following collection of semen the male dog is kept in the examination room. If his swollen penis does not start to become smaller and less erect within 5 minutes, the dog should be walked slowly. This exercise usually results in return of the penis into the sheath. If it does not, the penis should be massaged gently with cotton and tepid water. If the erection persists, the dog's penis should be immersed in ice water. This becomes especially important for dogs with an unusually large penis for their body size. Such dogs are often Bulldogs, Basset Hounds, Afghans, and other hounds. A stud dog should never be put in a cage or in a confined area with other dogs when his penis is still erect.

Evaluation of Semen

The tube of semen should be placed in a test-tube rack and its open end should be covered with parafilm. A warmed Pasteur pipette is used to obtain a representative drop of the semen and place it on a warmed glass slide. The drop is then covered with a warmed cover slip and examined promptly for sperm motility. At a minimum 80 to 85% of the sperm should be motile and have a progression speed of 5 (the speed of progression is based on a scale of 0 to 5). At a rate of 0 the sperm are motionless; at a rate of 5 they move rapidly across the microscope stage. This initial observation of sperm motility should be recorded.

The volume, pH, and color of the semen are noted next and recorded along with ejaculation time and evidence of libido. Semen of good quality is milky in color. A yellow color reflects the presence of urine. A red or brown color may reflect the presence of fresh or hemolyzed blood. In such cases the cause should be investigated.

To inspect the morphology of sperm cells an eosin-nigrosin stain is useful. This stain is prepared by adding 1 gram of eosin and 5 grams of nigrosin to a 3% solution of sodium citrate dihydrate. This mixture remains stable for a year.

If the ejaculate is to be inseminated, this should be done promptly after the initial examination. A bitch should never be inseminated, however, without examining the semen under a microscope. If this is not done, a bitch may be inseminated with immobile sperm and thus be legally bred to the infertile stud.

Sperm Abnormalities

Primary Abnormalities: Primary abnormalities (Fig 5) are considered to reflect disturbances of spermatogenesis. The different forms include:

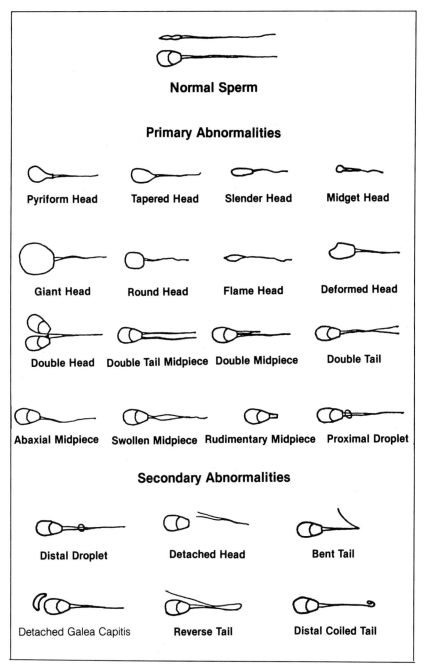

Fig 5. Sperm morphology. (Adapted from Van Camp in *Medical Nursing for Animal Health Technicians,* American Veterinary Publications, Santa Barbara, 1985.)

Head abnormalities
    Giant heads (Megalosperm)
    Slender and small heads (Microsperm)
    Tapered heads
    Abnormal acrosome
    Bicephalic

Midpiece abnormalities
    Abaxially attached midpiece
    Double midpiece
    Coiled midpiece
    Bent midpiece

Tail abnormalities
    Tightly coiled tails
    Double tails

Secondary Abnormalities: These forms (Fig 5) are believed to arise after spermatogenesis is completed, *ie,* after the spermatozoa have left the seminiferous tubules. They may be caused by too rapid passage through the epididymis because of over-use or disuse and dysfunction of the epididymis. The secondary sex glands may be responsible. Adverse influences on the collected semen, such as contamination with urine or water, exposure to adverse temperatures and chemicals, and rough mechanical handling, can produce some of the abnormal forms. The secondary forms are listed as follows:

Separation of acrosome

Presence of protoplasmic droplet
    Proximal: present high on the midpiece
    Distal: present distal on the midpiece, often accompanied
    by a bent tail. The appearance of the droplets indicates
    immaturity of the sperm cells.

Detached head and Galea Capitis.

Bent tails and bent midpieces: present in sperm cells with and without distal droplets. The bent tails and midpieces observed in sperm cells with distal droplets reflect adverse environmental influences.

Miscellaneous Abnormalities: Unusual numbered spermatids and spermatocytes: indicates testicular function.

White blood cells: indicates purulent inflammation somewhere in the genital tract.

Red blood cells: these ordinarily originate from lesions involving penile and preputial surfaces.

The incidence of each abnormality is determined by a differential count of the abnormal forms. Each abnormal form is recorded. In cases in which two abnormalities are observed in the same cell, the more serious is recorded. All abnormal and normal cells in a field are counted. This is repeated until 100 cells have been counted. Counting of several hundred cells may be advantageous. Recognition of the abnormal forms is not difficult provided that the abnormalities can be visualized. When in doubt, compare with normal cells. If in doubt, examine different fields in several slides, especially in borderline cases, before the results are accepted as final.

Abnormal forms are present in all animals' semen to some degree. In animals that are known to have normal fertility, the number of primary abnormal forms might reach 10 percent. It is generally accepted that the incidence of abnormal forms should not exceed 20 to 30 percent.

Counting Sperm

After inverting the tube containing the semen sample several times, a white blood cell Unipette tube is filled with semen and labeled with the dog's and owner's names and the date. A drop of the semen is then put on a slide for staining.

Sperm cells can be counted efficiently with a hemacytometer. The counts for semen of a fertile dog range from 300×10^6 to 2.0×10^9. The fertility of a medium-sized dog with a sperm count below 300×10^6 is suspect. If the dog has not been bred for more than 2 months, as many as 3 semen collections and examinations may be needed over a period of 10 days to obtain reliable results. If the sperm count is essentially normal but the sperm are immobile, a flaw in the collection technic should be suspected and another sample should be collected.

Artificial Insemination

To restrain a bitch for AI, an assistant stands with his back to a wall or counter for support and holds the dog's head and neck between his knees. The bitch's hindquarters are then elevated to an angle of about 60° from the floor. If the bitch attempts to escape, the assistant can restrict her movements by applying pressure with the knees. The bitch's hindlimbs are then rotated outward slightly and her tail (if long-tailed) is held to one side to expose the vulva. A small bitch (5 to 20 pounds) can be inseminated in this position on an examination table.

The AI equipment includes an 18-inch bovine insemination rod that has been broken in half, a short rubber connector, and a disposable syringe. Surgical or disposable gloves should be worn.

Before aspirating the fresh semen into the syringe, 1 ml of air is drawn into the syringe. The semen is then aspirated slowly to prevent air bubbles from rising through the seminal fluid and thus damaging the sperm cells. A small amount of lubricating jelly is spread on an index finger and the insemination rod and the finger are gently inserted into the bitch's vagina. A little finger is used in very small dogs. The finger is then moved dorsally over the brim of the pelvis. The insemination rod is moved beside the finger until it clears the pelvic brim. At this point the rod is tipped almost vertically and gently pushed into the cervix. If there is any resistance to movement of the rod, it should be withdrawn 1 or 2 inches and redirected at a slightly different angle. If resistance to movement of the rod persists, a small amount of semen can be deposited at this point, which will often enable deeper insertion of the rod. When moderate resistance indicates that the cervical area has been reached, the semen is deposited slowly. (Insertion depth should be 8 to 9 inches in large breeds, 6 to 7 inches in medium breeds, 4 to 6 inches in small dogs.)

The rubber connector is then closed with the left thumb and forefinger and the syringe is detached. After drawing 1 ml of air into the syringe the rubber connector is left open and the remaining semen is expelled from the rod. The insemination rod is then withdrawn from the vagina. The bitch's hindquarters are kept elevated for 6 minutes after the insemination.

Many authors recommend "feathering" the vagina by inserting a finger and gently massaging the vulva and clitoris. This can be done in medium-sized and large bitches by restraining her head and elevating her hindlimbs. After insemination of semen, the bitch should be returned to her cage, being careful that her vagina is not tipped in a way that would result in loss of the semen. If she must be carried, she should be cradled with one arm around the chest and the other arm around the hindquarters, with her head lower than her hindquarters. The bitch should be left in a holding cage with insufficient head room to prevent her from jumping or standing on her hindlimbs for 1 to 2 hours after the insemination.

Further Reading Material

Andersen, AC and Wooten, E in *Reproduction in Domestic Animals*. 1st ed. New York Academic Press, 1959, p 359.

Asdell, S: *Dog Breeding*. Little, Brown & Co, Boston, 1966.

Bane, A: Sterility in male dogs. Nord Vet **22** (1970) 561.

Boucher, JH *et al:* The evaluation of semen quality in the dog and the effects of frequency of ejaculation upon the semen quality, libido and depletion of sperm reserves. Cornell Vet **48** (1958) 67-86.

Hafez, E. *Reproduction and Breeding Techniques for Laboratory Animals.* Lea & Febiger, Philadelphia, 1970.

Harrop, A: *The Semen of Animals and Artificial Insemination.* Central Press Ltd, London, 1962.

McDonald, LE: *Veterinary Endocrinology and Reproduction.* Lea & Febiger, Philadelphia, 1975.

Seager, S: Successful pregnancies utilizing frozen dog semen. AI digest **17** (12) (1969) 6.

Seager, SWJ and Platz, CC: Artificial Insemination and Frozen Semen in the Dog. Vet Clinics of N Am Vol 7, No 4, 1977.

Von Krause, D, II: Examination of fertility in the dog. Dtsch Tierarztl Wschr, 72:3, 1965.

MANAGEMENT OF MISMATING
BY THOMAS J. BURKE

Introduction

Avoiding an unwanted pregnancy is best accomplished by preventing the occurrence of estrus or by preventing access of fertile males to a bitch or queen in estrus. Should these measures fail, as they often do, the owner of a mismated female is apt to seek an "abortion shot" for the animal.

Prior to initiating any therapy it is important to determine that mismating did occur. For this purpose a detailed history is imperative because many owners are ignorant about the reproductive biology of animals. The owner should be asked whether or not the animal had been given treatment for mismating. After obtaining the history, a physical examination should be performed to assess the probability that mating did occur. The back of a queen's neck should be inspected carefully for scratches or small bite wounds that would indicate a tom cat had grasped her there with his teeth during coitus. Vaginal cytology is also useful. If there is cytologic evidence that the patient is in estrus and had the opportunity to be exposed to fertile males, it is likely that coitus occurred. The absence of spermatozoa does not rule out this likelihood because sperm disappear from the vagina in 1 to 3 hours following mating and they are rarely seen.

Treatment Procedures
Surgery

If the animal is not to be used for breeding, an ovariohysterectomy is the treatment of choice. It is most effective and has the fewest side effects. The surgery should be performed during the first 30 days of metestrus. Because estrogen and progesterone are known to affect platelet function, it is recommended that a platelet count and a test for clotting function be performed prior to surgery.

Medical Treatments

If preservation of the animal's reproductive function is important, the owner should be counseled to allow the unwanted litter to be born because there are considerable risks associated with medical therapy for mismating. It should be pointed out that having a mongrel litter will not affect the pedigree of future litters by the involved bitch or queen.

Estrogens are useful because they affect the ovum's (zygote's) passage through the oviducts and they alter the endometrium. The effect of estrogen on ovum transportation is dose-dependent. Lower doses enhance passage and the normal ampullary-isthmic delay is abolished. Higher doses delay passage of the ovum into the uterus and result in degeneration of embryos. Estrogens also alter the biochemistry of the uterus and oviducts by depressing carbonic anhydrase. In addition, they tend to prevent the normal endometrial glandular changes for nidation.

Estrogens have been associated with serious side-effects, including myelosuppression and pyometritis. Their toxicity is related to the estrogen itself as well as the vehicle, dose, and route of administration. The age of the patient may also be important because dogs under 2 years of age had less myelosuppression than did older dogs given estradiol cypionate (ECP) in either single or multiple doses. Esterification of the estrogen molecule (valerate, cypionate, benzoate) prolongs its absorption and slows the rate of metabolism. It appears to be advantageous for the drug to have a prolonged low-level effect.

Myelosuppression appears to be dose-related and most cases of fatal aplastic anemia have been associated with gross overdosage. The occurrence of pyometritis, however, does not appear to be dose-related. Its incidence cannot be predicted, but it may be as high as 30%.

The efficacy of all estrogens is also dependent on the time between mating and administration of the drug. The sooner the hormone is given after mating the better is the result because the morulas enter the uterus 4 to 5 days after fertilization. The efficacy will decline when the drug is given after about 72 hours following fertilization. Because ovulation has usually occurred by the time the patient is presented, it should be stressed that the treatment (except for diethylstilbestrol) must be administered only once during an estrus. It should also be explained that the treatment will prolong the signs of estrus and that breeding may occur again without any need for retreatment. Many cases of fatal myelosuppression that I have seen resulted from repeated treatments given by different veterinarians during the same estrus. Such mistakes can be prevented by discovering that the animal has been treated previously.

Injectable, repositol diethylstilbestrol is virtually unavailable. The dosage of oral stilbestrol is 0.1 mg/kg daily for 5 days beginning within 48 hours of mating. Estradiol-17-cyclopentyl propionate (ECP) should be given IM at a dosage of 0.02 mg/kg for bitches. The recommended dose for a queen is 0.25 mg. Estradiol benzoate or valerate should be given IM at a dosage of 0.1 mg/kg (not to exceed a total dosage of 3.0 mg.)

Megestrol acetate has a contraceptive effect if given at a dosage of 2.2 mg/kg orally at least 3 days prior to coitus. This is presumably due to its anti-ovulatory effect. Post-coital treatment with progestogens is not effective in preventing pregnancy.

Pregnancy could be prevented if the corpora lutea could be destroyed prior to nidation. Corpora lutea are resistant, however, to the effects of dexamethasone and prostaglandin F_2 until well after pregnancy is established.

INDUCED ABORTION IN DOGS
BY JENAAY M. BROWN

Introduction
Abortifacients differ from drugs used to prevent conception in that they are used to terminate an established pregnancy rather than prevent implantation.

It unquestionably is better to prevent a pregnancy than to abort one, but abortion of an unwanted litter is preferable to adding more unwanted puppies or kittens to the existing surplus.

Physiology
The most fertile period in the bitch is from 4 days prior to 3 days after ovulation.[1] Ovulation may occur from 0 to 96 hours after the luteinizing hormone (LH) reaches its peak level. It thus might occur in late proestrus, but it occurs most often during early estrus.[1] From 6

to 7 days after fertilization (day 2 or 3 of diestrus) the fertilized eggs enter the uterine horn as morulas.[2,3] The morulas become blastocysts and float freely until about day 15 or 16 after fertilization. They then implant in the uterine wall after shedding their zonae pellucidae; embryonic differentiation begins at this time. From this point on, abortifacients have their effect.

Serum concentrations of progesterone begin to increase in late proestrus.[4-6] The most rapid increase occurs around ovulation and continues for about 10 days.[4,5] The peak levels of serum progesterone have been observed to occur between days 20 and 40 of gestation.[4,6] The serum progesterone levels return to baseline levels (<2 ng/ml) by parturition.[4,6]

Contrary to the opinion held for years, the bitch requires an ovarian source of progesterone throughout gestation in order to maintain pregnancy.[7] If the corpus luteum (CL) is removed, as in a bilateral ovariectomy, the pregnancy will terminate within 8 days.[7] To end a pregnancy, therefore, one must lower the level of circulating progesterone to below the baseline level required for maintenance of pregnancy.

Mechanical Abortion

Neither enucleation of the corpus luteum nor decapitation of the fetus is performed to stimulate abortion in the bitch because the relative small size of the dog makes either procedure too difficult or impossible.

Chemical Abortion

Initiation of abortion has been attempted with many different types of drugs, including estrogens, antiestrogens, corticosteroids, fermentation by-products, colchicines, and prostaglandins (Table 1).

Estrogens

Very small doses of estradiols (0.1 to 1.0 mg/dog) are being used to prevent conception, but such doses are not effective for inducing abortion in the bitch.[8] It should be noted that estrogens can cause gradual anemia and a profound leukocytosis followed by leukopenia.[9] Thrombocytopenia may occur and result in failure of the clotting mechanism.[9]

Antiestrogens

Antiestrogens are mostly nonsteroidal antagonists of estrogen. They are weak estrogens that have the ability to inhibit the effectiveness of other estrogens. None of these agents has been reported to be an effective abortifacient. Several antiestrogens have been effective, however, in preventing implantation in rats, rabbits, and bitches.[10,11]

Corticosteroids

Large doses of corticosteroids given near term to pregnant females of some species (bovine, ovine) can initiate parturition. When dexamethasone was given IM to pregnant Labrador Retrievers at a dosage of 5 mg BID for 10 days, fetal resorption occurred if the injections were started on day 30 of gestation.[12] The same dosage of dexamethasone caused abortion on about the 58th day of gestation when it was started on day 45.[12] The eventual effect of this treatment on future fertility is unknown. Other corticosteroids (hydrocortisone, triamcinolone, methylprednisolone) have not been observed to induce abortion.

Colchicines

Colchicine and its derivatives have been shown to have antimitotic activity and to relax smooth muscles. N-desacetyl thiocolchicine caused abortion in bitches when given at a dosage of 2 mg/kg either IV or IP after day 30 of gestation.[13,14] Shortly after injection of the drug, the animals salivated excessively, vomited, and had diarrhea. Their rectal temperature and leukocyte count decreased for 24 to 48 hours after the injection.[13] Expulsion of fetuses began 24 to 48 hours after injection of colchicine in bitches that were 30 days pregnant. Fetal expulsion occurred from 15 to 40 hours after injection in bitches that were between 40 and 53 days pregnant.[13,14] Subsequent fertility of these animals did not seem to be affected.[13,14]

Though the use of colcemide, a compound closely related to colchicine, has not been reported in the bitch, it has been studied in rabbits and rats.[15] Injection (SC) of this drug in pregnant rabbits was followed by death of rabbit fetuses. Further studies indicated that colcemide is extremely toxic to fetuses when started on day 9 of gestation and given in doses of 0.1 mg/kg to 5.0 mg/kg. At doses of 5.0 mg/kg, half of the does died.[15] Because of the high toxicity of colchicine compounds,[16] they apparently are unsatisfactory as abortifacients.[16]

Malucidin

This by-product of a beer-brewing process has been reported to induce abortion in the bitch.[17,18] A 3% solution given IV to a bitch at a dosage of 1 ml/3 lb of body weight during the last trimester of pregnancy caused abortion of the fetuses and fetal membranes within 21 to 25 hours.[17] When given at a dosage of 1.0 ml/3½ lb during the first

Table 1. Abortifacients Used in the Bitch

Drug	Dose	Date Effective	Interval to Abortion	Side Effects
Estrogen	Not established	Not established	Not established	Bitches may develop leukocytosis, leukopenia, thrombocytopenia, endometritis, pyometritis, and cystic endometrial hyperplasia
Antiestrogens		Not effective		
Dexamethasone	5 mg given IM BID for 10 days	Day 30 (resorption) Day 45 (abortion)	24-72 hrs after last injection	Unknown Polydipsia, polyuria, and adrenal suppression
N-desacetyl Thiocolchicine	2 mg/kg given IV or IP	Day 30 Days 40-53	24-48 hrs 15-40 hrs	Negative effects on multiple body systems reported in man and rodents
Malucidin	1 ml/3 lb IV 1 ml/3.5 lbs IV	Last trimester (abortion) First and 2nd trimester (reabsorption)	21-25 hrs	Transient drop in blood pressure, occasional prostration, and occasional pseudopregnancy
PGF$_2$	20-30 mcg/kg IM BID or TID	After day 25	56-80 hrs	Vomiting, diarrhea, hyperventilation, salivation, and hypothermia
	250 mcg/kg SC BID for 5 days	After day 30	3-5 days	Hyperpnea, hyper-salivation, vomition, defecation, and hypothermia
	25-50 mcg/kg SC BID or TID	After day 25	5-7 days	Minor side effects (hyperventilation, salivation)
	Approximately 1.0 mg/kg SC daily	Not effective		Hypothermia, vomiting, diarrhea, hyperventilation, and salivation
Fluprostenol	25 mcg/kg IM BID for 2 days	Not reported	Not reported	None reported
	12.5 mcg/kg (slow-release injection)	Day 35	Not reported	Mild side effects
	15 mcg/kg (slow-release injection)	Day 14	Not reported	Mild side effects
	20 mcg/kg (slow-release injection)	Day 28	Not reported	Mild side effects
	10 mcg/kg (intravaginal device)	Day 25 or 26	Not reported	None
	25 mcg/kg (intravaginal device)	Day 25 or 26	Not reported	Vomiting and diarrhea
Cloprostenol	10 mcg/kg (aqueous)	Not reported		Less severe side effects than with the higher dose
	10 mcg/kg (slow-release injection)	Day 14 or 28	Not reported	Mild side effects
	20 mcg/kg (slow-release injection)	Day 14	Not reported	Mild side effects
	40 mcg/kg (slow-release injection)	Not reported	48-168 hr (cervical dilation)	Tachycardia, tachypnea, vomiting, salivation, and severe diarrhea

Table 1, Con't.

	10 mcg/kg (intravaginal device)	Day 27 or 28	Not reported	Mild side effects
TPT	20 mcg/kg SC	Days 30-43	3-10 days	Hypothermia, hyperthermia, salivation, vomiting, diarrhea, and digging response
PG synthesis inhibitors		Not effective	Not effective	
L10503	50-150 mg/kg SC	Day 42, 45 or 48	1 week after expected shelping	Decreased appetite, loss of body weight, and diarrhea (sometimes blood-streaked)
L10492	25 mg/kg SC	Day 20	Resorption	Decreased appetite, loss of body weight, and diarrhea (sometimes blood-streaked, but less intense than with L10503
Uraria lagopoides DC	60 mg/kg	Unknown	Activity on canine uterus *in situ* — no abortion *per se*	Unknown
Azaserine	25 mg/kg IP	Days 19-23	Resorption	Anorexia, weight loss, mild diarrhea, and emesis
Isoquinoline (derivative)	1.0-2.0 mg/kg SC	Day 20	Not reported	No toxic effects noted
Triazole isoindole (derivative)	0.5-1.0 mg/kg SC	Day 20	Not reported	No toxic effects noted

43 days of pregnancy, it caused resorption of the fetuses.[17] Malucidin also produced a transient drop in blood pressure and occasionally prostration. This could be prevented by giving a "desensitizing" dose (10% of the total dose) approximately 10 minutes before the remainder of the calculated amount.[17,18] Milk production in the treated bitches was not affected. Pseudopregnancies often occurred after resorption of fetuses. Similar results have been observed in cats.[17] The results of these initial studies of malucidin have not been reproduced, however.[19]

Prostaglandins

Though serum progesterone levels dropped temporarily in pregnant bitches in response to prostaglandin injections, abortion did not occur.[20-22] The dosages of PGF2 alpha used in these 3 separate studies were 5 mg/animal given IM (3 injections at intervals of 1 to 24 hours), 1 to 4 mg/animal given IV, and 1 mg/kg given SC. Abortion or resorption did occur, however, in another experiment in which a bitch was given 1.25 mg/kg SC 24 days after breeding.[18] Subcutaneous injections of 250 mcg/kg BID for 5 consecutive days, starting on day 31 of pregnancy, caused abortion in 5 of 5 bitches.[23] The same dosage regimen did not cause abortion when given on days 1 to 5 of pregnancy. Lower doses, such as 25 to 50 mcg/kg given SC BID or TID for 3 to 5 days in the latter half of pregnancy, have been reported to cause abortion.[24] Dosages of 20 mcg/kg given IM TID and 30 mcg/kg given IM BID after day 25 of pregnancy have caused abortion in 4 of 7 and 7 of 10 bitches, respectively.[24]

PGF2 alpha causes significant side effects, including vomiting, diarrhea, hyperventilation, excessive salivation, and hypothermia, at most dosage levels.[20-23,25] Though subsequent fertility has not been definitively studied following the use of PGF2 alpha for abortion, there have been reports that litters were whelped by bitches that had been given PGF2 alpha as a treatment for uterine disease.[26]

PGF2 alpha has been used to induce abortion in the queen at dosages of 0.5 to 1.0 mg/kg given twice SC at a 24-hour interval after day 40 of gestation.[27,28] Efforts to reproduce those results failed and it was later determined that queens must either be stressed or given an injection of ACTH prior to injection of PGF2 alpha.[18] Doses of 0.5 to 5.0 mg/kg of PGF2 alpha were found to be non-luteolytic during the early luteal phase in the queen.[29] Side effects in queens are similar to those that occur in the bitch.[28]

Analogs of PGF2 alpha also have abortifacient activity in the bitch. An aqueous solution of fluprostenol given IM at a dosage of 25 mcg/kg BID for 2 days caused luteolysis and abortion (rate of success was unspecified). The same drug at 10 and 25 mcg/kg dosages produced similar results when given in a vaginal implant.[30,31] When given as a slow-release injectable preparation at doses of 12.5, 15, and 20 mcg/kg, fluprostenol terminated pregnancies in 1 of 11, 1 of 4 and 1 of 1 bitches, respectively. Toxic reactions occurred in bitches given 25 mcg/kg doses of cloprostenol, another prostaglandin analog. Lower doses of cloprostenol (10 mcg/kg) still caused hyperventilation, tachycardia, salivation, vomiting, and severe diarrhea.[30] A dose of 40 mcg/kg of cloprostenol in a slow-release implant induced abortions with fewer side effects.[30,32] When used as a slow-release injectable preparation at doses of 10, 20, and 40 mcg/kg, cloprostenol terminated pregnancies in 6 of 8, 1 of 3, and 2 of 3 bitches, respectively.[32]

Another synthetic prostaglandin, TPT, given at a dosage of 20 mcg/kg in a single SC injection induced resorption of fetuses in 2 of 4 bitches treated between days 20 to 22 of gestation. Abortion was induced by the same dosage in 5 of 5 bitches that were 30 to 43 days pregnant. All treated bitches, including those treated prior to 30 days of gestation, had reduced serum progesterone levels that remained low only in the bitches that aborted. Typical side effects were hypothermia followed by hyperthermia, salivation, vomiting, diarrhea, and a "digging response."[31]

A very limited amount of work has been done with prostaglandin $E_2(PGE_2)$ in the bitch. A slight, but not lasting, decrease in plasma progesterone levels followed infusion of 30 mcg over a 6-hour period.[21] In another study the use of PGE_2 as a vaginal suppository caused abortion or parturition in 3 of 5 bitches that were more than 45 days pregnant.[33]

Prostaglandin Inhibitors

Such drugs as aspirin, indomethacin, ibuprofen, and naproxen are prostaglandin synthetase inhibitors. Aspirin given to human females during the last 6 months of pregnancy prolonged gestation by interfering with production of endogenous prostaglandin and subsequent induction of labor.[34] Indomethacin has lengthened pseudopregnancy in rabbits, rats, and hamsters.[35,36] It has delayed implantation in the rat and caused nearly complete inhibition of fetal development in the rabbit when administered during early pregnancy.[37,38] Induced abortion has been delayed in laboratory animals by administering naproxen.[39] It thus is obvious that prostaglandin inhibitors have no value as abortifacients, but may be useful in preventing pregnancy.

Other Compounds

Other drugs are currently being assessed for their abortifacient activity in bitches.[40] The chemical identity of some is unknown. A compound called Azaserine has caused fetal resorption in bitches when given in a single IP injection of 2.5 mg/kg.[41] It was most effective when given between 19 and 23 days of pregnancy.

An isoquinoline derivative and a triazole isoindole derivative have also been found effective as abortifacients in bitches.[42]

On the basis of current information, it appears that the requirement of a successful abortifacient in dogs is the ability to reduce the serum progesterone level to below 2 ng/ml for at least 48 hours. Unfortunately, all attempts to date have not produced a safe and effective abortifacient for clinical use. The results with serial injections of prostaglandins and their analogs are encouraging, however.

Acknowledgment: Drs J. W. Lauderdale and J. H. Sokolowski are thanked for their advice and constructive criticism.

References

1. Nett, TM and Olson, PN: *In Textbook of Veterinary Internal Medicine,* 2nd ed, pp 1698-1710. WB Saunders, Philadelphia, 1982.
2. Holst, PA and Phemister, RP: Biol Reprod **5** (1971) 194.
3. Holst, PA and Phemister, RP: Amer J Vet Res **36** (1975) 705.
4. Smith, MS and McDonald, LE: Endocrin **97** (1974) 404.

5. Nett, TM *et al:* Proc Soc Exp Biol Med **148** (1975) 134.
6. Concannon, PW *et al:* Biol Reprod **13** (1975) 112.
7. Sokolowski, JH: Lab Anim Sci **25:5** (1971) 696.
8. Olson, PS: Lecture at Short Course on Canine Reproduction and Artificial Insemination. Colorado State Univ, Fort Collins, 1981.
9. Crafts, RC: Blood **3** (1948) 276.
10. Morris, JM *et al:* Fertil Steril **18** (1967) 18.
11. Hershberger, LG: Amer J Vet Res **23** (1962) 168.
12. Austad, R: J Reprod Fertil **46** (1976) 129.
13. Thiersch, JB: JAVMA **151** (1967) 1470.
14. Ruckstuhl, B: Kleintierpraxis **21:8** (1976) 302, 304.
15. Morris, JM *et al:* Fertil Steril **18** (1967) 7.
16. Goodman, L and Gilman, A: In *The Pharmacological Basis of Therapeutics,* 4th ed, p 340. The Macmillan Co, New York, 1970.
17. Whitney, LF: Vet Med **55** (1960) 57.
18. Whitney, LF: Vet Med **54** (1959) 25.
19. Sokolowski, JH: Personal communication.
20. VanDerHorst, CJG and Vogel, F: Tijschr Diergen **102** (1977) 117.
21. Jochle, W *et al:* Prostaglandins **3** (1973) 209.
22. Baker, BA *et al:* Theriogenol **14** (1980) 195.
23. Paradis, M *et al:* Canad Vet J **24** (1983) 239.
24. Lein, D: Presented at S.A. Theriogenology section, AVMA meet, 1981.
25. Concannon, PW and Hansel, W: Prostaglandins **13** (1977) 533.
26. Sokolowski, JH: JAAHA **16** (1980) 119.
27. Nachreiner, RF and Marple, DN: Prostaglandins **7** (1974) 303.
28. Schille, VM and Stabenfeldt, GH: Biol Reprod **21** (1977) 1217.
29. Wildt, DE *et al:* Prostaglandins **18** (1979) 883.
30. Jackson, P: Lecture at Conf Assn Vet Teachers and Research Workers, United Kingdom, 1980.
31. Vickery, B and McRae, G: Biol Reprod **22** (1982) 438.
32. Jackson, PS *et al:* J Small Anim Pract **23** (1982) 287.
33. Root, RG: Personal communication.
34. Lewis, RB and Schulman, JD: Lancet Nov 24, 1973, pp 1159-1161.
35. O'Grady, J *et al:* Prostaglandins **1** (1972) 97.
36. Lau, JF *et al:* Acta Endocrinol **78** (1975) 343.
37. Phillips, CA and Poyser, NL: J Reprod Fertil **62** (1981) 73.
38. Hoffman, LH: Biol Reprod **18** (1978) 148.
39. Csapo, AI *et al:* Prostaglandins **7** (1974) 39.
40. Galliani, G and Lerner, L: Amer J Vet Res **37** (1976) 263.
41. Friedman, MH: JAVMA **130** (1957) 159.
42. Galliani, G and Omodei-Sale, A: J Small Anim Pract **23** (1982) 295.

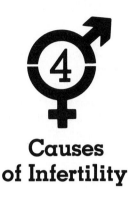

Causes
of Infertility

ANATOMIC ABNORMALITIES
BY THOMAS J. BURKE

Introduction
Anatomic defects may interfere with copulation, parturition, or the transport of gametes. They may be congenital or acquired. Little is known about the heritability of congenital defects, except for cryptorchidism. Acquired defects are usually the result of trauma or neoplasia. Cats are either affected less often than dogs or their abnormalities are often unrecognized.

Diagnosis of anatomic defects requires a thorough history, careful physical examination, and, in some cases, exploratory surgery or vaginoscopy. Correction, when possible, usually requires surgery (see Chapter 6).

Female Abnormalities
Strictures
Strictures of the lower reproductive tract are common in bitches. They appear to be rare in queens. The strictures may be congenital or acquired, presumably a result of trauma at birth. The most common location for genital strictures is the junction of the vulva and vestibule. They may also be found in the vagina at the level of the urethral meatus or, less commonly, more anteriorly. A tough, non-distensible fibrous band is palpable or visible by vaginoscopy. If one performs a proper pre-breeding physical examination, such strictures are readily found. The clinician may wish to reconfirm such a diagnosis at the time of the first estrus when prepuberal bitches are involved. Bitches of the giant breeds should be palpated with 2 digits.

Clinicians should be aware that some bitches may have more than one stricture. I found 3 in a German Shepherd. For this reason, vaginoscopy is indicated in all cases.

If a vaginal stricture is not discovered prior to mating, the history will usually reveal that the male was incapable of intromission (lower strictures) or could not achieve a complete tie. Pain will usually be manifested by both animals and minor bleeding may have been noticed.

Treatment of genital strictures requires episioplasty and/or vaginoplasty. Because post-operative cicatrization may occur, the patient should be re-examined prior to each planned breeding. The surgery is usually performed when the bitch is in metestrus or anestrus. If mating has occurred or artificial insemination was performed prior to diagnosis of a stricture, then surgery must be done prior to whelping because dystocia will occur otherwise.

The heritability of genital strictures is unknown. I have examined several daughters of affected bitches (Great Dane, German Shepherd, West Highland White Terrier, and Scottish Terrier), however, that did not have the condition.

Vaginal Hyperplasia

This condition is often referred to as vaginal prolapse. It reflects an abnormal response of vaginal and vestibular tissue (usually the floor of the posterior vagina and vestibule) to normal levels of estro-

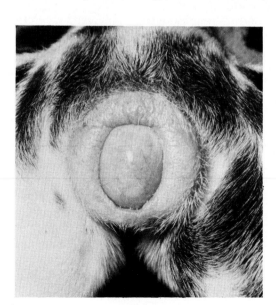

Fig 1. Vaginal hyperplasia in a Dalmatian.

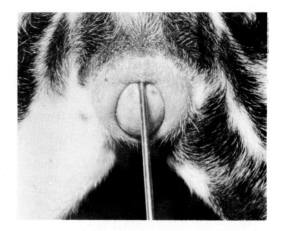

Fig 2. Urinary catheter placed in the bladder of bitch in Figure 1 showing that the floor of the vestibule is involved.

gen in proestrus and estrus. Spontaneous regression occurs with the onset of the luteal phase of the cycle and the condition is not present during metestrus or anestrus. The hyperplasia recurs to some degree with each estrus.

Physical examination reveals a smooth, pink mass protruding from the vulva (Fig 1). It cannot be reduced manually. Catheterization of the urinary bladder will enable one to determine which segment of the vagina is involved (Fig 2). True prolapses of the vagina involve its entire circumference and the urethral meatus is either located centrally or can be seen externally on the ventral surface of the prolapsed tissue. Prolapses are almost always associated with parturition or, rarely, with false pregnancy. They do not regress spontaneously and are usually reducible manually (at least partially).

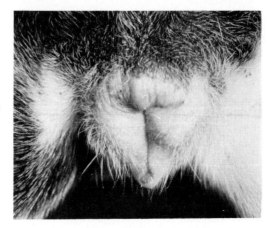

Fig 3. Same bitch as in Figures 1 and 2 after 5 days of therapy with megestrol acetate.

Vaginal hyperplasia prevents normal copulation. An affected bitch must be inseminated artificially. The tissue will not be hyperplastic at whelping. Medical treatment involves keeping the exposed tissue from desiccating. Artificial tears should be applied frequently to the protruding tissues until the swelling subsides. An antibiotic and glucocorticoid may be administered topically if superficial inflammation or infection is present. Recovery may be hastened by oral administration of megestrol acetate at a dosage of 2.2 mg/kg given once daily for 5 to 7 days (Fig 3). Breeding should not be planned if megestrol is used. The protruding tissue may also be protected by lacing the lips of the vulva together to cover some or all or it. Permanent correction requires resection of the portion of vagina that becomes hyperplastic. Ovariohysterectomy prevents recurrence.

The heritability of this condition is unknown though a familial tendency has been reported in Dalmatians.[4]

Vaginal Septa

Pillars of tissue of varying thickness extending from the ceiling to the floor of the vaginal vault are found occasionally in bitches (Fig 4). They do not interfere with copulation, but will cause dystocia. These septa are usually too far cranial to palpate, but they can be seen through a vaginoscope. The treatment involves surgical resection. Gaining adequate exposure to the surgical site can be difficult.

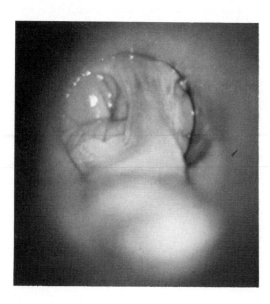

Fig 4. Vaginal septum in a bitch. Normal vaginal mucosa can be seen on either side of the septum.

Abnormal Angulation of the Vulva

This condition varies in severity. Affected bitches have an abnormal angulation of the vulva causing it to become horizontal at too acute an angle to allow normal intromission by the male. The condition can be diagnosed by careful digital examination of the lower genital tract. The presenting history may be similar to that of an animal with a vaginal stricture because the male's penis hits the dorsum of the vestibule, causing pain. I am unaware of any published reports of successful correction of this defect.

Vulvo-vaginal Cleft

Congenital absence of the dorsal vulvar commisure and ceiling of the vestibule is usually noticed early in the animal's life by either the owner or veterinarian at the time of the first physical examination (Fig 5). There is a concomitant clitoritis and vaginitis that could

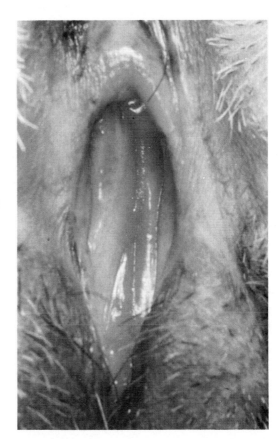

Fig 5. Vulvo-vaginal cleft in a German Shepherd. Note exposure of the vestibular floor.

cause infertility. The defect can be corrected with an inverted "U" episioplasty.[1] The heritability of this defect is unknown.

Ovarian Agenesis

Unilateral agenesis of an ovary will not result in infertility per se. It may or may not be accompanied by agenesis of the ipsilateral uterine horn. The diagnosis is usually made by chance during surgery or at necropsy. Bilateral ovarian agenesis will result in continued anestrus that does not respond to the administration of exogenous gonadotropins. There is no treatment.

Segmental Aplasia of the Tubular Tract

Aplasia of one segment of either uterine horn or either oviduct may not interfere with fertility. If multiple aplastic areas are bilateral, ovum transport and nidation will be obstructed, leading to apparent infertility though estrous cycles and breeding activity are normal. A similar condition may be caused by chronic inflammatory disease and scar formation following cesarean section.

The diagnosis can be made by hysterosalpingography, but it is advisable to confirm the diagnosis by performing an exploratory laparotomy. Following the laparotomy an organic dye, such as Evans blue, is injected into each uterine horn near its junction with the body of the uterus and is milked cranially until it can be seen in the ovarian bursa. Interruption of passage of the dye is abnormal. Surgical correction requires microsurgical technic.

I am unaware of documented cases of total uterine aplasia. Unilateral aplasia has been reported and it does not interfere with fertility. The heritability of the condition is unknown.

Cervical Stenosis

Cervical stenosis causes infertility by interfering with the transport of sperm. It is diagnosed more often in queens than bitches. If there is total closure of the cervix, the uterus may fill with fluid associated with normal endometrial function, producing so-called mucometra, hydrometra, or sterile pyometra.[2] The estrous cycles of affected animals are normal except that in the bitch there is no sanguineous discharge associated with proestrus. This defect can presumably be either congenital or acquired. Its diagnosis requires direct inspection after a laparotomy, revealing the inability to pass a urinary catheter retrograde through the cervix through an incision made cranially to the body of the uterus. To my knowledge there are no reports of correcting this defect.

Male Abnormalities

Cryptorchidism

Cryptorchidism is the failure of one (unilateral) or both (bilateral) testes to descend and be maintained in the normal scrotal position. The term monorchid is applied most correctly to unilateral failure of development of a testis. Unfortunately, the term is often used in reference to unilateral cryptorchidism.

In the newborn puppy the testes are just inside or within the internal inguinal ring and they reach the scrotal area at 10 to 14 days of age.[4] As the scrotum develops the testes are carried with it and assume a normal intrascrotal position. Further somatic growth by the neonate draws the inguinal rings further away. The testes are normally above the scrotal area until the scrotum develops, but their palpation may be difficult in well-nourished puppies because of fat deposits in this area. Scrotal development should be evident by 10 to 16 weeks of age. Similar changes are thought to occur in kittens, except that scrotal development may be delayed in some breeds, notably the Persian where it may require most of a year.

In some puppies the testes or a testis may seem to come and go from the scrotum. The reason is unclear, but this has been blamed on the slackness of the inguinal tissues in prepuberal dogs. In my experience such "yo-yo" testes almost always become cryptorchids and they usually are palpable next to the penis or in the inguinal area.

Rarely a testis is found in the perineal region. This condition has been referred to as ectopic testis and it is thought to occur when a testis is displaced during its descent outside the inguinal ring.[4]

Testes retained outside the scrotum are incapable of spermiogenesis because of their exposure to normal body temperature. They are much smaller than a descended testis and may be difficult to find when located intra-abdominally (Figs 6-8).

In most species cryptorchidism is thought to be a simple autosomal, recessive genetic defect. It is obviously sex-linked, although females can be carriers. This appears to be true in the dog. The relative infrequency of cryptorchidism in the cat suggests that it may have a different genetic pattern or that genetic dilution prevents its expression. It may also be unnoticed in the cat. Because true monorchidism is rarely diagnosed, its genetics are unknown. This condition may be more common than realized because it is rare that the detailed pathologic studies necessary to confirm its diagnosis are performed. It appears to be common that the tissue removed at surgery for monorchidism is discarded rather than submitted for microscopic examination.

[handwritten marginal note: See pp. 386]

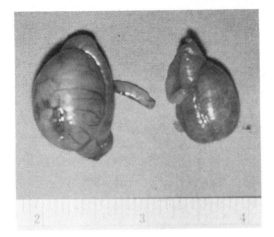

Fig 6. Gross appearance of a normal, descended testis (left) and cryptorchid testis (right from a Schipperke.

Medical therapy for cryptorchidism, including the use of gonadotropins and/or testosterone, is usually unsuccessful, and orchiopexy is a contravention of veterinary ethics. The preferred treatment is surgical castration because the retained testis is at higher risk for development of neoplasia and torsion. When the cryptorchidism is unilateral, I recommend that the scrotal testis also be removed be-

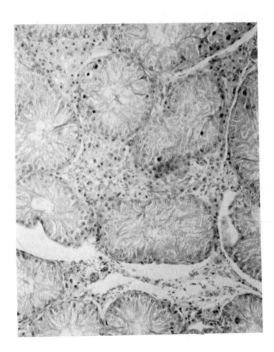

Fig 7. Microscopic appearance of the cryptorchid testis shown in Figure 6. Notice the absence of spermatogenesis.

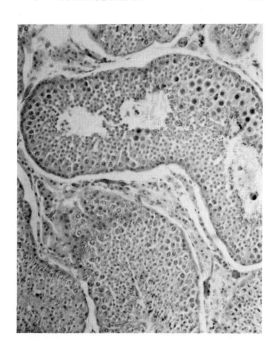

Fig 8. Microscopic appearance of the normal testis shown in Figure 6. Notice the normal sequence of spermatogenesis.

cause it also appears to be at higher risk of developing a tumor. This practice also eliminates the chance that the affected male will be bred and further disseminate this defect. It is also significant that tumors of retained testes are more often malignant than those of descended ones.

Aplasia of the Excurrent Duct System

Segmental aplasia of the epididymis or vas deferens has been reported.[3] If the condition is bilateral, the patient will be infertile and consistently azoospermic. Biopsy of affected structures reveal normal testicular tissue and stages of spermiogenesis. The diagnosis can be confirmed by radiographic studies using a radiopaque dye following cannulation of the epididymis. In man such defects are repaired with microsurgical technics.

Blockage of the excurrent duct system may also occur as a result of trauma or infection. In such cases the occluded area may be palpable as a hard, fibrotic mass.

The heritability of segmental aplasia is unknown.

Urethral Abnormalities

Hypospadias (failure of fusion of the ventral urethra) is the most common urethral abnormality in dogs. Dorsal openings (epispadias)

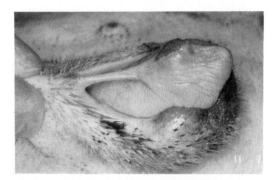

Fig 9. Persistent penile frenulum in a German Shepherd puppy.

are rare. In animals with hypospadias involving the urethra cranial to the preputial fornix, the prepuce is also involved. Hypospadias has also been seen in intersex animals.

The diagnosis is based on physical examination. Affected animals are obviously incapable of fertilization because semen will not be transported normally. The heritability of this defect is unknown.

Small hypospadias may close spontaneously. The treatment of choice is perineal urethrostomy and amputation of the distal structures.

Persistent Penile Frenulum

Persistence of the frenulum between the glans penis and prepuce causes an inability to extend the penis (Fig 9). Affected puppies may show signs of discomfort prior to reaching puberty as evidenced by persistent licking of the sheath. The diagnosis is based on physical examination. The treatment involves surgical removal of the frenulum. The heritability of this defect is also unknown.

Deviation of the Penis

Lateral or ventral deviation of the erect penis is uncommon. It supposedly is a result of a malformed os penis and results in aberrant thrusting during attempts to mate. Most affected males will be able to accomplish intromission with minimal assistance. This condition should not be confused with clumsy attempts at mating by inexperienced, yet vigorous, males.

References
1. Burke, TJ and Smith, CW: JAAHA **11** (1975) 774.
2. Burke, TJ: Vet Clin No Amer **6** (1976) 317.
3. Copland, MD and Maclachlan, NL: J Sm Anim Pract **17** (1976) 443.
4. Jones, DE and Joshua, JO: In *Reproductive Clinical Problems in the Dog*. Wright PSG. Bristol, England. 1982.

LESIONS OF THE SCROTUM AND SCROTAL STRUCTURES
BY ROLF E. LARSEN & FRANCES O. SMITH

Signs of Scrotal Disease

Except for acute injuries, lesions of the scrotum and its contents seldom cause well-defined syndromes. Clinical problems involving these structures are reflected by 1) the presence of fluid in the scrotum; 2) the occurrence of pain in the scrotum; 3) abnormal consistency, size, or shape of scrotal contents; and 4) reduced fertility or semen quality. Scrotal dermatitis may accompany any of the other changes. Though it is true that all of these signs may be concurrent, it is useful to consider each in turn when making a differential diagnosis.

Excess Fluid

Excess fluid in the space between the vaginal tunics is usually from one of 3 possible sources. It may be serous fluid associated with inflammation or secretion of the peritoneal lining of the vaginal space or peritoneum (called hydrocele). It may be blood resulting from trauma or a vascular defect within the spermatic cord or testis (called hematocele). Or it may be the fluid within a section of intestine herniated through the inguinal canal. Though any of these 3 conditions may exist without pain or loss of fertility, pain is often associated with traumatic and infectious causes of hydrocele and hematocele.

Pain

Pain associated with scrotal lesions often causes the affected animal to walk stiffly with the hindlimbs spread. Occasionally, an affected dog will seek a cool, wet place on which to sit. Severe scrotal pain may be accompanied by increased thirst, poor appetite, and vomiting. Certain resting positions are avoided to prevent stretching of tissues in the inguinal area. Dermatitis and lick granulomas are often sequelae to scrotal pain. Nearly every lesion of the testis, epididymis, and scrotum may be accompanied by pain except for the congenital anomalies.

Changes in Shape or Consistency

The consistency, size, and shape of the testes of show and working dogs are inspected regularly by their owners. Small changes are often brought to the attention of the veterinarian. In the absence of scrotal pain or detection of an abnormality by the owner, many changes in scrotal structures will be found only by a thorough physical examination. Injuries, infections, and granulomas account for changes in scrotal size, consistency, and symmetry. Neoplasia, primary autoimmune orchitis, and hormonally mediated changes are usually chronic processes that often are noticeable only when the shape or size of an affected testis has changed visibly or when the animal is found to be infertile.

Infertility

Animals presented because of infertility are unlikely to be in the acute stage of an inflammatory process. The majority of these stud dogs, if they are truly infertile, have fewer sperm in their semen due to blockage of a duct or hypoplasia of the seminiferous tubules that may be congenital or acquired. Libido is seldom affected. The cause of infertility in male dogs is often unknown.

Scrotal Dermatitis

Scrotal skin is thinner and more easily irritated than skin over most of the body. Insect bites, chemical irritants, minor trauma, and licking are the most common causes of scrotal dermatitis. The lesions develop rapidly and with continued licking they soon resemble a "hot spot." The affected area becomes firm and thickened and in some cases blood oozes from petechiated areas.

Treatment of scrotal dermatitis generally involves measures that are appropriate for contact dermatitis. If the cause of pain is intrascrotal, the treatment should include an attempt to remove the lesion. Administration of antihistamines, corticosteroids, and/or tranquilizers may be helpful. Application of an Elizabethan collar is often indicated. The treatment should be vigorous to prevent thermal injury to the testes. Though the prolonged administration of corticosteroids has been found to be detrimental to spermatogenic function in a number of species, their use in cases of scrotal dermatitis is justified. In chronic cases, surgical removal of the scrotal lesion may be necessary.

Inguinal Hernia

Whenever the scrotum or spermatic cord is enlarged, the possible causes include inguinal hernia. These lesions range from small portions of omentum that are herniated through the inguinal ring to loops of intestine within the cavity surrounding the testis. In adult animals the condition is usually unilateral. Breeds of dogs with an apparently greater risk for this condition include the Basenji, Basset Hound, Cairn Terrier, Pekingese, and West Highland White Terrier.[1,2]

A diagnosis of inguinal hernia is suggested by the presence of a substance in the vaginal cavity that resembles spermatic fluid that often can be squeezed back into the peritoneal cavity. The cord and inguinal ring should be palpated for evidence of unusual thickness. We have seen cases in 2 related Basset Hounds in which herniated omentum caused apparent thickening of the spermatic cord. In one of the dogs the herniated omentum surrounded the testis and this animal was infertile due to a high proportion of morphologically abnormal spermatozoa. The other dog was fertile but he suffered discomfort when attempting to rest in the frog-leg position because of omental adhesions to the inguinal canal. Herniorrhaphy was reparative in both dogs. When inguinal hernia is a possible diagnosis, the scrotum should be incised carefully during surgical exploration. A blind needle biopsy is contraindicated. If the scrotal cavity is opened, the surgeon should be prepared to perform a herniorrhaphy. In most cases the herniated tissue will have become adhered to the inguinal canal. If there are extensive adhesions to the vaginal tunics, unilateral castration on the affected side may be indicated to avoid excessive manipulation of the testis and spermatic cord.

Lesions of the Epididymis

Though in many cases of orchitis the epididymis is also affected, the epididymis can be the primary site of lesions. Aplasia or segmental aplasia of the epididymis and ductus deferens has been reported.[3,4] This is unlikely to be detected in most affected animals. If the condition is unilateral, it is not associated with infertility.

A spermatocele is a cyst-like structure that may obstruct a ductus epididymidis. These lesions occur following rupture of a duct and result in blockage of spermatozoa. The incidence of these lesions is unknown, due to the difficulty of identifying them. When they occur unilaterally, fertility is not impaired.

Adenomyosis of the canine epididymis has been described as a condition that may lead to formation of granulomas.[5] It is characterized by epithelial invasion of the muscle layers of the epididymis and the surrounding connective tissue of the epididymal tubule. Spermatozoa migrate into ducts formed by the epithelium and subsequently cause granulomas. Prolonged stimulation by estrogen may contribute to the development of adenomyosis. This condition has been found in dogs treated with estrogens and in dogs with Sertoli cell tumors.[6]

Infections of the epididymis are usually abscesses caused by bacteria. Retrograde migration of infectious organisms causing prostatitis may result in abscesses and sperm granulomas in the epididymis with little involvement of the testis. Epididymitis occurs in sexually mature dogs with canine distemper; both cytoplasmic and intranuclear inclusion bodies are found in the epithelial cells.[7] In dogs with brucellosis both epididymitis and orchitis are common and testicular atrophy and infertility are common sequelae.[8]

Scrotal Injuries

Because of their mobility within the scrotum, the testes are better protected from injuries than their exposed position may suggest. They are occasionally injured, however. Scrotal injuries may go unnoticed in long-haired dogs and they may become the sites of lick dermatitis.

Contusions of the testes are commonly caused by kicks and motor vehicles. Intracapsular hematomas create pressure and enlargement of the testis with resultant pain. The tunica albuginea usually remains intact, even with total maceration of a testis.[9] In some cases a testis is totally replaced by blood clots and may have a fluid consistency for months. Though atrophy is a typical sequel of testicular injuries, recovery of apparently normal size and consistency does occur. In such cases of apparent recovery, the testicular ducts may remain obstructed. When an injured testis remains enlarged and filled with fluid, its removal is indicated. This should involve removal of all tunica vaginalis tissue surrounding the testis to minimize contamination resulting from spillage of infected fluid.

Lacerations of the scrotum caused by bites, bullets, and automobiles should be regarded as contaminated. In cases in which the tunica vaginalis has been opened for less than 24 hours and the damage is only moderate, the vaginal cavity should be flushed with physiologic saline solution containing an antibiotic, the tunica vaginalis parietalis sutured, and the scrotal wall repaired. When such injuries are older than 1 day and the exposed tissues are obviously infected, they may be treated best as an open wound. With severe damage to the scrotal wall and testes, the latter should be removed.

Penetrating wounds that extend through the tunica vaginalis visceralis-tunica albuginea should generally be closed only at the tunica vaginalis parietalis and skin level. If the tunica albuginea has been ruptured and testicular parenchyma has been extruded, the testis should be removed. When the testicular capsule retains its shape and contents, the tunica albuginea will heal rapidly if infection is controlled.[10] Though adhesions may form between the visceral and parietal layers of the tunica vaginalis, this is preferred to pressure damage associated with suturing injured tissues following testicular injuries. Prompt administration of a systemic antibiotic is critical to the success of scrotal laceration treatment. If castration is performed, the incision should be made through nonscrotal skin in the caudal prepuce-inguinal area unless there are local infections that may contaminate surgically exposed tissues. Generally, removal of all vaginal tunics (closed castration) is indicated.

Vascular damage to the testes occurs following malicious placement of rubber bands or string at the base of the scrotum; it also is associated with torsion and thrombosis. Foreign objects that constrict the scrotum should be removed and treatment given to reduce the edema. The patient should be monitored for pyrexia and evidence of thromboembolism. If the swelling is not reduced within 24 hours, castration along with scrotal ablation is indicated.[11] Following surgery the patient should be given a broad-spectrum antibiotic.

Testicular torsion occurs most commonly in dogs with intra-abdominal testes. It may be associated with neoplastic enlargement of a retained testis.[12] Torsion usually causes acute pain, anorexia, and vomiting. Intrascrotal torsion accompanied by swelling and edema of the affected testis has been reported; in some cases the scrotal changes are slight.[12-15] Affected animals usually stand and walk stiffly. Orchidectomy is usually indicated. In dogs used to study the effects of testicular torsion it was found that a torsion of 360 degrees must exist for 24 hours to produce infarction.[16] Complete interruption of blood flow for 10 hours causes complete destruction of the testis and fibrotic replacement of testicular tissue.[17] Ischemia for 1 to 2 hours is sufficient to produce irreversible damage.[18] Though correction of the torsion and replacement of the testis in the hemiscrotum may be possible in an affected dog, unless cosmetic considerations are paramount the affected testis should be removed.[19]

Infections of Scrotal Structures

The principal causes of orchitis and epididymitis are trauma and infection. Trauma may also intensify an infectious process that is already present. Orchitis and epididymitis are often sequelae of urinary tract infections. Such organisms as *E coli, Proteus vulgaris,* streptococci, and staphylococci are common causes. *Mycoplasma* have been isolated in cases of unilateral epididymo-orchitis. *Mycoplasma* may also occur in association with other organisms.[20] Extensive involvement of the tunica vaginalis propria with fibrinous adhesions between the visceral and parietal layers may reflect extension of infection from the peritoneum. Such spread of peritoneal infections is rare, however. Sequelae to epididymo-orchitis are duct blockage, spermatoceles, sperm granulomas, abscesses, hydrocele or hematocele, fistulous tracts, atrophy, and fibrosis.

Environmental Influences on Testicular Function

Nonspecific environmental and psychological influences may be reflected by the testes. Healthy, well-fed dogs that are placed in cages often develop atrophic changes in the testes within 8 to 60 days.[9] Such atrophic changes are reversible after continued confinement for 4 months or longer and the testes usually return to normal. This testicular change was not prevented by administration of testosterone proprionate. Exogenous testosterone would not be the drug of choice in any case because of its negative feedback effects on the pituitary and hypothalamus.

Mild hyperthermia of the canine testis will result in reduced motility of sperm, but this effect seems to be reversible. Repeated warming of the scrotal sac of dogs to 38-40 C has resulted in reduced sperm motility within 5 days.[21] After 10 days of scrotal hyperthermia, sperm are no longer motile. Within 10 days after stopping the scrotal warming, motile sperm are present again in the semen and after 30 days the sperm are normal.

Autoimmune Orchitis

Orchitis and lymphocytic infiltration of the testis has been diagnosed in dogs suffering from autoimmune thyroiditis. As do the brain and testes, the thyroid gland contains antigens not recognized as self by the immune system. Thyroiditis has been produced experimentally by injecting dogs with homologous thyroid extracts emulsified in Freund's adjuvant.[22-24]

Lymphocytic thyroiditis was found in 0.4% of 4500 Cocker Spaniels, Corgis, and Beagles, suggesting the existence of a genetically linked autoimmune etiology.[25] The influence of inherited genes on the incidence of thyroiditis has been studied in a closed breeding colony of Beagles. In this colony a high rate of male infertility and lymphocytic orchitis was found to occur spontaneously.[26,27] Occurrence of the orchitis was genetically influenced and related to the incidence of lymphocytic thyroiditis. Three forms of cellular infiltration were found in the testes: nodular, diffuse, and aggregative. More than one form was often present. The lymphocytic infiltrations were located in the epididymis and in all portions of the testes, including the interstitium, and within the seminiferous tubular epithelium and tubular lumina. The pathologic changes in the testes resulted in reduction in their size and weight as well as sterility or reduced fertility. Degenerative changes were generally localized and accompanied by aggregations of spermatozoa, cytoplasmic and nuclear debris, and giant cells within the lumina or adjacent interstitium. Testes with diffuse tubular atrophy had only Sertoli cells within the intact tubules.

A focal peritubular orchitis has been described in related Black Labrador Retriever dogs. It has been associated with infertility, spermatogenic arrest, and azoospermia.[28] In some cases the orchitis was characterized histologically by localized inflammatory infiltrates surrounding a portion of degenerated seminiferous tubules while apparently normal spermatogenesis was occurring in much of the testes. Despite the presence of some normal testicular tissue, there were no spermatozoa in the rete testes, the epididymides, and the semen. Though thyroiditis was not apparent in these cases, an immune-mediated pathogenesis was suggested.

Fertility Subsequent to Epididymo-Orchitis

Dogs with epididymo-orchitis due to trauma and/or urogenital infection are often presented late in the course of the disease. Although the infection may be controlled, relatively few animals regain their fertility when the involvement has been bilateral. This is probably due to fibrous scarring and ductal obstruction. At least 12 weeks sexual rest is recommended following epididymo-orchitis before an evaluation of fertility is made. When the inflammation is unilateral, normal fertility is often regained.

References

1. Fox, MW: JAVMA **143** (1963) 602.
2. Hayes, HM: Amer J Vet Res **35** (1974) 839.
3. Majeed, ZZ: J Small Anim Pract **15** (1974) 263.
4. Copland, MD and MacLachlan, NJ: J Small Anim Pract **17** (1976) 443.
5. McEntee, K: Nuovo Veterinaria **50** (1974) 194.
6. McEntee, K: Proc Ann Meet Soc Theriogenology, 1979.
7. McEntee, K: Pathology of Domestic Animals. Academic Press, New York, 1970.
8. Carmichael, LE: Canine Brucellosis. In Current Veterinary Therapy VI. WB Saunders, Philadelphia, 1977.
9. Bloom, F: Pathology of the Dog and Cat. American Veterinary Publications, Santa Barbara, CA, 1954.
10. Larsen, RF: Vet Clinics No Amer **7** (1977) 747.
11. Burke, TJ and Reynolds, HA: The Testis. In Pathophysiology in Small Animal Surgery. Lea and Febiger, Philadelphia, 1981.
12. Pearson, H and Kelly, DF: Vet Rec **97** (1975) 200.
13. Hulse, DA: VM/SAC **68** (1973) 658.
14. Young, ACB: J Small Anim Pract **20** (1979) 229.
15. Zymet, CL: VM/SAC **70** (1975) 1330.
16. Sonda, LP, Jr and Lapides, J: Surg Forum **12** (1961) 502.

17. Smith, GI: J Urol **73** (1955) 355.
18. Hinman, F and Smith, GI: Fertil Steril **6** (1955) 443.
19. Moyad, R *et al:* Invest Urol **12** (1975) 387.
20. Lein, DH: Canine Orchitis. In Current Veterinary Therapy VI, WB Saunders Co, Philadelphia, 1977.
21. Chomiak, M *et al:* Ann Marie Curie Sklodoska, Lublin, Sec DD9 (1954) 223.
22. Beierwaltes, WH and Nishiyama, RH: Endocrinol **83** (1968) 501.
23. Mawdesley-Thomas, LE: J Small Anim Pract **9** (1968) 539.
24. Tucker, WE: Amer J Clin Path **38** (1962) 70.
25. Musser, E and Graham, WR: Lab Anim Care **18** (1968) 58.
26. Fritz, TE *et al:* Exp Mor Path **24** (1976) 142.
27. Fritz, TE *et al:* Exp Mor Path **12** (1970) 14.
28. Allen, WE and Longstaffe, JA: J Small Anim Pract **23** (1982) 337.

INJURIES TO THE EXTERNAL GENITALIA
BY THOMAS J. BURKE

Introduction

Physical trauma to the external genitalia of dogs and cats occurs mostly in males. Fight wounds are encountered in both dogs and cats and foreign body injuries are common in dogs, especially the sporting breeds. Chemical and thermal injuries are more serious in males than females.

Management of Injuries

The guiding principle in wound management is to minimize inflammation. Scrotal hyperthermia can result in either temporary or permanent loss of spermatogenesis. Scrotal wounds should be debrided and sutured as soon as possible and the technic used should be as aseptic and atraumatic as possible. Administration of antibiotics depends on the cause and duration of the wound, but most wounds can be considered to be infected. Until the results of bacterial culture and sensitivity testing are known, a broad-spectrum antibacterial agent should be given because wound contamination by soil will tend to result in Gram-positive aerobic and anaerobic infections and fecal contamination predisposes to Gram-negative infections of the scrotum. Scrotal cellulitis may result if treatment is delayed (Fig 1). Every effort should be made to minimize inflammation, including the application of cool compresses and the judicious use of glucocorticoids.

Postoperative self-multilation of genital wounds is not uncommon. Elizabethan collars and similar restraint devices should be used

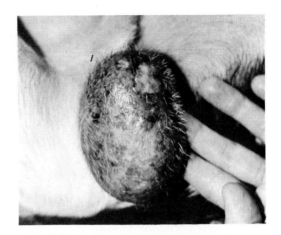

Fig 1. Scrotal swelling associated with cellulitis. This inflammation was painful and hyperthermic.

whenever necessary, but aromatic-based wound dressings should not be applied because they may induce local irritation. Diphemanil sulfate cream has been used to reduce self-mutilation and causes no apparent local irritation. Bandaging the wounded area is difficult and should probably not be attempted because it tends to retain heat.

A wounded testis should usually be removed because primary healing is virtually impossible and leakage of sperm from traumatized tubules into the interstitium leads to formation of sperm granulomas. In addition, exposure to testicular antigen may lead to development of immune-mediated orchitis that could affect both testes. One should be aware, however, that present AKC rules do not permit removal of a testis for any reason in animals to be shown in conformation competition. The owner may thus have to decide whether to maintain the animal for show purposes and risk his future as a stud or to improve his breeding future but lose his show potential. Postoperative considerations for testicular wounds are the same as for scrotal wounds.

Wounds of the penis and prepuce should be managed similarly to scrotal wounds. Inflammation of these structures is not as serious, however, as scrotal inflammation unless it results in urethral changes that impede ejaculation. When necessary to maintain patency of the urethra, an indwelling catheter may be inserted. Proper procedures to guard against ascending infection must be employed.

Fractures of the os penis are uncommon. They are usually simple transverse fractures that require minimal treatment because the fibrous tissue surrounding the os usually provides adequate stability. Hematoma formation, local edema, and comminuted fractures may occlude the urethra, which usually can be managed by inserting an in-

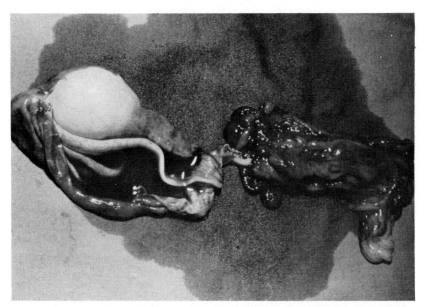

Fig 2. Intrascrotal hematocele resulted from thrombosis of the pampiniform plexus. The swelling was fluctuant and normothermic when the dog was presented.

dwelling catheter. In some cases, however, a perineal urethrotomy may be necessary. The penis should be amputated only as a last resort.

Though painful, blunt trauma to the testis usually does not result in permanent changes that would decrease fertility. There is always the danger of hematoma formation, however, that could occlude the duct system or disrupt seminiferous tubules and lead to formation of sperm granulomas or immune-mediated orchitis. Therefore, the prognosis for testicular injuries should be guarded.

The treatment of testicular injuries should be designed to minimize inflammation, including the use of glucocorticoids and cool compresses. Trauma to the base of the scrotum or inguinal area may disrupt the vas deferens or blood vessels, especially the pampiniform plexus (Fig 2). If disruption of a vas deferens persists, the wound can be repaired by vasovasostomy, which involves using microsurgical techniques. Disruption of blood supply is irreparable, however, and will result in loss of spermatogenesis in the affected testis.

Chemical and thermal injuries of a testis can result in either permanent or temporary loss of spermatogenesis. Following removal of

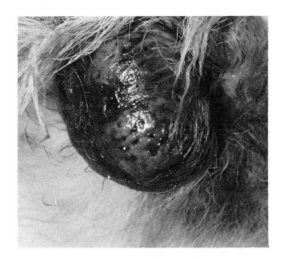

Fig 3. Scrotal swelling caused by a constrictive foreign body (twine). The scrotum exuded serum and was discolored and hypothermic.

the offending substance, anti-inflammatory therapy should be instituted. The prognosis should be guarded.

A cool, swollen scrotum is usually due to a constrictive foreign body (eg, rubber band, string) that has been placed around the base of the scrotum. The scrotal skin in such cases becomes discolored and serum oozes from it (Fig 3). By the time that the animal is presented, the changes are nearly always permanent. Castration and scrotal ablation are recommended.

Vulvar injuries are usually not serious, although the owner is often alarmed by the amount of hemorrhage. Lacerations should be treated as described for scrotal tears except that anti-inflammatory therapy is not necessary. Puncture wounds are best left open and flushed frequently with hydrogen peroxide. Antibiotic liquids or lotions are also indicated. Lacerations at or near the dorsal commissure of the vulva may result in cicatrization that can impede intromission by the male or normal delivery of fetuses if pregnancy ensues. In such cases a permanent episiotomy should be performed.

Injuries of the uterus are usually not serious unless they occur when the uterus contains fluid or pus or is gravid. Rupture at that time can lead to extrauterine pregnancy, sterile peritonitis, or septic peritonitis. Radiographs and abdominal paracentesis assist a diagnosis. The treatment is surgical, including unilateral hysterectomy. An attempt should be made to preserve uterine function if the animal's owner wants to preserve the female's fertility. Suture patterns should be chosen that minimize the chance of annular cicatrization.

INTERSEXUALITY
BY THOMAS J. BURKE

Introduction

Intersexuality or hermaphroditism is a term that generally applies to individuals whose sexual identity is obscure. The term has been used for individuals who are phenotypically normal but whose nuclear or chromosomal sex is opposite to their gonadal sex (sex-reversed individuals).[1] In this section we will consider only those animals whose genitalia have both male and female elements because karyotyping is not widely practiced by veterinary clinicians.

Etiology

The gonads, urethra, and external genitalia of mammals arise from bipotential anlagen, but the internal genitalia arise from sex-specific tissue: Wolffian ducts for the male and Mullerian ducts for the female. Maleness must be induced by secretions from the fetal testes whereas femaleness is basic and will develop regardless of the state of the fetal ovaries.

The etiology of hermaphroditism includes (1) abnormal sex chromosomes, (2) exposure to virilizing agents *in utero*, (3) in utero

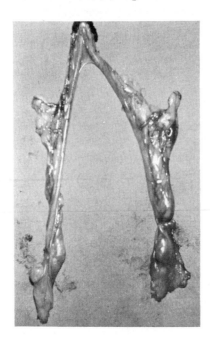

Fig 1. Uterus and ovotestes from a true hermaphrodite (Afghan Hound).

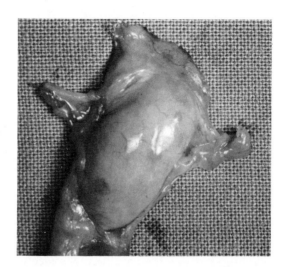

Fig 2. Ovotestis from a hermaphroditic Afghan Hound.

trauma that damages the reproductive organs, and (4) single-gene mutations that interfere with normal biochemical events in the fetus (*eg,* androgen synthesis). Abnormal sex chromosomes, such as XXY (Klinefelter's syndrome), does not induce intersexuality. Affected individuals are sterile, however. This is extremely rare in the dog. Single X females (Turner's syndrome) has not been reported in the bitch. In one review of 100 cases of intersexuality in dogs, 52 were in-

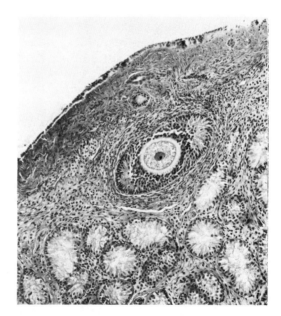

Fig 3. Photomicrograph of ovotestis in Figure 2.

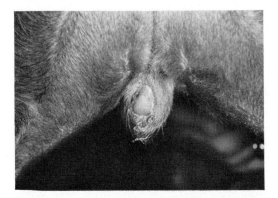

Fig 4. Clitoral hypertrophy and ventral displacement of the vulva in a male pseudo-hermaphroditic Weimaraner. Notice discharge associated with clitoritis.

duced *in utero* by administration of virilizing agents (testosterones or norethindrone with progesterone) and 48 arose spontaneously.[2] Karyotyping was done in 21 of the latter and XX was found in all forms of intersexuality, while XY was found in only male pseudohermaphrodites and unclassified intersexes. Mosaicism was found only in true hermaphrodites.

Clinical Types

Hermaphrodites are classified by the histology of their gonads. True hermaphrodites possess both testicular and ovarian tissue in the form of one ovary and one testis or both in one gonad (an ovotestis) (Figs 1, 2, 3) or any combination (*ie,* a testis and an ovotestis). Male pseudohermaphrodites have non-scrotal testes and may have external characteristics resembling either a male or female (Fig 4). Female pseudohermaphrodites have ovaries and are masculine in external appearance (Figs 5, 6). The external appearance of true hermaphrodites is that of a female with clitoral hypertrophy. The clitoris may even resemble a small penis and contain an os.

Male pseudohermaphroditism is the most commonly encountered of the intersexes and female pseudohermaphroditism is the least common. There does appear to be breed-associated incidence of intersex, suggesting a genetic basis. This is especially the case for Cocker Spaniels that are true hermaphrodites and is highly suspected in Chinese Pugs and Beagles. Breed-associated male pseudohermaphroditism has been reported in Cocker Spaniels and Miniature Schnauzers and is suspected in Chinese Pugs.[3] Though intersex dogs are usually infertile, there is one report of a true hermaphrodite Cocker Spaniel whelping a litter of 3 pups, one of which was an XX male.[4]

True hermaphrodites and feminine-form male pseudohermaphrodites are usually presented at a young age because of the clitoral

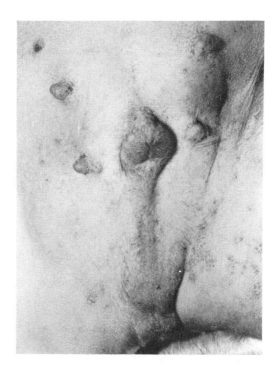

Fig 5. External genitalia of
a female hermaphroditic
Miniature Schnauzer.
Notice underdevelopment
of prepuce and scrotum.

hypertrophy and associated clitoritis. The owner usually desires that
the pet appears to be normal. Amputation of the clitoris will usually
resolve the major problem, but excretory urography must be performed prior to surgery to determine where the urethra empties. Gonadohysterectomy is recommended because there may also be internal anatomic defects that can fill with fluid. Removal of the gonads
will not result in atrophy of the clitoris.

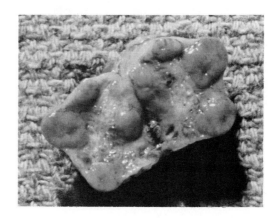

Fig 6. Sectioned ovary from
female pseudohermaphro-
ditic Miniature Schnauzer.
Notice corpora lutea.

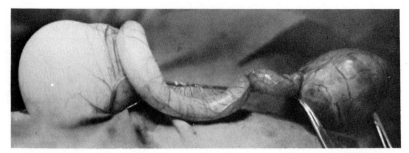

Fig 7. Sertoli-cell tumor in retained testis (right) and cystic uterus masculinus in prostate gland (left).

Masculine-form male pseudohermaphrodites and female pseudo-hermaphrodites are usually presented as adults with signs referable to the reproductive tract. Sertoli cell neoplasia and either mucometra or pyometra may be seen in male pseudohermaphrodites (Fig 7). Female pseudohermaphrodites may have gynecomastia, lactate, bleed from the "penis," or have pyometra (Fig 8). The bleeding may be cyclic and coincide with normal ovarian activity. The treatment for all of these anomalies is gonadohysterectomy.

References
1. Hare, WCD: Cytogenetics. In *Current Therapy in Theriogenology.* Ed by DA Morrow. WB Saunders, Philadelphia. 1980. p. 119.
2. Hare, WCD: Can Vet J **17** (1976) 7.
3. Selden, JR: Compendium Cont Ed for SA Pract **1** (1979) 435.
4. Selden, JR, *et al:* Science **201** (1978) 644.

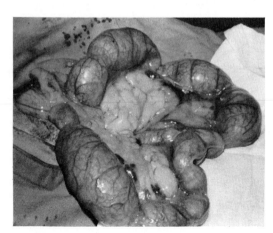

Fig 8. Pyometra in pseudo-hermaphroditic Miniature Schnauzer.

HORMONAL IMBALANCES
BY THOMAS J. BURKE

Introduction

Subfertility can be associated with most major hormonal imbalances. Such conditions as diabetes mellitus, Cushing's disease, and Addison's disease may be accompanied by disturbances in gamete production and they usually are associated with infertility until controlled with appropriate medication or surgery. For example, I recommend ovariohysterectomy for animals with diabetes mellitus because of the extreme difficulty in regulating the dosage of insulin for the intact females due to the anti-insulin effects of estrogen and progesterone. The normal daily output of testosterone in intact males does not seem to appreciably alter insulin requirements.

Hypothyroidism is the most common condition that directly affects the reproductive tract in dogs. This condition is extremely rare in cats. The signs referable to the reproductive tract are variable and in males include decreased libido, slight to moderate decrease in testicular size, palpable softening of the testicular parenchyma, and hypospermia. In the female the most common sign is an abnormal estrous cycle (prolonged anestrus, abbreviated proestrus and estrus, "weak" estrus). I have seen a few affected bitches, however, with apparently normal estrous cycles but unable to conceive. The only detectable abnormality in these animals was hypothyroidism. Administration of synthetic thyroxine resulted in conception and successful pregnancies. It is thus recommended that appropriate laboratory evaluation of thyroid function be an integral part of the examination of all patients presented because of infertility.

Hormonal Infertility in Females

Prolonged Anestrus

Prolonged anestrus may be either congenital or acquired. It is thought that the congenital form arises from a lack of normal function of the hypothalamo-hypophyseal axis. The cause is unknown. These animals have juvenile vulvas and no evidence of mammary development. Microscopic examination of ovarian tissues reveals primary follicles but no evidence that ovulation has occurred. The thyroid function of affected animals is normal. Plasma estradiol and progesterone are at baseline levels. Because some females do not attain puberty until 18 to 20 months of age, I am reluctant to make a diagnosis of prolonged anestrus until the patient is 24 months old.

After the initial examination and prior to giving exogenous hormones, the patient should be confined with another female in heat and close to a vigorous male. Under such conditions the patient is exposed to the pheromones of other animals. Such exposure has resulted in estrus and conception in some cases.

Exogenous hormone therapy involves the administration of gonadotropins to induce a normal fertile estrus. Although the administration of estrogens will result in overt signs of estrus, follicles are not developed. Among the various regimens for gonadotropin administration, most involve the use of pregnant mare serum gonadotropin (PMSG) as a source of follicle stimulating hormone (FSH) and human chorionic gonadotropin (HCG) as a source of luteinizing hormone (LH). I have had mixed results with PMSG, presumably because of variation in potency among the batches of this product. I have had more consistent results with pituitary-derived FSH (FSH-P).

The dosage of FSH-P for bitches is 0.75 mg/kg given IM daily for 10 days. HCG is then given IM for 2 days at a dose of 500 IU/kg. Mating is allowed at any time during the treatment. A few patients will stand for the male as early as the 8th day of treatment. Some bitches will not accept the male until the 17th day after initiation of treatment. Gonadotropin-releasing hormone (GnRH) may be given instead of HCG. It appears to be equally effective in inducing ovulation. The dose of GnRH is 5 to 50 mcg per patient given IM.

Some animals given this therapy will have normal estrous cycles within a few months of the treatment if conception does not occur. Others will require the therapy whenever they are to be mated. Conception rates have averaged about 75% in otherwise normal bitches.

This treatment may be used to schedule a litter in normal bitches. It is expensive, however. Prior to initiation of such therapy, the animal's plasma progesterone should be at baseline level. The bitch's normal estrous cycle will not be permanently altered by this treatment.

Acquired anestrus can be caused by cystic ovaries; neoplasia of the pituitary gland, midbrain, or ovary; hypothyroidism; and any other disease that severely affects homeostasis. Prior to giving exogenous hormones a thorough clinical examination is mandatory. If no other cause can be found for the prolonged anestrus, the described therapy may result in a fertile estrus.

To induce estrus in an otherwise normal queen, I have given FSH-P at a dosage of 1 mg/cat/day for 5 days. It is administered IM. Following mating an exogenous source of LH (HCG-500IU or GnRH-10 mcg) IM is given to help ensure ovulation.

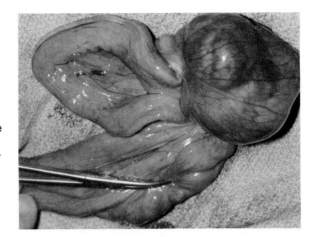

Fig 1. Estrogen-producing ovarian cysts in a Mastiff caused prolonged estrus. The normal ovary is grasped by a forceps.

Cystic Ovaries

Ovarian cysts may produce estrogens that result in prolonged proestrus-estrus (nymphomania), progesterone, or no hormones (Fig 1). When progesterone or no hormones are produced, anestrus is prolonged. Progesterone-producing cysts may cause cystic endometrial hyperplasia (Fig 2). They cannot be differentiated from estrogen-producing cysts by gross examination, but by microscopic examination of uterine tissues and plasma hormone evaluations the biochemical activity of ovarian cysts can be determined.

Estrogen-producing cysts will cause an estrus-like state that persists longer than 21 days. The vulva becomes edematous and a

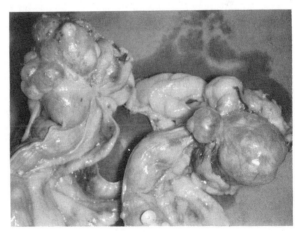

Fig 2. Progesterone-producing ovarian cysts. Also notice the endometrial cysts. This is a formalin-fixed specimen.

vaginal discharge may be pink-tinged to clear or nonexistent. Vaginal cytology will reveal evidence of estrogen stimulation (all cells are either fully or partially cornified and white blood cells are absent) that does not change from week to week. These cysts are large and may be palpable or visible in radiographs.

Treatment of estrogen-producing cysts involves an attempt to induce ovulation with LH. Intramuscular injections of HCG (500 IU/kg) or GnRH (10 to 100 mcg/patient) are given daily for 3 days. If there is no clinical or cytologic change in a week, the treatment is repeated at double the initial dose. If this fails, the cyst is drained surgically with a needle and syringe after a laparotomy. Animals that are treated successfully usually return to a normal estrous cycle within a few months and may then be bred. Conceptions have occurred on the first post-treatment mating. I am unaware of any recurrence of these cysts.

Cysts that result in prolonged anestrus may also be large enough to be palpated or visualized radiographically. Because they appear to be resistant to exogenous LH therapy, surgery (drainage or ovariectomy) is recommended.

Frequent Estrus

Some bitches have an apparently normal estrus every 3½ to 4 months. They are almost always infertile. The cause may be lack of ovulation (unsubstantiated by the author) or it is possible that the endometrium does not have an opportunity to undergo complete involution and is unsuitable for implantation (nidation). In such cases, the patient is given mibolerone for 6 to 12 months and then allowed to have an estrus. If this occurs within 60 days after therapy, breeding should be postponed until the next estrus.

Failure of Ovulation

Failure of ovulation is often suspected by the owner, but it is seldom confirmed. Gross and microscopic examinations of corpora lutea do not reveal that they are functional. Plasma progesterone levels should be measured 21 and 30 to 50 days after cessation of estrus. They should be significantly elevated above baseline levels if functional luteal tissue is present, thus confirming that ovulation had occurred. If ovulation has not occurred, the animal can be given HCG or GnRH at her next mating. The hormone is given at the doses used to treat cystic ovaries beginning on the day after her first mating.

Hormonal Infertility in Males

The precise physiology of spermatogenesis, ejaculation, and erection is still poorly understood in the dog and cat. For this reason, few syndromes of infertility with a hormonal basis have been identified in males.

Lack of Libido

Because the major cause for lack of libido seems to be psychologic, affected male animals should be placed with trainers who excel at training studs. Lack of libido has been associated with low levels of testosterone in a few dogs. Brain tumors and estrogen-producing tumors of the testes have also been incriminated. Plasma testosterone should be measured and if it is below baseline level then replacement therapy may be considered. Because testosterone may stimulate a negative feedback through the hypothalamo-gonadal axis, the dosage must be carefully selected. The empirical use of testosterone in any male that refuses to breed should be discouraged.

The normal 24-hour production of testosterone in the dog has been estimated to be 0.1 to 0.25 mg/kg. I have prescribed methyltestosterone to be given orally at this dose for 21 to 30 days and then attempted to ejaculate the dog in the presence of a teaser bitch. Plasma testosterone is also re-evaluated and the dose is altered accordingly.

Hypospermia and Gonadal Atrophy

These conditions could presumably be caused by lack of appropriate amounts of endogenous gonadotropins. In the majority of cases, however, they appear to be due to some other cause, such as trauma, hyperthermia, neoplasia, hypothyroidism, or drugs. If after a complete examination no other cause can be found, a testicular biopsy should be performed. In a few cases, non-inflammatory changes have resulted in arrest of spermiogenesis and/or Leydig cell hypoplasia. One might assume that animals with Leydig cell dysfunction are lacking in LH, while those with primary tubular hypoplasia have a deficiency of FSH. Therapy has been based on these suppositions. Successful treatments have not been found, however, and the prognosis for these cases is poor. I have observed one case in which a Collie with spermatogenic arrest and Leydig cell hypoplasia was treated with 250 IU of HCG twice weekly for 60 days. This dog sired a litter shortly after the treatment was completed. Other cases in my experience have been failures and until more is known about the physiology of male reproduction in dogs, they will probably continue to be so.

INFECTIOUS CAUSES OF ABORTION AND STILLBIRTH IN CATS
BY GREGORY C. TROY AND MARY A. HERRON

Introduction

During the last 10 years additional information has been obtained about the infectious causes of prenatal and postnatal mortality in kittens. In this section we will discuss the role of bacteria and viruses as causal agents of abortions, stillbirths, and neonatal deaths.

Bacterial Infections

Bacteria can enter the uterus when the cervix is open during breeding and parturition. Organisms entering at breeding are likely to cause abortion because the progesterone-influenced environment of the pregnant uterus is ideal for bacterial growth. *E coli,* staphylococci, streptococci, salmonella, and mycobacteria may be involved, but no specific disease, such as canine brucellosis, has been identified in the cat.[1]

Signs preceding abortion include pyrexia, malaise, abdominal discomfort, straining, inappetence, and vaginal discharge. The discharge may have a fetid odor and be yellow to brownish-red. If the pregnancy is advanced, recognizable fetuses or portions of fetuses in various stages of decomposition and shreds of fetal membranes may be seen in the discharge. Infections that persist without treatment may result in weakness, dehydration, hypothermia, and death. In acute infections the hemogram is characterized by neutrophilic leukocytosis and the vaginal smear contains bacteria, numerous neutrophils, and possibly placental and uterine cells. In more persistent or chronic cases, hemograms reflect toxic changes.

Treatment is designed to eliminate the causal agent and empty the uterus. Initially, material taken from the cervix is used for culturing and antibacterial sensitivity testing. Until results of sensitivity testing are known, a broad-spectrum bactericidal antibiotic should be administered along with fluids and other supportive measures.

Administration of drugs to stimulate uterine contraction may be useful in evacuating this organ. Injection (IM) of 0.1 mg of ergonovine maleate (Ergonil) followed by oral administration of the same drug (0.05 mg BID for 2 to 3 days) may stimulate uterine contraction.[2] Prostaglandin F_{2a} (Lutalyse) has also been found efficacious for stimulating uterine contractions. Subcutaneous injection (0.5 mg/kg) of this agent has caused abortion in cats after the 40th day of gestation.[3] Dosages of 0.1 to 0.25 mg/kg have been used to empty the uterus of female dogs with endo- and pyometritis.[4] Prostaglandin F_{2a} has only been used experimentally in the cat, however, and has not yet been approved for clinical use in this species.

The uterus may be emptied by lavage through the cervix combined with external manipulation of the uterine horns through the abdomen. Inherent in this procedure is the risk of rupturing the uterus because it is difficult to assess damage caused by palpation or passage of a lavage catheter. For these reasons exposing the uterus surgically has definite advantages. It enables direct observation of the uterus and facilitates manipulation of the tissues and lavage catheter.

If necessary, a hysterotomy can be performed to thoroughly empty and clean the uterus. Though it must be done carefully to prevent contamination of the peritoneal cavity, this surgery provides an opportunity to obtain a biopsy sample and inspect the endometrium. Ovariohysterectomy is an acceptable treatment for metritis when the tissue damage is beyond repair and when the queen will not be used for breeding.

When medical therapy is provided for metritis in queens, the antibacterial medication should be continued for at least 2 to 3 weeks and the queen should be monitored through the next breeding period. Cervical swabs may be cultured during the succeeding estrus to determine whether or not infection persists. Recovery of breeding potential after eliminating a bacterial infection depends on regeneration of an adequate endometrium.

Prevention of bacterial abortion involves proper management of cats used for breeding. Tomcats should not be allowed to breed queens that have genital discharges or histories suggesting genital infection. The genitalia of both the male and female should be examined before every breeding. Animals with any bacterial infection should be isolated from breeding cats.

Viral Infections

Feline Herpesvirus 1

Feline herpesvirus 1 causes infectious rhinotracheitis and a wide variety of other clinical manifestations. This is an enveloped DNA virus and is highly species-specific.[5-7] The virus survives only for hours in a moist environment and is sensitive to heat, acids, and a variety of disinfectants.[6,8,9]

Herpesvirus 1 infection usually is reflected by signs of upper respiratory disease. The organism may be transmitted intranasally, orally, or conjunctivally through direct contact with contaminated secretions.[5-7,10-12] The clinical signs of infection include fever, anorexia, depression, sneezing, coughing, ocular and nasal discharges, and keratitis. Infection of pregnant animals may result in abortion or infection of the fetuses.[7,11,13-15]

Inapparent infections with herpesvirus 1 and chronic carrier animals are known to exist.[6,10-12,16,17] In one survey it was found that 80% of infected animals became carriers and that 45% of these animals were involved in transmission of the infection.[18] Carriers of the virus may shed it intermittently after periods of stress.[18] Generalized infections occur in neonatal animals and are commonly accompanied by high mortality. Fibrinosuppurative rhinitis, tracheitis, bronchopneumonia, keratitis with secondary panophthalmitis, and focal hepatic necrosis are commonly observed in infected neonates.[12-14,19]

The pathogenesis of abortions due to feline herpesvirus 1 depends on the route of infection. Following intravenous or intranasal inoculation, abortion occurs during the 5th to 6th week of gestation.[13] Lesions within the placental vasculature occur with IV inoculation. Virus and viral antigen can be isolated from the placenta and uterus, but not from fetuses. Lesions include multiple infarcts and thromboses in the placenta, endometrium, and maternal vessels.[13] Lesions are not found in the placenta, uterus, or fetuses of animals infected intranasally.

In pregnant queens that were infected IV, the clinical signs included sanguineous vaginal discharge, fever, and serous nasal discharge 24 hours prior to aborting. Intranasal exposure to the virus caused severe upper respiratory disease, but not vaginal discharges, in pregnant queens.[13]

Intravaginal instillation of the feline herpesvirus 1 did not produce abortion.[7,19] It did result in vaginal hyperemia, serous vaginal discharges, and signs of upper respiratory disease.

Diagnosis of herpesvirus 1 infection is based on the associated clinical signs and isolation of the virus. When isolated in feline kidney cell cultures, herpesvirus 1 produces characteristic cytopathic effects that include cellular lysis, multinucleated giant cells, and type-A intranuclear inclusion bodies.[5,20] Serum neutralization titers and direct immunofluorescent tests may also be used as diagnostic aids. Nasal, pharyngeal, and tonsillar swabs provide adequate specimens for viral isolation.

Because of the high incidence of herpesvirus 1 in catteries, viral isolation is the best method of detecting infected animals. Though the absence of clinical signs in carrier animals may lead to a false impression, viral isolation studies enable their proper identification. Chronic carriers may shed the virus when given a glucocorticoid for 2 to 3 days.[16,21]

Prevention of feline rhinotracheitis has been difficult. Injectable vaccines have not provided adequate immunity to prevent infection or the carrier state. A more recently developed vaccine (Rhinolin-CP) that is given intranasally may provide more rapid and complete protection against feline herpesvirus 1 than the injectable products.[11,16,17] The development of chronic carriers may also be prevented by using the intranasal vaccine.[16,17] Kittens respond to vaccination by 8 weeks of age. Giving them 2 doses of vaccine 4 weeks apart should provide adequate immunity. Booster vaccinations should be administered annually. In catteries and breeding colonies in which viral respiratory diseases are prevalent, biannual boosters may be indicated.

Feline Panleukopenia

Feline panleukopenia is caused by a small non-enveloped, single-stranded DNA virus of the genus parvovirus. This organism is very stable and is resistant to alcohol, phenol, ether, quaternary ammonium compounds, iodines, and increased temperature.[9] Effective disinfectants for it are sodium hypochlorite, formaldehyde, and glutaldehyde.[9] Feline panleukopenia is an acute, highly contagious disease and it primarily affects animals less than one year of age. A greater incidence has been observed in late summer and early fall. High morbidity and mortality rates, sometimes approaching 100%, may occur in susceptible populations.

The virus is transmitted by direct contact of susceptible animals with saliva, feces, urine, and vomitus from infected animals.[22,23] Neonatally infected kittens may shed the virus in urine for as long as 57 weeks.[24]

The disease is characterized by anorexia, depression, fever, vomiting, diarrhea, and dehydration. Sudden deaths occur. Infection of pregnant queens can result in neonatal death, abortion, stillbirths, and teratogenic effects, including cerebellar hypoplasia.[23,25]

When a pregnant queen becomes infected, the virus passes the placental barrier and infects the fetuses. Viral replication is demonstrable within placental cells, but histopathologic lesions are not evident.[24] Transplacental passage of the virus does not necessarily result in infection of all the fetuses in a litter. The tissues most severely affected in neonatal animals are those with a high degree of mitosis, such as the external granular layer of the cerebellum, thymus, small intestinal epithelium, lymphoid tissue, and hematopoietic tissue.[5,8,22]

Infection of pregnant queens may be reflected by mild to severe clinical signs. When the signs are severe, they primarily reflect gastrointestinal disease. Subclinical infections may result in abortion, stillbirths, or cerebellar ataxia of one or more littermates.[12,23,25]

Neonatal kittens with cerebellar hypoplasia exhibit ataxia, hypermetria, intentional head tremors, rolling, and spasticity. These signs are not progressive, which helps to differentiate cerebellar hypoplasia from other central nervous disorders that are inheritable and progressive. All of the kittens in a litter are not affected.[23] Cerebellar size may be reduced to a fifth of its normal size; the degree of hypoplasia is not directly proportional to the severity of the clinical signs, however.[25]

The diagnosis of feline panleukopenia is based on the history, clinical signs, demonstration of leukopenia, histopathology, and isolation of the virus. Urine, feces, and vomitus are used to demonstrate the virus.[20] Typical histopathologic lesions include cerebellar hypoplasia, collapse of intestinal crypts, hypoplasia of bone marrow, and depletion of T-dependent areas of lymphoid tissue.[5]

Losses caused by panleukopenia virus can be prevented by vaccination. Vaccinated queens pass from 80 to 90% of their antibody titers to their offspring via colostrum within 24 hours after birth.[26] The half-life of these antibodies is 9.5 days and protective titers are 1:80 or greater. Kittens then become susceptible to infection by 8 to 12 weeks postpartum. A modified-live-virus vaccine should be given to kittens at 8 to 10 weeks of age and a booster vaccination should be given a month later.[27] Available vaccines may be given IM, SC or intranasally. When kittens are older than 3 months when first vaccinated, a single injection will be adequate.[27] Killed-virus vaccines can be given to pregnant queens, but the use of modified-live-virus vaccines may result in cerebellar hypoplasia in the kittens.

Strict sanitation should be practiced to prevent transmission of panleukopenia virus. Sodium hypochlorite (1:32 dilution) has been found to be an economical and effective disinfectant. Susceptible cats entering households or catteries where outbreaks of panleukopenia have occurred should be vaccinated 2 weeks before being exposed.

Feline Infectious Peritonitis
Feline infectious peritonitis (FIP) is caused by a coronavirus. This enveloped RNA virus is fragile and is susceptible to most common

disinfectants.[5] Another coronavirus has recently been isolated from cats and it is ubiquitous among cats, causes enteritis, and is antigenically similar to FIPV.[28] It has been suggested that this virus may mutate to FIPV.

Transmission of FIPV is thought to be by oral or nasal routes.[29-30] Infection with FIPV was once thought to be common, but because of its serologic relationship to enteric coronavirus, past surveys of FIPV prevalence may be misleading.

FIPV has recently been incriminated as a possible cause of a variety of clinical syndromes characterized by reproductive failures and high neonatal and kitten mortality. The syndrome has been referred to as the "kitten mortality complex" (KMC).[30-32] Whether or not other infectious agents are involved in KMC is not known. Studies to date have implicated FIPV as a cause of infertility, repeat breeding, stillbirths, endometritis, abortion, chronic upper respiratory infections, fetal resorption, fading kittens, and cardiovascular disease. This pathogenicity is in addition to the classical forms of FIP, which include peritoneal effusions, pleural effusions, and pyogranulomatous lesions within single or multiple organs.

KMC has been reported in the Himalayan, Persian, Siamese, Domestic Shorthair, and Burmese breeds.[31-33] The highest incidence has been in Himalayans. Young and old queens have been equally affected. The role of male cats in the disease complex is not known. Breeding colonies in which KMC has occurred have been relatively free of feline leukemia virus, feline herpesvirus 1, feline calicivirus, feline panleukopenia virus, and *Toxoplasma.*

Reproductive failure in queens may be the result of conception failure, fetal resorption, abortion, stillbirths, or fetal mummification.[30,31] Queens do not exhibit severe signs of disease during abortion or fetal resorption.[31-33] The abortions occur within the last half of gestation; the majority occur during the last 2 weeks.[32] The partially formed fetuses have subcutaneous hemorrhages. Excessive vaginal bleeding may be observed in some queens following an abortion. Some or all kittens of a litter may be stillborn.

Kitten mortality in catteries with KMC may approach 40%. Fading kittens usually succumb within the first few weeks of life. Anorexia, failure to gain weight, and emaciation are characteristic.

A variety of cardiovascular lesions has been found in kittens that die suddenly with acute respiratory distress. Stress may precipitate the development of clinical signs. Congestive cardiomyopathy has been diagnosed by histologic examination; acute degeneration of muscle fibers and subendocardial fibroelastosis have been the most prominent lesions. Other common lesions include septal defects, chronic interstitial pneumonia, thrombosis, hemorrhage of pulmonary parenchyma, and endocarditis.[32]

The clinical signs exhibited by adult animals in KMC colonies are variable. Signs of chronic respiratory disease are common, however. Unexplainable fever is frequently detected. Cats may become depressed and anorectic for several days and then behave normally. Endometritis is a major problem among queens in the colony. As many as 41% of the queens in one cattery had signs of endometritis.[32]

Diagnosis of FIPV infection is based on clinical signs, appropriate clinical pathologic tests, histologic examinations, and serology.[35] Technics for viral isolation have only recently been perfected and are not widely available for routine application. Serologic tests are perhaps the best method of detecting FIPV infection. The results of such tests must be considered in the light of the clinical signs, other clinical pathologic tests, and histopathologic lesions. Both indirect immunofluorescent and enzyme-linked immunosorbent (ELISA) tests are available; the latter is more sensitive and reproducible. These tests detect only antibody to FIP virus and not the virus. At present, there is no way of differentiating immune cats from asymptomatic carriers.

The recent identification of enteric coronavirus (EC) has caused problems concerning the serologic tests used to detect antibodies to FIPV. These 2 viruses are antigenically similar, and thus are inseparable by current tests. Antibody titers greater than 1:1600 are uncommon in cats infected with EC, but such titers are common in cats with FIP.[28]

Feline Leukemia

Feline leukemia virus (FeLV) is a member of the family Retroviridae, genus Oncovirus. It is a single stranded RNA virus that contains the enzyme called reverse transcriptase.[35] This virus is shed in the urine, feces, and saliva of infected cats.[36] It is very unstable and seldom survives more than a few hours at room temperature. It is inactivated by most disinfectants.

Because FeLV is labile in the environment, infection probably occurs by direct contact between infected and susceptible cats. The incidence of infection in the general population of cats is about 2%. In certain catteries it is 30 to 50%.[37,38] The high incidence of FeLV infection in some catteries may be related to the exchange of cats for breeding, overcrowding, and use of common utensils. Dissemination of infection is always favored by the congregating of cats.

Clinical manifestations of FeLV infection are varied. Lymphosarcoma, leukemia, aplastic anemia, glomerulonephritis, fetal thymic atrophy, abortion, and fetal resorption have all occurred in infected cats.[35,37-39]

Abortion and fetal resorption associated with FeLV infection usually occur between the 3rd week of gestation and term. Surveys of cats presented because they don't conceive, have aborted, or suffered fetal resorption have revealed that 68 to 92% were positive for FeLV.[37,40] Queens that are involved usually show no signs of infection. Examination of their uteri reveals retention of fetal placental tissue without signs of inflammation and degenerated fetuses.[37] It is thought that the FeLV damages the maternal-fetal attachment.[40]

Diagnosis of abortion or fetal resorption associated with FeLV should be based on the results of the direct immunofluorescent test or the enzyme-linked immunosorbent test. These tests determine the presence or absence of virus or viral antigen in blood components or in serum. Differences in their results have been observed. The ELISA test may be positive during the incubation of an FeLV infection before platelets and neutrophils are infected. Cats that fail to develop an adequate immune response will usually become positive to both tests.

In catteries it is essential that all animals be tested for FeLV. Cats that are positive should be isolated or euthanized. Before animals are added to a cattery, they should have 2 negative tests. It is preferable that new animals not be added to a "clean" colony of cats.

Protozoal Infection

Toxoplasmosis

Most infections by *Toxoplasma gondii* in cats are subclinical, as demonstrated by the results of serologic surveys.[41-43] Infections have also been reported in most of the domestic animals and man. The cat is the only known definitive host in which the sexual phase of the organism exists.[44,45]

Transmission of *Toxoplasma* has been found to occur through ingestion of infected intermediate hosts or sporulated oocysts and transplacentally.[41,42-50] In the cat, ingestion of infected hosts or sporulated oocysts are the primary ways of acquiring infections. In a recent article, however, what might be the first cases of transplacental transmission in the cat were reported.[48] Experimental transmission of toxoplasmosis in the cat has not been reported.[52]

Clinical signs of toxoplasmosis in the adult cat usually reflect acute respiratory disease. Anorexia, depression, dyspnea, peripheral lymphadenopathy, and hepatosplenomegaly are common.[43-46,48] Signs of central nervous system disorder, such as incoordination and seizures, have also been described.[45,46] Ocular involvement is common in both experimental and naturally occurring cases.[43-48,51] Infections in neonatal kittens have been reflected by anorexia, depression, dyspnea, ocular discharges, incoordination, and death.[48] In these cases the queens did not have clinical signs related to the infection.

The diagnosis of toxoplasmosis is based on finding oocysts in fecal preparations, serologic tests, and histopathologic examination of infected tissues. Fecal specimens should be examined when fresh. Because cats may shed oocysts intermittently, several specimens should be examined.

A variety of serologic tests have been used to diagnose toxoplasmosis, including complement fixation, indirect hemagglutination, indirect immunofluorescent, Sabin-Feldman dye test, and enzyme-linked immunosorbent assays.[41,42,44,46,48] They all have proved reliable in clinical situations. A 4-fold increase in antibody titer indicates recent infection. The titer level should be measured at least twice, 2 to 4 weeks apart, because 15 to 64% of domestic cats carry *Toxoplasma* antibodies.[41,42] It has been reported that most infected cats are negative on serologic tests during the period that they are shedding oocysts.[48]

In clinical cases a diagnosis of toxoplasmosis may be suggested by thoracic radiographs. In many cases there is a pattern of nodular densities with ill-defined margins throughout the lungs.[43] Air bronchograms are usually present also.

In suspected cases it may be possible to demonstrate the presence of *Toxoplasma* by microscopic examination of tissue fluids obtained from the lungs, lymph nodes, or liver. Histopathologic changes include pneumonitis, hepatitis, lymphadenitis, myocarditis, myositis, encephalitis, and retinitis.[43-48,51] Multifocal areas of necrosis with infiltration of mononuclear cells and tachyzoites containing cysts are prominent findings.

The drugs of choice in the treatment of toxoplasmosis are sulfadiazine and pyrimethamine.[43,46] Dosages suggested for cats are 100 mg/kg/day of sulfadiazine, divided into 4 doses, and 1 mg/kg/day of pyrimethamine. Some success has been experienced in the treatment of toxoplasmosis with a sulfadiazine-trimethoprim combination (Tribrissen).

Preventing toxoplasmosis involves good sanitation, confinement to prevent carnivorism, and feeding dry, canned, or well-cooked food.[43,44,46] In catteries, serologic testing can detect active infections when they occur and infected animals can be removed. Cats with

Table 1. Infectious Causes of Abortion and Stillbirth in Cats

Causal Agent	Disease	Diagnostic Tests	Material For Laboratory Examination
E coli Staphylococci Streptococci Salmonellae Mycobacteria	Bacterial endometritis	Complete blood count Vaginal or cervical cultures Vaginal cytology	EDTA blood Vaginal Swabs
Toxoplasma gondii	Toxoplasmosis	Fecal flotation Radiography Serology Histopathology	Fresh fecal specimen Serum Lungs, liver, brain, spleen, eyes, muscle, and small intestines
Herpesvirus 1	Rhinotracheitis	Virus isolation Fluorescent antibody test Serum neutralization Histopathology	Nasal, ocular, throat and lung swabs Nasal and conjunctival scrapings Serum Nasal mucosa, turbinates, lung, trachea, aborted fetus
Parvovirus	Panleukopenia	Complete blood count Virus isolation Electron microscopy Histopathology Serum neutralization	EDTA blood Urine, feces. vomitus, ileum, spleen, lymph nodes Fresh fecal specimen Ileum, liver, thymus, and cerebellum Serum
Coronavirus	Feline infectious peritonitis Kitten mortality complex	Complete blood count Biochemical profiles Electrophoresis Fluid analysis Serology Histopathology	EDTA blood Serum Serum Ascitic or thoracic effusions Serum Kidney, liver, lymph nodes, peritoneum, CNS, aborted fetus
Oncovirus	Feline leukemia complex	CBC, reticulocyte count Biochemical profiles Bone marrow exam Radiography Cytology Serology Histopathology	EDTA blood Serum Bone marrow aspiration Chest, abdomen Tumor, lymph nodes, blood, fluids Serum Tumor, lymph nodes, bone marrow

stable antibody titers may be immune to infection, however, and thus need not be removed.[46]

Prevention of Infections

Abortions and neonatal deaths in a cattery cause immediate concern because the causal agent may spread throughout the group and cause a severe loss of animals. In such cases the history becomes important. It is useful in defining the nature of the immediate problem, identifying past problems, and helping to identify animals that may be carriers of infection. The history of an abortion should include a detailed description of the clinical signs shown by the queens, the appearance of the fetuses, and identification of involved individuals. Males associated with the breeding should also be identified.

Animals that are the source of a problem or are carriers of an infectious agent may be difficult to identify. By tracing the movement of animals within a colony, however, and comparing it with the occurrence of the abortions it may be possible to establish an association with certain animals.

Though owners and managers of catteries are often sensitive about their management practices, needed information can usually be obtained by tactful questioning and careful observation. This involves information about isolation facilities and practices, grouping of animals by age, sharing of food utensils, use of disinfectants, type of diet(s), and record systems.

Table 1 is presented as a summary of the procedures used to diagnose infectious causes of abortion and stillbirths in cats.

References
1. Hemsley, LA: Vet Rec **68** (1956) 152.
2. Herron, MA and Stein, B: *Current Veterinary Therapy VII,* Small Animal Practice. pp 1231, 1237. WB Saunders Co, Philadelphia, 1980.
3. Nachreiner, RF and Marple, DN: Prostaglandins **7** (1974) 303.
4. Sokolowski, JH: JAAHA **16** (1980) 119.
5. Brunner, DW and Gillespie, JR: *Hagan's Infectious Diseases of Domestic Animals.* 7th ed, pp 484, 490; 574, 577. Cornell University Press, Ithaca, 1981.
6. Crandall, R: Adv Vet Sci Comp Med **17** (1973) 201.
7. Kahn, DE and Hoover, EA: Vet Clinic North Amer **6** (1976) 397.
8. Gillespie, JH and Scott, FW: Adv Vet Sci Comp Med **17** (1973) 163.
9. Scott, FW: Amer J Vet Res **41** (1980) 410.
10. Povey, RC: Canad Vet J **17** (1976) 93.
11. Ford, RB: Comp Cont Educ **1** (1979) 337.
12. Scott, FW and Gillespie, JH: Scope **17** (1973) 2.
13. Hoover, EA and Griesemer, RA: Amer J Path **65** (1971) 173.
14. Spradbrow, PG *et al:* Vet Rec **89** (1971) 542.
15. Hoover, EA and Griesemer, RA: JAVMA **158** (1971) 929.
16. Orr, CM *et al:* Vet Rec **106** (1980) 164.
17. Clark, WB *et al:* VM/SAC **75** (1980) 415.

18. Gaskell, RM and Wardley, RC: J Small Anim Pract **19** (1977) 1.
19. Bittle, JL and Peckman, JC: JAVMA **158** (1971) 927.
20. Weiss, RC and Scott, FW: Feline Pract **11 (1)** (1981) 31.
21. Gaskell, RM and Povey, RC: Vet Rec **93** (1973) 204.
22. Timoney, JF: Vet Clinic North Amer **6** (1976) 385.
23. Kilham, L *et al:* JAVMA **158** (1971) 888.
24. Csiza, CK *et al:* Amer J Vet Res **32** (1971) 419.
25. Csiza, CK *et al:* Infection and Immunity **3** (1971) 838.
26. Scott, FW *et al:* JAVMA **156** (1970) 439.
27. Feline Infectious Disease Colloq, JAVMA **158** (1971) 835.
28. Pedersen, NC *et al:* Amer J Vet Res **42** (1981) 368.
29. Sherding, RG: Comp Cont Educ **2** (1980) 95.
30. Norsworthy, GD: Feline Pract **9 (2)** (1979) 57.
31. Scott, F *et al:* Feline Pract **9 (2)** (1979) 44.
32. Norsworthy, GD: Feline Pract **4 (6)** (1974) 34.
33. Pedersen, NC and Madewell, BR: *Current Vet Therapy VII,* pp 404, 409. WB Saunders Co, Philadelphia, 1980.
34. Scott, FW *et al:* Feline Pract **8 (6)** (1978) 31.
35. Hardy, WD, Jr *et al:* Nature **244** (1973) 266.
36. Jarrett, WF *et al:* Nature **202** (1964) 567.
37. Cotter, SM *et al:* JAVMA **166** (1975) 449.
38. Hardy, WD, Jr *et al:* Cancer Res **36** (1976) 482.
39. Anderson, LJ *et al:* J Nat Cancer Inst **47** (1971) 807.
40. Hardy, WD, Jr: JAAHA **17** (1981) 941.
41. Jones, FE *et al:* Amer J Trop Med Hyg **6** (1957) 820.
42. Behymer, RD *et al:* JAVMA **162** (1973) 959.
43. Farrow, BRH and Love, DA: In: *Textbook of Veterinary Internal Medicine,* p 225. WB Saunders Co, Philadelphia, 1975.
44. Curridge, MJ: Comp Cont Ed **11(3)** (1980) 233.
45. Petrak, M and Carpenter, J: JAVMA **146** (1965) 728.
46. Frenkel, JK: Comp Immunol Microbiol Infect Dis **1** (1978) 15.
47. Dubey, JP and Frenkel, JK: J Protozool **19** (1972) 155.
48. Dubey, JP and Johnstone, I: JAAHA **18** (1982) 461.
49. Larsen, JW: Teratology **15** (1977) 213.
50. Watson, WA and Beverley, JKA: Vet Rec **88** (1971) 120.
51. Couvreur, J and Desmonts, G: Dev Med Child Neuro **4** (1962) 519.
52. Dubey, JP and Hoover, EA: JAVMA **170**(1977) 538.
53. Bartels, JE: Feline Pract **2 (3)** (1972) 11.

CANINE BRUCELLOSIS
BY LELAND E. CARMICHAEL

Introduction

Canine brucellosis is an important contagious disease that is characterized by testicular atrophy, epididymitis, and infertility in males; 3rd-trimester abortion in females; and generalized lymphadenopathy in either sex. It has special importance to breeders because infection with *Brucella canis* essentially ends a dog's reproductive ability. Most breeders are very aware of the disease and seek professional advice regarding it. The disease is insidious and difficult to diagnose. Treatment generally has been unsuccessful and no vaccine is available. Because the potential for rapid spread of the disease within a kennel is great, clinicians must be well-informed about the diagnosis, prevention, treatment, and control of canine brucellosis.

B canis was first isolated in 1966 from the placental and fetal tissues of aborted pups.[1,2] It was subsequently identified as the cause of widespread abortions and reproductive failures in dogs.[3,4] Initially believed to be widespread only in Beagles, the disease was subsequently diagnosed in other breeds and has been recognized throughout the US and several other countries.[4-6] Although the better-known *Brucella* species (*B abortus, B melitensis,* and *B suis*), can infect dogs, the disease in dogs caused by these species is self-limiting and the organisms do not appear to persist.[7] Canine brucellosis is more common in kennels with a high turnover of breeding dogs, but an ever-increasing number of infected pets have been found.

The reported prevalence of canine brucellosis varies depending on the area sampled and/or the diagnostic procedures employed.[4,8-11] Human infections with *B canis* have been recognized, but the disease in man usually is mild and the duration of illness is short compared with human brucellosis caused by the classical species.[4,12,13] Cats have been infected experimentally with *B canis,* but natural cases have not been reported.

Clinical Signs

Canine brucellosis is insidious in onset and its clinical manifestations vary greatly. The clinical signs are not sufficient evidence to diagnose the disease, but brucellosis should be considered in dogs with epididymitis, orchitis, or prostatitis, and in bitches that abort or are infertile.[4,15,16] The principal signs are generalized enlargement of lymph nodes, abortion, early embryonic death, epididymitis, and testicular degeneration. Although canine brucellosis is a systemic disease, there usually is no pyrexia.

Abortions usually occur between the 45th and 55th days of gestation, but they may occur earlier.[15] An important characteristic of canine brucellosis is the prolonged bacteremia, often persisting 1 to 2 years or longer.[15,17] The bacteremia may be intermittent, especially during the chronic stage.

Infection can occur by penetration of all mucous membranes. The pathogenesis of *B canis* resembles that of *Brucella* infections in other animals.[15] Dogs exposed orally usually developed a bacteremia within 2 to 3 weeks. Clinical signs were not evident during this period. The organisms become localized in lymph nodes, spleen, and the reproductive tract. Generalized enlargement of lymph nodes due principally to

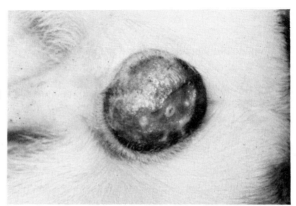

Fig 1. Scrotal ulceration
in dog infected with
B canis.

reticular cell hyperplasia is common in both sexes. [1,19] There is no
fever. In the pregnant bitch the first indication of infection is often
spontaneous abortion late in gestation. Early embryonic deaths with
resorption, however, may occur within 10 to 20 days after a mating.
Some litters may include both living and dead pups. One group of
pups exposed experimentally at birth had a bacteremia that persisted
more than 36 months.[17,18] Infected bitches generally abort once or
twice, but as many as 4 consecutive abortions have occurred as long
as 1 year apart.

Though clinical signs may be absent in males, epididymitis and orchitis with varying degrees of prostatitis and testicular atrophy are
observed commonly.[15,20] Scrotal ulceration has been observed (Fig 1).
Prostatitis may be particularly severe and persistent. Examination of
semen usually reveals abnormal spermatozoa and severe reduction in
their motility. Male infertility is due partly to isoimmune reactions
resulting from local and systemic immune responses to sperm antigens that reach the general circulation via macrophages.[20]

Signs of canine brucellosis also include fatigue, reduced appetite,
weight loss, malaise, and behavioral abnormalities. Discospondylitis
in dogs with *B canis* infection is accompanied by pain, inappetence,
and recurring fever.[21,22] This condition was observed during the 4th
year of infection in 2 of 8 Beagles exposed experimentally to *B canis*
during their 1st week of life.

Microscopic lesions include reticular cell hyperplasia of all lymphoid tissues.[15,19] Splenomegaly and focal hepatitis occur along with
mononuclear cell infiltration of the prostate and epididymides. Microscopic granulomas may be found in various organs, including kidneys, brain, and uterus. Chronically infected dogs may have meningitis and focal nonsuppurative encephalitis. Hyalin deposits, thicken-

ing of basement membranes, and "wire loop" lesions have been observed occasionally in the renal glomeruli of infected dogs. Anterior uveitis has been seen in some chronically infected animals; B canis has also been isolated from an eye of an infected dog.[23,24]

Transmission

The most important mode of B canis transmission is via placental tissues and vaginal discharges following an abortion.[4-15] Organisms may be shed in vaginal fluid for several weeks after an abortion. Transmission by contaminated urine or other body excretions is less common because the number of organisms shed by these routes is often less than required to establish infection. Nevertheless, transmission through contact has been observed between male dogs after 3 to 4 months of cohabitation in isolation units. Venereal transmission is also important because male dogs have been found to harbor the bacteria in the epididymides and prostate gland for long periods (>5 years). Excretion of Brucella in semen is unpredictable, however, because organisms may be isolated consistently from ejaculated semen only during the 1st to 2nd month after initial infection.[21] The organism has been cultured from the prostate gland and epididymal tissues of infected males up to 2 years after the bacteremic stage had ended.

Though carrier males may appear normal, examination of semen usually shows abnormalities. Transmission of infection did not occur when infected, nonpregnant, and uninfected females or infected and uninfected prepuberal males were housed together in isolation units for several months. Because of the prolonged bacteremia (in some animals more than 5 years), infection may be transmitted via transfused blood or contaminated needles.

Diagnosis

Clinical signs are not sufficient for the diagnosis of canine brucellosis. The disease must therefore be considered whenever there is a history of abortion in females or poor reproductive performance in either sex.

There are presently 3 widely used serologic tests for the diagnosis of canine brucellosis: the rapid slide agglutination test (SAT), the tube agglutination test (TAT), and the modified mercaptoethanol-tube agglutination test (ME-TAT).[4,16,17] The SAT was developed to provide presumptive diagnosis relatively quickly and it is available commercially. This test has been found highly accurate in identifying noninfected dogs; "false negative" reactions have been detected, though rarely. On the other hand, "false positive" reactions are common. The SAT was recently modified to include an additional step that involves a brief reaction of undiluted sera with 2-mercaptoethanol (0.2 M) prior to adding the test antigen. This modification does not reduce the test's sensitivity, but it improves its specificity. When SAT results are positive, more specific serologic tests and bacteriologic examinations should be performed.

The TAT and ME-TAT are widely used. In both tests an antigen suspension of *B canis* is used, but the antigens are prepared differently. In a protracted study of experimentally infected, specific-pathogen-free dogs, the TAT and ME-TAT titers were similar.[17,18] A titer of 1:200 in both tests is generally considered presumptive evidence of infection. Occasionally, dogs with normal reproductive histories and negative bacteriologic examinations have diagnostically "significant" or "suspicious" titers of 1:50 to 1:100, sometimes with incomplete agglutination. Such reactions have been perplexing when investigation ruled out brucellosis but failed to determine the cause of the reaction. False-positive reactions are caused by cross-reacting antibodies provoked by other bacteria. Such antibodies are not readily distinguished from antibodies against *B canis*.

A useful serodiagnostic regimen involves the use of an agglutination test for screening in combination with an agar-gel diffusion (AGD) test. With the AGD test, a reference serum must be used, to interpret the results correctly. Sera with "suspicious" levels of agglutinating antibody have often been found nonspecific by the AGD test, especially when "soluble" cytoplasmic extracts of brucella cells are used as antigen. Such "soluble antigens" are specific for antibodies against *Brucella* organisms.

Blood cultures should always be done when canine brucellosis is suspected.

Additional diagnostic procedures should include examination of semen from suspected male dogs. As mentioned previously, the sperm from infected males is usually abnormal.

Prevention and Control

There is no vaccine for canine brucellosis. Control measures in an infected kennel include the elimination of all infected animals.[25-27] Commercial disinfectants, such as ammonium compounds and halogens, should be used whenever an abortion has occurred.

All female dogs that have aborted or failed to conceive after successive matings and males with genital disease should be considered to be possibly infected. These dogs should be isolated and specimens taken for serologic and bacteriologic examinations. Positive-reactors to these tests should be destroyed and at least 3 monthly tests of all dogs should be negative before a kennel can be considered uninfected.[25]

Dogs to be introduced into a kennel, especially pregnant females and all animals to be used for breeding, should be admitted only after they have had 2 negative tests at a 30-day interval. Animals with low ("suspicious") titers should be considered to be potentially infected until their status has been confirmed by repeated tests. Males may shed organisms in the semen for long periods after the bacteremia has terminated and agglutinin titers have fallen below diagnostically significant levels.

Because the infection is spread principally by vaginal discharges and seminal fluids, castration and spaying should reduce its transmission. Dogs usually recover spontaneously after 1 to 4 years and are then immune.

Treatment

At the present time the prognosis for *Brucella*-infected dogs is grave. As in other *Brucella* infections, a practical and uniformly effective treatment is not available. Brucellosis is not life-threatening, but an infected dog should not be used for breeding because it will continue to be a source of infection for other dogs, and possibly humans.

B canis is susceptible *in vitro* to streptomycin, tetracyclines, ampicillin, erythromycin, gentamicin, rifampin, spectinomycin, and chloramphenicol.[16] Of these drugs, ampicillin and tetracycline, often in combination with streptomycin, have been used successfully in the treatment of *B canis* infection in man.[12,13] In contrast, the administration of tetracycline, Tribrissen, streptomycin, rifampin, and Declomycin, alone and in combinations, was unsuccessful in eliminating *B canis* from dogs.[17] Several agents, including tetracycline alone and in combination with streptomycin, eliminated during the period of therapy the bacteremia that characterizes the disease.[17,28] None of these treatments completely eliminated the organism from the tissues, however, and bacteremia commonly recurred 1 to 3 months after therapy was discontinued. This recurrence indicates that claims for "cures" of canine brucellosis must be viewed with caution. Negative results of blood cultures during or shortly following therapy cannot be interpreted as a cure (complete elimination of the organism). Likewise, a decrease in antibody titers that may accompany prolonged treatment is a poor indicator of its effectiveness unless dogs become seronegative and remain so.[16,17]

In limited experimental and field trials, a combination of streptomycin and tetracycline has been found especially effective, and further study is indicated.[29] A high success rate (>90%) has been achieved with intensive treatment of dogs that had not been infected for over 2 months. Treatment for a 1-month period consisted of dihydrostreptomycin (10 mg/lb q12h during weeks 1 and 4) plus tetracycline hydrochloride (25 mg/lb q8h during weeks 1 through 4).

In the course of treatment trials it has been discovered that animals cleared of *B canis* during treatment became susceptible to reinfection within 1 month. It thus appears that cured animals are not subsequently immune and may be readily reinfected.

Presently a clinician has only 2 options when a dog is diagnosed as infected with *B canis*. One is euthanasia. This should be recommended when there are valuable uninfected breeding animals in a kennel or when there is concern about infection of humans, which is rare. When the infected dog is a treasured pet, a second option may be chosen. It involves spaying or castration followed by treatment with a combination of oxytetracycline and streptomycin. If the latter course is selected, the owner should be told that the therapy is expensive and not always successful. Successful treatment has been more frequent with infected females, possibly because of the difficulty in eliminating foci of infection from the male genitalia, especially the prostate gland.

References

1. Carmichael, LE and Kenney, R.M: JAVMA **152** (1968) 605.
2. Moore, JA: JAVMA **155** (1969) 2034.
3. Hill, WA *et al:* Lab Anim Care **20** (1970) 205.
4. Carmichael, LE: CRC Handbook Series in Zoonoses, section A, vol 1, pp 185-194. J. H. Steele, Ed. CRC Press Inc, Boca Raton, 1979.
5. Ueda, K *et al:* Jap J Vet Sci **36** (1974) 359.
6. Flores-Castro, R *et al:* J Clin Microbiol **6** (1977) 591.
7. Morgan, WJB: J Dairy Res **37** (1970) 303.
8. Fredrickson, LE and Barton, CE: JAVMA **165** (1974) 987.
9. Lewis, GE: JAAHA **8** (1972) 102.
10. Brown, J *et al:* JAVMA **169** (1976) 1214.
11. Flores-Castro, R and Segura, R: Cornell Vet **66** (1976) 347.
12. Swenson, RM *et al:* Annals Int Med **76** (1972) 435.
13. Munford, RS: J Amer Med Assoc **231** (1975) 1267.
14. Pickerill, PA: JAVMA **156** (1970) 1741.
15. Carmichael, LE and Kenney, RM: JAVMA **156** (1970) 1726.
16. Pollock, RVH: Compend Cont Educ **1** (1979) 255.
17. Flores-Castro, R and Carmichael, LE: 27th Gaines Vet Symp, 1977.
18. Zoha, SJ and Carmichael, LE: Serological responses of dogs to cell wall and internal antigens of *B canis*. Vet Microbiol **7** (1982) 35.
19. Gleiser, CA *et al:* Lab Anim Sci **21** (1971) 540.
20. George, LW *et al:* Amer J Vet Res **40** (1979) 1589.
21. Henderson, RA *et al:* JAVMA **165** (1974) 451.
22. Hurov, L *et al:* JAVMA **173** (1978) 275.
23. Saegusa, J *et al:* Jap J Vet Sci **39** (1977) 181.
24. Reike, JA and Rhodes, HE: JAVMA **165** (1975) 1734.
25. Pickerill, PA and Carmichael, LE: JAVMA **160** (1972) 1607.
26. Moore, JA *et al:* JAVMA **153** (1968) 523.
27. Yamauchi, C *et al:* Jap J Vet Sci **36** (1974) 175.
28. Jennings, PB *et al:* JAVMA **164** (1974) 513.
29. Lewis, GE *et al:* JAVMA **163** (1973) 239.
30. Zoha, SJ: JAVMA **180** (1982) 1474.

VAGINITIS
BY THOMAS J. BURKE

Introduction

Vaginitis may be the most common disease of the female genital tract in dogs. It appears to be uncommon in the cat, but this may not be true due to failure of owners to observe the signs and/or to the queen's grooming habits. Chronic recurring vaginitis is not uncommon and it can be a frustrating clinical problem.

Besides causing signs that the owner considers objectionable or cause patient discomfort, vaginitis can result in infertility. The infertility has been related to spermicidal activity of the vaginal exudate.

Cause

The term vaginitis is not synonymous with bacterial vaginitis. Although bacterial infection is apparently the most common cause, others include neoplasia, herpesvirus infection, foreign bodies, and androgen-induced hypertrophy of the clitoris.[1-3] Yeast infection is rarely a cause.

Studies have been made of the normal bacterial flora of the canine vagina.[4-11] In several of them an attempt has been made to compare culture results of normal versus abnormal bitches, namely those with vaginal discharge or a history of infertility.[4,6,9-11] These studies have revealed that 1) bacteria normally inhabit the canine vagina; 2) many of the isolated bacteria are anaerobes; 3) the bacterial populations are usually mixed; 4) there are more bacteria in the caudal than the cranial vagina; 5) though the types of organisms isolated from bitches with vaginitis do not vary significantly from the organisms found in normal bitches, higher numbers of only 1 or perhaps 2 types of bacteria are often present in cases of primary bacterial vaginitis; 6) the stage of the estrous cycle does not affect the microflora; 7) the onset of puberty does affect the flora in that prepuberal females harbor significantly more coagulase-positive staphylococci; and 8) up to 30% of normal females may harbor the "breeder-dreaded" B-hemolytic streptococci.

It thus appears that contamination of the vagina with bacteria considered to be pathogens is not sufficient to cause disease. The reason that so many cases of so-called "puppy" vaginitis have disappeared spontaneously at puberty is also unclear. The pathogenesis of bacterial vaginitis is thus unsolved.

I have recently measured immunoglobulin levels in a few cases of chronic recurrent vaginitis in postpuberal bitches and observed a consistent deficiency of IgA. One bitch was also deficient in IgG and IgM. Perhaps the bitches with persistent vaginitis lack the ability to produce protective levels of secretory antibodies. Other factors associated with host-defense mechanisms must also be considered.

Canine herpesvirus can cause a vesicular vaginitis with petechial hemorrhages.[2,3] The vesicles become sunken and regress in a few weeks. They then become lymphoid follicles. This is probably the condition described as "dog pox."[12] Its recurrence is common, especially during proestrus.[3] In one kennel the disease was associated with a 50% decrease in fertility as well as a decline in the number of puppies whelped per litter and the number reared to weaning.[3] This herpesvirus also causes abortion, early fetal death, and mummification.[13] It can have a disastrous effect on an infected bitch's reproductivity.

Clinical Signs

The most common reason for presentation of a bitch is vaginal discharge. Other signs include frequent licking of the vulva, pollakiuria, and evidence of discomfort when the animal is sitting. The signs associated with herpesvirus infection are minimal (mild serous discharge and sensitivity to vaginal palpation); the infection may be asymptomatic.[2,3] In the assessment of a vaginal discharge, other causes of a discharge at the vulva should be considered, including those that occur at proestrus and after parturition and the discharges associated with other genital tract diseases, such as pyometritis.[1] Other signs may occur with diseases of the lower urinary tract, vulva, perineum, and with anal sac disease.

In a bitch with vaginitis the discharge may be serous, sanguinopurulent, or purulent. Vaginoscopy enables direct observation of the congested mucosa and small pools of the exudate. Focal lesions, such as pustules, vesicles, and petechial hemorrhages, may be observed. Culture of the exudate is essential for diagnosis and a biopsy is often helpful, especially in cases of suspected viral or neoplastic disease.

Cytologic examination will reveal cells that vary with the stage of the estrous cycle. Although neutrophilia is characteristic of vaginitis, these cells may be found in normal bitches during anestrus and metestrus, especially early metestrus. They may also originate from the uterus or cervix. The morphology of neutrophils may be affected somewhat by infectious organisms. In another cellular change associated with vaginitis the epithelial cells tend to desquamate and appear

CHAPTER 4

in clusters.[14] These cells will often have large or even multiple nuclei. Bacteria are nearly always present in smears from the canine vagina, whether or not vaginitis is present.[1] Lymphocytes may be present in cases of follicular vaginitis.[14]

Treatment

Prepuberal vaginitis often subsides without therapy. Bacterial vaginitis in adult bitches usually responds well to administration of a combination of local and systemic antibacterial drugs. The selection of a systemic antibacterial drug should be based on a sensitivity test and the treatment should be continued at least 72 hours after disappearance of the clinical signs.

Local treatments include administration of infusions and suppositories. Useful antibacterials for infusion include chlorhexidine, povidone-iodine, Furacin, neomycin, and gentamicin solutions. They are administered with a bulb syringe or soft rubber catheter twice daily. Enough solution should be administered to fill the vagina. Antibiotics should be diluted so that the amount infused does not exceed the average therapeutic dose for a particular patient. The instruments used for administration should be lubricated. A patient's resistance to local treatments may necessitate the use of a lubricating jelly containing a local anesthetic.

It has been recommended that bitches not be bred during the 1st estrus following the treatment of infectious vaginitis.[1] This is not always possible, however, because some bitches will have some degree of vaginitis during each estrus. In these cases the treatment should be started as early as possible prior to breeding. Because the antibacterial infusions are probably spermicidal as well as bactericidal, they should either not be used or not given 72 hours prior to mating. This recommendation is made even though it is not known how long the infusion solution remains in the vagina and uterus. Radiographic dyes used to perform vaginography or hysterosalpingography are not detectable, however, after 24 to 36 hours.

There is no effective treatment for herpesvirus infection at this time, but recently developed anti-herpes drugs will hopefully be tested in bitches with this infection.

Vaginitis associated with tumors, foreign bodies, and androgen-induced clitoral hyperplasia should be treated by removing the inciting cause. The infusion of a glucocorticoid solution following removal of a foreign body or resection of a tumor may hasten the subsidence of clinical signs, but may delay healing.

The use of estrogens as adjunctive therapy appears to have little basis because it has been shown that the stage of the estrous cycle has no effect on vaginal bacterial flora.[4,5,9] In addition, these hormones may have severe side-effects, such as bone marrow suppression and increasing the susceptibility to pyometritis.

Prognosis

A guarded prognosis for a permanent cure is indicated for all cases of infectious vaginitis. The animal's owner should be advised that recurrence is common and that the need for additional treatment is the rule rather than the exception.

References

1. Olson, PS: In *Current Veterinary Therapy VII.* WB Saunders, Philadelphia, 1980.
2. Hill, H and Mare, CJ: Amer J Vet Res **35** (1974) 669.
3. Poste, G and King, N: Vet Rec **88** (1971) 229.
4. Allen, WE and Dagnall, GJR: J Small Anim Pract **23** (1982) 325.
5. Baba, E *et al:* Amer J Vet Res **44** (1983) 606.
6. Hirsh, DC and Wiger, N: J Small Anim Pract **18** (1977) 25.
7. Ling, GV and Ruby, AL: Amer J Vet Res **39** (1978) 695.
8. Olson, PNS and Mather, EC: JAVMA **172** (1978) 708.
9. Osbaldiston, GW *et al:* JAAHA **8** (1972) 93.
10. Osbaldiston, GW: JAAHA **14** (1978) 363.
11. Platt, AM and Simpson, RB: Southwestern Vet **27** (1974) 76.
12. Joshua, JO: Vet Rec **96** (1975) 300.
13. Hashimoto, A *et al:* Amer J Vet Res **44** (1983) 610.
14. Roszel, JF: Vet Scope **19** (1975) 2.

METRITIS, PYOMETRITIS
BY JAMES H. SOKOLOWSKI

Introduction

Pyometra can be described as an acute or chronic disease that occurs frequently during diestrus or metestrus in mature intact bitches and less frequently in mature intact queens.[1] It may be reflected by a variety of clinical signs related to disease in both genital and extragenital areas. The genital lesions are in the uterus; the extragenital lesions are primarily in the bladder and kidneys.

The etiopathogenesis of the genital lesions includes the effects of estrogenic and then progestational activity along with bacterial infection. Although it occurs during the peak of endogenous progesterone production, the development of pyometra depends on estrogen-priming of the uterus during proestrus and estrus. It has been demonstrated that uterine changes induced by progesterone (progestogen) do not occur after ovariectomy, which eliminates the influence of estrogen. It has also been observed that administration of estrogen alone to ovariectomized bitches will not result in cystic endometrial hyperplasia and pyometra.

Although metritis and pyometritis occur frequently in older nulliparous bitches, they also occur in bitches and queens of all ages. Though the precise incidence of uterine disease in the bitch and queen is unknown, it is agreed that the incidence increases with the age of susceptible animals. It may be as high as 15 to 50% in intact bitches that are more than 8 years old.

Classification of Pyometra

A 4-part classification of pyometra has been based on histologic changes in the uterus.[2] Type 1 was described as a cystic glandular hyperplasia of the endometrium with no evidence of inflammation. The clinical signs associated with Type 1 are minimal, and irregularities in the estrous cycle are the predominant ones. The average age of affected bitches is 7.1 ± 2.4 years, with a range of 3 to 12 years of age.

The Type 2 category includes bitches that are 7.2 ± 1.9 years of age, with a range of 4 to 11 years. Affected animals have a marked cystic hyperplasia of the endometrium, plasma cell infiltration, and evidence of degenerative changes in the endometrium. Bitches with Type 2 have a mucoid vaginal discharge, a swollen vulva, and some uterine enlargement about 60 days after estrus.

An acute inflammation along with cystic hyperplasia of the endometrium characterizes Type 3. This type is the classic clinical form. Affected animals are depressed, anorectic, and febrile. They have a distended abdomen, enlarged uterus, leukocytosis, and an increased sedimentation rate. These clinical signs generally occur 10 to 50 days following estrus in bitches that are 8 ± 2.2 years of age (range 4 to 13 years).

Animals with Type 4 constitute a smaller group and they are difficult to recognize under clinical circumstances. In some affected females in this group, subclinical pyometritis, possibly Type 1, has been occurring for years. These animals are typically 11.8 ± 1.7 years of age. They have a history of post-estrual abnormalities and have myometrial and endometrial atrophy with fibrosis. As a consequence of these changes, the uterus becomes friable.

Etiopathogenesis

It was once speculated that estrogen was not important in the etiology of pyometra, but that progesterone released by corpora lutea was responsible. It is known now, however, that estrogen primes the uterine mucosa for the sequence of subsequent changes.[3]

After ovulation occurs and the corpora lutea are functional, the uterus is under the influence of progesterone. Polycystic endometritis results and, if bacteria are present, pyometritis may develop. Frequently, however, a non-infectious mucometra develops rather than a true pyometra.

Animals with pyometritis, especially chronic cases, accumulate large quantities of fluids in the uterine lumen. The animal's body responds with an increase in the number of leukocytes in peripheral blood and the release of prostaglandins.[4] Though the prostaglandins stimulate activity of the uterine musculature, fluid usually tends to accumulate in the uterus.

The uterine changes at this point may affect renal function. The dysfunction may be due to prerenal disease, primary glomerular disease, or a reduction in the ability of renal tubules to concentrate urine. The glomerular lesions that can occur with pyometritis may result from immunologic reactions. It has also been suggested that the polydipsia/polyuria associated with pyometritis is caused by *E coli* endotoxins.[5,6]

Progestogens given perorally or parenterally have been implicated in the production of uterine disease in bitches of all ages.[7] The induced condition mimics the natural disease in its progression and clinical signs with the major exception being that there is no relationship to the stage of the estrous cycle. Another form of pyometritis results from the injudicious administration of estrogens. If they are given during the luteal phase of the estrous cycle, uterine disease may result.

Clinical Signs

The clinical signs of metritis/pyometritis vary with the condition's severity and duration, the occurrence of bacterial infection, the existence of endotoxemia, the patency of the cervix, and the animal's general health. Prime suspects are identified by the occurrence of depression, mild fever, anorexia, polydipsia and polyuria in an intact female that is more than 6 years old and has recently been in estrus or has been given estrogen. In some cases there is only a history of irregular estrous periods or infertility. In chronic cases the animal may be presented because of her lethargy and the development of abdominal distention.

Bitches with subclinical pyometra have been observed for months under experimental conditions before they developed obvious signs of the disease. These animals may periodically have a vaginal discharge.

They may also have an increased sedimentation rate and a mild leu-kocytosis.

Digital palpation of the uterus through the abdominal wall may reveal a uniform, non-segmented enlargement of the uterus. When the uterus is grossly enlarged, palpation is less helpful. Because of the friability of an affected uterus, palpation must be performed gent-ly. During palpation, evidence of dehydration may be noticed.

In animals with acute pyometra, some hematologic changes are very significant and useful in diagnosis. White cell counts in excess of 30,000/mm³ are common. Some affected animals with severe toxemia have lower white cell counts. An increase in the rate of red cell sedi-mentation is another common finding associated with pyometra. It must be remembered, however, that the sedimentation rate also in-creases during pregnancy. Anemia occurs in some affected animals and impaired renal function may be reflected by an elevated BUN, reduced serum protein, and proteinuria.

Radiographs can be helpful in the diagnosis of some obscure cases of pyometra. Injection of contrast media, such as air, will often delineate the swollen uterus.

Treatment

The most satisfactory treatment for the majority of animals with pyometritis, and for many cases of metritis, is ovariohysterectomy. In most cases, surgical intervention should not be delayed. Suppor-tive therapy is indicated to maintain hydration and to prevent shock and infection. The selection of fluids should ideally be made on the basis of electrolyte and acid-base analyses. When these assessments are not available, reasonable options include lactated Ringer's solu-tion and whole blood. Soluble steroids can be given IV to control shock, and a broad-spectrum antibiotic, such as gentamicin, can be used to control infection.

Another surgical procedure that has been used is hysterotomy with curettage of the endometrium. This has not proved to be very successful because it does not remove the causes of the disease. However, concomitant removal of corpora lutea from the ovaries has been advocated with satisfactory results.[11]

Drugs that would be useful in the treatment of pyometritis, ex-cept that they require estrogen-priming, include the ergot alkaloids, especially ergonovine maleate. Oxytocin also can stimulate activity of the uterine smooth muscle, but priming with estrogen is necessary for maximum response. As noted earlier, estrogens are contraindi-cated in the treatment of uterine disease.

Testosterone and its derivatives have been used in the treatment of uterine disease. Although success has been reported for such therapy, the number of successful cases is small and the potential for hepatocellular necrosis and masculinization is relatively high.

The use of an indwelling uterine catheter and infusion of various drugs has been reported. Such therapy should be attempted only when the cervix is open. The cervix is very difficult, if not impossible, to cannulate, and the danger of uterine puncture is great. Such therapy may require tranquilization of the patient. Drainage of the uterus has also been combined with curettage of the endometrium.

Although the use of prostaglandins is still considered an experimental treatment in the dog and cat, good results have been reported following their use in animals with endometritis, metritis, and pyometritis.[8-10] Different natural prostaglandins and prostaglandin analogues have been used and it is important to note that the analogues are much more potent than the naturally occurring prostaglandins.

Prostaglandin F_2-alpha* appears to be the most reliable. The recommended dose is 0.25 mg/kg given subcutaneously once daily. The treatment is administered daily until there is minimal or no discharge within the first hour following the injection.[12] This varies from 3 to 15 days. The patient should be returned 3 to 5 days later for another injection to ensure that the uterus is not filling up with pus again. The side effects reported following prostaglandin therapy are transitory and include vomiting, loose stool, tachypnea, hypersalivation, staggering, collapse, hypothermia, and pupillary dilation or constriction. They may occur in any combination and are not consistent in a given patient during a treatment regime. Unpublished in vitro studies have shown that PGF_2-alpha dilates the cervix and thus can be used in cases of closed pyometra.

Post-treatment fertility approximates 75%. Presumably those not fertile have irreversible endometrial disease resulting from chronic inflammation. Cultures and, if necessary, appropriate antibacterial therapy should be performed at the first post-treatment proestrus. Breeding at the first post-treatment estrus has been recommended.[9]

References
1. Dow, C: Vet Rec **69** (1957) 1409.
2. Hardy, RM and Osborne, CA: JAAHA **10** (1974) 245.
3. Teunissen, GHB: Acta Endocrinol **9** (1952) 407.
4. Heap, RB and Poyser, NL: Brit J Pharm **55** (1975) 515.
5. Borresen, B: Nord Vet Med **27** (1975) 508.
6. Sandholm, M et al: JAVMA **167** (1975) 1006.
7. Sokolowski, JH: Amer J Vet Res **35** (1974) 1285.
8. Sokolowski, JH: JAAHA **16** (1980) 119.
9. Nelson, RW and Feldman, EC: 31st Gaines Veterinary Symposium, 1981.
10. Sokolowski, JH: JAVMA **170** (1977) 536.
11. Herron, MR and Herron, MA: Vet Clin NA **5** (1975) 471.
12. Burke, TJ: Personal communication, 1984.

*Prostaglandin F_2-alpha THAM salt: the Upjohn Co., Kalamazoo, MI.

PROSTATIC DISEASES
BY JEANNE BARSANTI & DELMAR FINCO

Introduction
The questions addressed in this section are: When a male dog is presented because of infertility, could prostatic disease be the cause? If so, which prostatic diseases are associated with infertility? What plan for diagnosis should be followed? What therapy should be tried and how successful is it likely to be? Unfortunately the relationship of canine prostatic disease to fertility has not been studied. Thus, to find answers for these questions, one must turn to the human literature. The similarity in prostate structure and physiology between the 2 species encourages extrapolation of data from human to dog.

Infertility Caused by Prostatic Disease
Diseases of the prostate gland can cause infertility by producing obstruction of the deferent ducts and by leading to bacterial infection.[1] The former mechanism is most clearly defined. The deferent ducts pass through the prostate to enter the urethra (Fig 1). With an expansive disease of the prostate, such as neoplasia, abscessation, acute inflammation, or cyst development, the ducts may become obstructed. All of these conditions can cause the prostate to be increased in size, changed in shape, or become painful and thus the abnormality can be detectable by physical examination. In fact, rectal and/or abdominal palpation of the prostate gland should always be part of the examination of an infertile dog. If the prostate gland is not palpable, radiographs should be obtained to determine its size and shape.

The relationship of bacterial prostatitis to infertility when large abscesses are absent is not well understood.[1,2] Bacteria do adversely affect sperm viability and motility, but only if they are present in large numbers ($>10^6$/ml).[3-8] Such large numbers of bacteria are not common in men with chronic bacterial prostatitis.[5-7] Infertility in affected men is thought to be due to secondary dysfunction of prostatic secretion rather than a direct effect of the bacteria. Normal prostatic fluid stimulates motility of spermatozoa in both man and dogs and albumin is one component of prostatic fluid that contributes to this effect.[5,7,9-11] Prostatic fluid also contains large amounts of zinc, calcium, and magnesium.[6,12-14] Chronic bacterial prostatitis results in decreased secretions and reduced concentrations of these substances

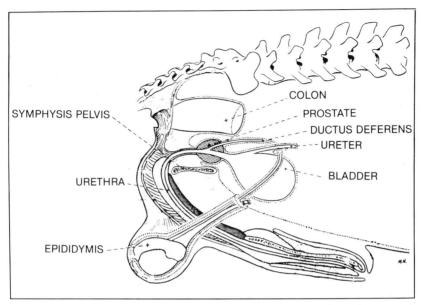

Fig 1. Diagram of structures in caudal abdomen of the male dog. From *Anatomy of the Dog.* WB Saunders CO, Philadelphia, 1968.

in semen.[6,13-15] Decreased sperm motility and viability may also occur. Changes in sperm morphology may or may not result.

The relationship of zinc to semen quality is not completely understood. Human and canine prostatic fluid is normally high in zinc, but prostatic fluid from men with chronic bacterial prostatitis contains lesser amounts.[13,16-23] Adding zinc to human sperm had no noticeable effects on sperm motility.[11,24] That the zinc concentration of prostatic fluid is closely correlated with semen quality is debatable. It is known that decreased concentration of zinc in prostatic fluid is associated with a higher concentration of the metal in spermatozoa.[9,13,14] Higher concentrations of zinc in intrasperm semen are associated with decreased viability and motility of spermatozoa. The decrease in zinc concentration in prostatic fluid from men with chronic bacterial prostatitis may be due to the absence of a factor in prostatic fluid that normally binds zinc. Without this factor, zinc could enter spermatozoa and reduce their viability.

The relationship of chronic bacterial prostatitis to clinical cases of infertility has not been studied in large numbers of infertile men because of the number of tests required to establish a definite diagnosis. In the one study in which careful technics were used to eliminate the possibility of bacterial contamination from the urethra, 3 of 21 infer-

tile men who were normal on physical examination were found to
have chronic bacterial prostatitis.[1] The number of spermatozoa increased and their morphology improved in the men whose infection
was eliminated. In most men with chronic bacterial prostatitis, there
is no evidence of infertility.

Secretory dysfunction of the prostate that is not associated with
infection has also been postulated to be a cause of infertility in
man.[5,16] The infertility is attributed to decreased viability of sperm.
The factors that cause a decrease in sperm viability are unknown, but
a relationship to decreased concentrations of zinc has been
suggested.[16]

Most dogs presented because of infertility have no discernible abnormalities on physical examination.[25] Chronic bacterial prostatitis
could be present, however, without abnormalities detectable by physical examination.[26] It is not known whether or not prostatic secretory dysfunction can occur in dogs without infection. The number of
infertile dogs that have chronic bacterial prostatitis or any prostatic
secretory dysfunction is also unknown.

In the remainder of this section one approach to the diagnosis and
treatment of chronic bacterial prostatitis will be described.

Chronic Bacterial Prostatitis in Dogs
Clinical Signs

One clinical sign of chronic bacterial prostatitis is an intermittent
hemorrhagic or purulent urethral discharge. This discharge probably
results from hemorrhage and/or exudation of pus from the prostatic
acini through the prostatic ducts into the prostatic urethra in sufficient quantities to not only reflux into the bladder but also to drain
through the urethral orifice. Whenever a urethral discharge is noticed, the prepuce should be carefully examined to determine whether
or not it is the origin. Though urethritis is a possible cause of a
purulent or hemorrhagic discharge at the urethral orifice, such inflammation that is not associated with primary inflammation of the
bladder or prostate is probably rare in the dog. Any prostatic disease
that results in inflammation or hemorrhage can cause urethral
discharge.

Rectal palpation of an infected prostate gland may reveal no abnormalities. In other cases, however, changes in consistency and symmetry of the prostate are detected. Fibrination in response to chronic
inflammation may result in small firm infiltrations. Small abscesses
that form may feel softer than normal prostate tissue. Chronic infection alone probably results in no change in the prostate's size, but if

chronic infection occurs in a hyperplastic prostate (common in older dogs) then the gland's size may be increased.

Chronic bacterial prostatitis is the major cause of recurrent infection in the lower urinary tract of adult men.[27-29] The same may be true for the male dog. Other causes of recurrent cystitis in male dogs are chronic pyelonephritis and urolithiasis. Recurrent cystitis may be the only abnormality associated with chronic bacterial prostatitis. This underlying cause of cystitis may not be suspected when routine antibiotic therapy results in elimination of bacteria in bladder urine and disappearance of clinical signs. The prostatic infection will persist, however, and cause recurrent cystitis after administration of antibiotics is stopped.

Semen Evaluation

The ejaculate is valuable in assessing prostatic disease because prostatic fluid is its largest component. The same sample can be used to assess fertility. Before collecting an ejaculate, we first obtain a urine sample by cystocentesis. The urine is divided and half is used for routine analysis and half for culture. A sample of urethral content is collected by inserting a small swab (Calgiswab: American Can Co) 2 to 4 cm into the distal urethra. This swab is then put into a sterile tube containing 4 to 5 ml of sterile saline. A qualitative culture is obtained from the swab and a quantitative culture can be obtained from the saline solution. We then place the dog in a quiet environment and collect semen by manual massage. Any preputial discharge is gently wiped from the erect penis with a sterile gauze sponge prior to ejaculation. The semen sample is collected in one or more sterile containers. The first 2 components of the ejaculate, the pre-sperm and sperm components, are collected together. When the milky component has been collected and clear prostatic fluid is discharged, it is collected in a different sterile container.

The first sample should be evaluated for number, motility, and morphology of spermatozoa. The 2nd sample should be assessed by cytologic examination and quantitative culture. If an ejaculate cannot be collected in this manner, a bitch in estrus or an anestrus bitch with the canine pheromone, p-methyl hydroxybenzoate (Kodak Chemical Co), applied to the vulva can be used as a teaser.[30]

Quantitative culture of the ejaculate is essential because the distal urethra has a normal bacterial flora.[31] Because of urethral contamination, ejaculates from normal dogs may contain up to 100,000 organisms per ml.[32] These urethral organisms are usually gram-positive, but occasionally gram-negative organisms are present.[31] Quantitative cultures can be performed by commercial laboratories, but the counts are probably reliable only if the sample is kept refrigerated and cultured within 8 hours. The dip slide technics may be more practical.

The results of an ejaculate's culture should be compared with the urine and urethral cultures. The urethral culture will indicate which organisms may have originated in that structure.

Cytologic examination of the ejaculate will assist in determining whether or not prostatic disease is present. Normal dogs occasionally have leukocytes in their semen.[32] Large numbers of leukocytes are abnormal, however, and they reflect inflammation if the semen has not been contaminated by preputial exudate. Blood may be found in ejaculates from dogs with prostatic infection, cysts, neoplasia, and possibly hyperplasia. Bleeding may occasionally occur during ejaculation of a normal dog due to rupture of a penile vessel. In such cases the bleeding site on the surface of the penis is usually observed.

Prostatic Massage

Although prostatic fluid is obtained most reliably from dogs by collecting the 3rd fraction of the ejaculate, it is not possible to obtain ejaculates from all dogs that may have prostatic disease because of the animal's pain, inexperience, or temperament. Abnormalities in the semen may also originate in the testes or epididymides as well as the prostate.

Another method of collecting prostatic fluid is to massage the prostate. In this procedure a urethral catheter is passed aseptically into the bladder and the bladder is emptied. A sample of the urine can be saved for subsequent analysis and culture. The bladder is then flushed several times with sterile saline solution to ensure that it is empty. From 5 to 10 ml of the last flushing is kept as the pre-massage sample. The catheter is withdrawn until its tip is just distal to the prostate as determined by rectal palpation. The prostate is then massaged per-rectum or per-abdomen or both for 1 to 2 minutes. From 5 to 10 ml of sterile physiologic saline solution are injected slowly through the urethral catheter while the urethral orifice is digitally occluded around the catheter to prevent reflux of fluid from the orifice and to prevent any change in the catheter's position. In this way the urethral content expressed from the prostate gland is washed into the bladder. The catheter is slowly advanced to the bladder as the urethral fluid is repeatedly aspirated. Most of the fluid will be aspirated from the bladder. The pre- and post-massage samples are then compared cytologically and by quantitative culture. It is very important that the 2 samples be compared because this enables identification of the source of abnormal cells or other material. Massage of a normal dog's prostate produces only a few erythrocytes and transitional epithelial cells.[32]

The main disadvantage of prostatic massage is the inability to assess abnormalities in prostatic fluid if the urine is abnormal. In such cases, antibiotics that reach the urine but not the prostatic fluid, such as ampicillin, can be administered for several days prior to prostatic massage.[33] The samples obtained must be cultured immediately because the antibiotic in the urine may kill bacteria in the sample of prostatic fluid. Alternatively, the urinary tract infection can be treated for several weeks prior to prostatic massage. The massage is given after the urinary infection has been eliminated and a few days after stopping the antibiotic medication. Collecting a sample of prostatic fluid at this time is very important even though the dog is asymptomatic. If one waits until clinical signs recur before collecting the sample of prostatic fluid, the same problem of determining the source of the abnormality will exist.

Prostatic Biopsy

The type of prostatic disease can also be determined by needle aspiration or biopsy. Needle aspiration can be performed perirectally or transabdominally depending on the location of the prostate.[34] The procedure is performed aseptically with a long needle and stylet. When done perirectally, the needle is guided by a finger inserted into the rectum.[34] It can be performed in most dogs after inducing mild tranquilization. Needle aspiration should probably not be performed when prostatic abscesses are present. We thus avoid the procedure in dogs with fever or leukocytosis related to prostatic disease and prefer to evaluate prostatic fluid obtained by ejaculation or massage before doing anything else. Despite these precautions we have discovered prostatic abscesses by aspiration in 4 dogs. Apparently the abscessed areas in these dogs were not communicating with the urethra. Two of the affected dogs were placed on antibiotics immediately and surgical drainage was performed within 24 hours after discovering the abscesses. No adverse effects were observed. The other 2 dogs were treated with antibiotics given perorally. Both animals became anorectic and febrile and showed signs of pain in the caudal abdomen. The pain was apparently related to localized peritonitis. Both affected dogs responded to fluid therapy and antibiotics given IV. The antibiotics were selected on the basis of sensitivity tests.

Because of the possibility of an occult abscess, we always perform a needle aspiration before doing a closed biopsy. A closed biopsy of the prostate can be performed perirectally or transabdominally in dogs after inducing tranquilization and local anesthesia.[34] We use a Tru-Cut needle (Travenol Lab). The only complication that has been associated with blind biopsy is mild hematuria.[32,35,36] Significant hemorrhage is possible, however, as it is after any blind biopsy. The patient should always be watched closely for several hours after a biopsy.

The biopsy material can be used for bacterial culture and microscopic examination. In men with chronic bacterial prostatitis, the number of bacteria in prostatic tissue is very low and the infection may be multifocal rather than diffuse.[6,15,37] Therefore, negative cultures do not eliminate the possibility of bacterial infection. Histopathologic evidence of prostatic inflammation in men does not confirm the presence of infection if cultures of prostatic tissues and fluids are negative. Non-infectious causes of prostatitis are recognized in men.

Prostatic biopsy can also be performed after opening the abdominal cavity to expose the gland. Applying traction on the bladder will bring the prostate into view. This surgical procedure can be performed fairly rapidly and it facilitates sampling any area of the prostate that appears or feels abnormal. Any resultant hemorrhage can be seen and controlled.

Radiography

Radiographs of the prostate have limited value in the diagnosis of most prostatic diseases. A better assessment of the gland's condition can often be made by digital palpation. Changes in size of the urethral lumen and reflux of contrast material into the prostate during retrograde urethrography were once associated with specific diseases of the prostate.[38] Subsequent observations of the same conditions in normal dogs have discounted their significance.

When the prostate cannot be palpated, radiographs may reveal some evidence of the gland's size and shape. Radiographs also enable an assessment of the effects of prostatic enlargement on the colon, bladder, urethra, ureters, and kidneys. Radiographs are also needed to examine the thorax, vertebral bodies, and sublumbar lymph nodes for evidence of metastasis when prostatic neoplasia is a possibility.

Treatment of Chronic Bacterial Prostatitis

Chronic bacterial prostatitis is difficult to cure because the blood-prostatic fluid barrier is intact. This barrier is due to the pH differences among blood, prostatic interstitium, and prostatic fluid; the characteristics of prostatic acinar epithelium; and the protein-binding characteristics of antibiotics.[29,40-43]

The pH of blood and prostatic interstitium is 7.4.[16,41,43] Although prostatic fluid pH in men with bacterial prostatitis becomes more alkaline, the pH in some dogs with naturally occurring bacterial prostatitis was acidic, as was prostatic fluid from dogs experimentally infected.[23,44-49,54] If infected prostatic fluid in dogs is acidic, then such antibacterial agents as erythromycin, oleandomycin, and trimethoprim will cross the barrier more effectively than other antibiotics. Distribution of chloramphenicol is not affected by pH differences because it is nonionizable.

Lipid solubility is also important in the passage of drugs across prostatic epithelium. Drugs with low lipid solubility cannot enter the prostatic acini. These drugs include penicillin, ampicillin, amoxicillin, cephalosporins, and the aminoglycosides. Chloramphenicol, the macrolide antibiotics, and trimethoprim are examples of lipid-soluble drugs.

Protein-binding in plasma determines the amount of drug that enters prostatic fluid. When protein-bound, less drug is available to cross the prostatic epithelium. Examples of drugs with significant protein-binding are clindamycin and chloramphenicol. This factor is probably less important than lipid-solubility or pH because biologic systems rarely reach equilibrium.

Current recommendations for treatment depend on whether a gram-negative or a gram-positive organism is the infecting agent. Gram-negative organisms are much more common.[50] In man, gram-positive organisms are considered questionable prostatic pathogens.[3,33] If the causal organism is gram-negative, chloramphenicol or trimethoprim is preferred. If the causal organism is gram-positive, then erythromycin, clindamycin, oleandomycin, chloramphenicol, or trimethoprim can be selected on the basis of sensitivity tests. Measurement of prostatic fluid pH would aid the selection of a potentially effective drug.

Antibiotic medication should be continued for at least 4 to 6 weeks. Urine and prostatic fluid should be re-cultured after 3 to 4 days of treatment and 1 month after discontinuing antibiotics to ensure that the infection has been eliminated and not merely suppressed.

Based on the experience in men, the prognosis for a cure by using antibiotics is only fair. The long-term cure rate in man is approximately 30%.[33]

If prostatic infection cannot be eliminated with antibiotics alone, other treatments have been used to reduce the prostate's size. Two of these treatments, castration and administration of estrogens, should not be recommended for breeding animals. It has been reported that a new anti-androgen, flutamide, reduces prostatic size without having adverse effects on libido or fertility in dogs.[51] Decreased spermatogenesis has been observed in men, however, who are treated with this drug.[52]

Prostatectomy can be performed to remove infected tissues. This will result in infertility, however, unless special care is taken to preserve the ductus deferens.

If the prostatic infection cannot be eliminated, antibiotics are used either intermittently or continuously.[2] Trimethoprim is preferred for long-term administration.[6] It can be given once daily in the evening to prevent recurrent infection of the bladder; it is occasionally given at 50% the usual daily dose after the urinary tract infection is eliminated.[2] Supplementation with folic acid will help to prevent a deficiency that might develop with long-term use of trimethoprim.

Summary

The prostatic diseases most frequently associated with infertility are those that cause obstruction of the deferent ducts (neoplasia, abscessation, cyst formation, acute inflammation). Bacterial prostatitis and prostatic secretory dysfunction are other potential causes of infertility.

When a dog is presented because of suspected infertility, the prostate gland should always be palpated. If it is not palpable, radiographs should be obtained to determine the gland's size and shape. If the prostate is abnormal in size and shape, the cause should be investigated by examining any urethral discharge, urinalysis, CBC, semen evaluation, examination of urethral fluid collected before and after prostatic massage, and aspiration or biopsy of the prostate. Treatment will depend on the cause.

When no prostatic abnormalities are detected on physical examination, chronic bacterial prostatitis should still be considered a possible cause of the infertility. Its presence should be investigated by urinalysis, semen evaluation, and culture of prostatic fluid. When chronic bacterial prostatitis is diagnosed, antibiotics that penetrate the blood-prostatic barrier must be given for an extended period. The prostatic fluid must be cultured repeatedly to monitor the status of the infection.

References

1. Ulstein, M et al: In Human Semen and Fertility Regulation in Men, pp 355-362. CV Mosby, St Louis, 1976.
2. Stamey, TA: Pathogenesis and Treatment of Urinary Tract Infections, pp 417-419. Williams & Wilkins, Baltimore, 1980.
3. Derrick, FC and Dahlberg, G: In Human Semen and Fertility Regulation in Men, pp 389-397. CV Mosby Co, St Louis, 1976.

4. Del Porto, GB *et al:* Urology **5** (1975) 638.
5. Meares, EM: *Accessory Glands of the Male Reproductive Tract,* pp 139-174. Ann Arbor Science Publishers, Ann Arbor, MI, 1978.
6. Meares, EM: J Urol **123** (1980) 141.
7. Meares, EM: Kidney Int **20** (1981) 289.
8. Teague, NS: Fertil Steril **22** (1971) 281.
9. Eliasson, R and Lindholmer, C: In *Human Semen and Fertility Regulation in Men,* pp 44-50. CV Mosby Co, St Louis, 1976.
10. Ivanov, II and Kassavina, BS: Nature **158** (1946) 625.
11. Lindholmer, C and Eliasson, R: Fertil Steril **25** (1974) 424.
12. Hommonnai, ZT *et al:* Fertil Steril **29** (1978) 539.
13. Lindholmer, C and Eliasson, R: Int J Fertil **17** (1972) 153.
14. Lindholmer, C and Eliasson, R: Int J Fertil **19** (1974) 45.
15. Caldamone, AA and Cockett, ATK: Urol **12** (1978) 304.
16. Marmar, JL *et al:* Fertil Steril **26** (1975) 1057.
17. Saito, S *et al:* Amer J Physiol **217** (1967) 749.
18. Saito, S *et al:* Invest Urol **4** (1967) 546.
19. Prout, GR *et al:* J Urol **78** (1957) 471.
20. Bartlett, DJ: J Reprod Fertil **3** (1962) 190.
21. Smith, E: *Normal and Abnormal Growth of the Prostate,* pp 530-533. Charles C Thomas Co, Springfield, IL, 1975.
22. Marmar, JL *et al:* Urol **16** (1980) 261.
23. Anderson, RU and Fair, WR: Invest Urol **14** (1976) 137.
24. Janick, J *et al:* Fertil Steril **22** (1971) 573.
25. Harrop, AE: J Small Anim Pract **7** (1966) 723.
26. Barsanti, JA and Finco, DR: Vet Clin No Amer **9** (1979) 679.
27. Meares, EM and Stamey, TA: Brit J Urol **44** (1972) 175.
28. Meares, EM: Ann Rev Med **30** (1979) 279.
29. Stamey, TA *et al:* J Urol **103** (1970) 187.
30. Goodwin, M *et al:* Nature **203** (1979) 549.
31. Ling, GV and Ruby, AC: Amer J Vet Res **39** (1978) 695.
32. Barsanti, JA *et al:* JAVMA **177** (1980) 160.
33. Meares, EM and Stamey, TA: Brit J Urol **44** (1972) 175.
34. Finco, DR: Vet Clin No Amer **4** (1974) 367.
35. Leeds, ER and Leav, I: JAVMA **154** (1969) 925.
36. Weaver, AD: J Small Anim Pract **18** (1977) 573.
37. Schmidt, JD and Patterson, MC: J Urol **96** (1966) 519.
38. Greiner, TP and Belts, CW: *Veterinary Internal Medicine,* pp 1274-1306. WB Saunders Co, Philadelphia, 1975.
39. Stone, EA *et al:* JAAHA **14** (1978) 115.
40. Stamey, TA *et al:* J Urol **103** (1970) 187.
41. Reeves, DS *et al:* Proc 2nd Nat Symp Urinary Tract Infect, London, pp 197-205, 1972.
42. Haveland, H: Prostatic Pharmacokinetics. Int Symp, Sardinia, pp 73-77. Churchill, Livingston, London, 1973.
43. Winningham, DG *et al:* Nature **219** (1968) 139.
44. Fair, WR and Cordonniere, JJ: J Urol **120** (1978) 695.
45. Fair, WR *et al:* J Urol **121** (1979) 437.
46. Baumueller, A *et al:* Invest Urol **15** (1977) 158.
47. Barsanti, JA: Studies in progress.
48. Baumueller, A and Madsen, PO: Urol Res **5** (1977) 211.
49. Baumueller, A and Madsen, PO: Urol Res **5** (1977) 215.
50. Hornbuckle, WE *et al:* Cornell Vet **68** (1978) 284.
51. Neri, RO and Monahan, M: Invest Urol **10** (1972) 123.
52. Stewart, BH: Drug Therapy. Dec, 1975, 42.
53. Barsanti, JA: AAHA Proc, 1982.
54. Ling, GV: Personal communication.

IMMUNOLOGIC INFERTILITY
BY ROBERT C. ROSENTHAL

Introduction

Infertility due to immunologic causes is recognized in human beings.[1-3] In both natural and experimental settings, immunologic infertility is also recognized in a number of other animal species. For example, a specific complement-fixing antibody to the acrosome of guinea pig spermatozoa exists in the serum of normal guinea pigs. It lyses spermatozoa and germinal cells and can cause damage if it enters the male reproductive tract.[4] Antisperm antibodies have also been detected in the rat. Naturally occurring antibodies that agglutinate sperm are occasionally found in low titers in the serum of aged male rats.[5] Studies on repeat breeder cows have demonstrated the presence of antibodies to seminal antigens in the cervical mucus.[6] Some turkey hens have a serum factor that may be causally related to their sterility.[7] Naturally occurring antisperm antibodies have been found in the serum of both male and female mink.[8] Immunologic infertility also has been observed in rabbits, mice, and monkeys.[9-11] To this date, however, immunologic infertility has not been clearly identified as a clinical entity in dogs or cats.

Immunologic Infertility in the Dog

The problem of canine infertility has attracted limited attention in the veterinary literature. In a "comprehensive book on reproduction in the dog," the problems of infertility were mentioned only briefly.[12] Improper timing of mating and other management errors have been frequently cited as causes of apparent infertility. In many cases the cause of canine infertility remains poorly defined.

Keeping good records and mating at the proper time on the basis of clinical signs, vaginal cytology, and semen evaluation are important factors in successful breeding.[13-17] Other important causes of canine infertility concern hormonal imbalances.[14,15,18] infections,[19-23] neoplasms,[24,25] and anatomic defects.[14,26-29]

Both the clinical and contraceptive implications of immunologic infertility in the dog have been discussed.[29-33] For example, some strains of Beagles that develop lymphocytic thyroiditis also seem to have a genetic predisposition for lymphocytic orchitis. The associated changes include decreased testicular size and weight and reduced fertility. Lymphocytes infiltrate the testes and epididymides and the testes atrophy.[30,34]

An attempt has been made to induce and assess antisperm antibodies in the bitch by injecting mixtures of spermatozoa and killed bacteria (*Streptococcus* spp and *Escherichia coli*) into the vaginal submucosa. Serum and cervical mucus were subsequently examined for evidence of antisperm antibodies by a microagglutination test. Serum also was examined by macroagglutination tests and cervical mucus by sperm immobilization tests. The results indicated that both serum agglutinating technics were of no value. The microagglutination test using cervical mucus was said to show "promise in providing a diagnostic aid for immunologically-caused infertility."[31]

Antisperm antibody has been induced and detected in male Pointers by injecting them with autologous sperm in Freund's complete adjuvant. A second injection of the autologous sperm was given without the adjuvant 2 weeks later. Indirect immunofluorescence was then demonstrated on the acrosome of autologous sperm at dilutions of up to 64 times baseline values. In a microagglutination test, sperm antibodies were demonstrated in dilutions 16 times that of baseline values.[35] Though a sperm-immobilization test failed to demonstrate sperm antibody reliably in the same study, such technics may be useful after problems of complement source are resolved.[32] Elevated sperm-agglutination titers have also been detected by a microtiter technic following injection of homologous sperm (repeatedly frozen to -60 C and thawed to rupture cell membranes) and Freund's complete adjuvant. Increases in titer were most evident 2 weeks after the injection.[36]

In a study of the effect of vasectomy and vasovasotomy in the dog, antibodies to testicular basement membrane and sperm were sought. They were not found following vasovasotomy. Antisperm antibodies were detected by indirect immunofluorescence in 5 of 8 dogs between 1 and 5 months after vasectomy. The antibodies persisted from 1 to more than 7 months in titers that ranged from 1:4 to 1:32 and were directed at acrosomal or tail antigens.[37]

Immunologic control of fertility has been attempted in dogs. Males immunized against bovine luteinizing hormone produced antibodies and were unproductive for as long as a year. Prostatic, epididymal, and testicular atrophy occurred among the treated animals. A single injection of ovine gonadotropin in dogs resulted in antibody production and inability to ejaculate for more than 20 weeks.[38] Repeating such injections did not consistently result in reproductive failure, however.[39] Both male and female dogs immunized with a single dose of human chorionic gonadotropin developed specific serum antibodies demonstrated by radioimmunoassay, but they suffered no reproductive dysfunction. It was believed that the absence of reproductive dysfunction was related to lack of cross-reactivity among antibodies to human chorionic gonadotropin and canine gonadotropin.

The possibility of immunologic control of fertility in dogs by inducing the development of antibodies against antigenic sites on gametes has been suggested.[29] Prevention of pregnancy has been achieved in dogs by injecting them with porcine zona pellucida antigens. In these studies, serum antizona antibody titers were demonstrated by indirect immunofluorescence and precipitation tests. Infertility was associated with high titers of antizona antibodies; fertility returned when the titers declined. Antizona antibodies appeared to interfere with the binding of sperm to receptor sites or the escape of the embryo from the zona at implantation.[40] There seem to be no clinical reports about the occurrence of antisperm or antiovary antibodies in infertile dogs.

References

1. Megne, AC and Behrman, SJ: Clin Obstetrics and Gynecology **22** (1979) 231.
2. Alexander, NJ: Contemp Ob/Gyn **14** (1979) 92.
3. Siegler, AM: Fertil Steril **33** (1980) 360.
4. Johnson, MH: J Reprod Fert **16** (1968) 503.
5. Rumke, P. and Titus, M: J Reprod Fert **21** (1970) 69.
6. Bhatt, GN *et al:* Indian Vet J **56** (1979) 184.
7. Yu, WCY and Burke, WH: Poult Sci **58** (1979) 1378.
8. Tung, KSK *et al:* Prog Reports, Mink Farmers' Research Foundation, 1981.
9. Kiddy, CA *et al:* J Immunol **82** (1959) 125.
10. Tung, KSK *et al:* J Reprod Immun **1** (1979) 145.
11. Alexander, NJ: Fertil Steril **28** (1977) 562.
12. Harrop, AD: *Reproduction in the Dog.* Bailliere, Tindall, and Cox. London, 1960.
13. Larsen, RE: Vet Clin No Amer **7 (4)** (1977) 735.
14. Johnston, SD: JAVMA **176** (1980) 1335.
15. Larsen, RE and Johnston, SD: In *Current Veterinary Therapy VII,* WB Saunders Co, Philadelphia, 1980.
16. Roszel, JF: Vet Clin No Amer **7 (4)** (1977) 667.
17. Saeger, JWJ and Platz, CC: Vet Clin No Amer **7 (4)** (1977) 765.
18. Rhoades, JD and Foley, CS: Vet Clin No Amer **7 (4)** (1977) 789.
19. Barton, CL: Vet Clin No Amer **7 (4)** (1977) 711.
20. Barton, CL: Vet Clin No Amer **7 (4)** (1977) 705.
21. Pollock, RVH: Compend Cont Educ **1** (1979) 255.
22. Flores-Castro, R and Carmichael, LE: In *Current Veterinary Therapy VII,* WB Saunders Co, Philadelphia, 1980.
23. Sokolowski, JH: JAAHA **16** (1980) 119.
24. Muller, G and Kirk, RW: *Small Animal Dermatology.* WB Saunders Co, Philadelphia, 1976.
25. Theilen, GH and Madewell, BR: *Veterinary Cancer Medicine.* Lea & Febiger, Philadelphia, 1979.
26. Cobb, LM: Vet Rec **71** (1959) 66.
27. Cobb, LM and Archibald, J: JAVMA **134** (1959) 393.
28. Reid, JS and Frank, RJ: JAAHA **9** (1973) 367.
29. Faulkner, LC: In *Current Therapy in Theriogenology.* WB Saunders Co, Philadelphia, 1980.

30. Larsen, RE: In *Current Therapy in Theriogenology*, WB Saunders Co, Philadelphia, 1980.
3l. O'Keefe, CM: Master's thesis, Kansas State University, 1977.
32. Wildt, DE *et al:* JAAHA **13** (1977) 223.
33. Wildt, DE and Seager, SWJ: Vet Clin No Amer **7 (4)** (1977) 775.
34. Fritz, TE *et al:* Exp Mol Path **24** (1976) 142.
35. Rosenthal, RC *et al:* AJVR **45** (1984) 37a.
36. Larsen, RE (Univ Minnesota): Unpublished data, 1982.
37. Lansac, J *et al:* J Gyn Obst Biol Reprod **5** (1976) 5.
38. Faulkner, LC: JAVMA **166** (1975) 479.
39. Faulkner, LC *et al:* In *Immunization with Hormones in Reproduction Research.* North Holland Publishing Co, Amsterdam, 1975.
40. Shivers, CA *et al:* JAAHA **17** (1981) 823.

ADVERSE EFFECTS OF DRUGS
BY LLOYD E. DAVIS

There probably is no area of veterinary therapeutics in which there is greater uncertainty than the use of drugs in breeding animals. Drugs can affect the development of gametes with resultant infertility. They can affect the blastocyst prior to implantation and cause embryonic death or they may interfere with development of the embryo and thus produce malformations. Later in gestation, drugs may cause functional abnormalities in the fetus and drugs administered during parturition may adversely affect the ability of the newborn puppy or kitten to adapt to its new environment.

In no phase of veterinary practice is the risk of treatment greater than in the treatment of pregnant females. There are several reasons for this: (1) the pregnant bitch or queen undergoes physiologic changes that alter the disposition and effects of drugs, (2) many drugs have not been studied specifically in pregnant dogs and cats, (3) though many adverse drug reactions are reversible in the adult animal they frequently are irreversible in the developing embryo, and (4) untoward effects of drugs on the conceptus or fetus are not immediately apparent to the clinician. In the following discussion an attempt will be made to provide a conceptual basis for planning the treatment of dogs and cats of breeding age.

Physiologic Changes During Pregnancy
The presence of fetuses in the uterus and change in hormonal secretion cause adjustments in the bitch or queen that compensate for the increased physiologic burden imposed by pregnancy. The uterus greatly enlarges, the basal metabolic rate increases, and there is an

increased requirement for nutrients. The increase in uterine size, development of the placenta, and increased metabolic rate require an increase in cardiac output, which is accomplished by retention of water and sodium and a concomitant increase in blood volume. The body weight of a dam increases throughout gestation and this can affect the dosage of drugs (Fig 1). This is due to the weight of fetuses, uterus, placenta, fetal membranes, amniotic fluid, mammary glands, and retained fluids.

Renal function is altered during pregnancy. Tubular resorption of sodium, chloride, and water is increased in response to the effects of steroidal hormones. This is offset by an appreciable increase in glomerular filtration rate, however, and there is little change in urine formation. These changes could alter the effects of certain drugs on the kidneys of a dam.

The effect of pregnancy on rates of excretion or biotransformation of various drugs by the bitch or queen is unknown. Increase in extracellular fluid volume undoubtedly affects the concentration of drugs. Pregnancy may predispose a dam to unusual toxic effects. For example, tetracycline given parenterally causes an acute hepatotoxicity that is characterized by fatty metamorphosis in the pregnant bitch. As this does not occur in the male dog or nonpregnant bitch, it prob-

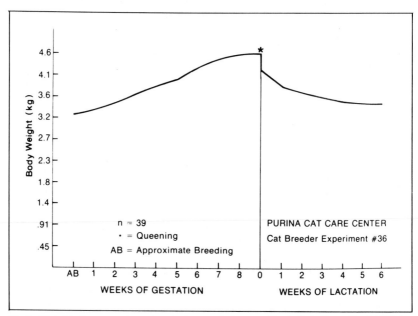

Fig 1. Weight changes of queens during gestation and lactation. From Kealy, RD: In *Current Therapy in Theriogenology*, p 858. WB Saunders Co, Philadelphia, 1980.

ably reflects some biochemical or physiologic difference in the pregnant animal.

Influence of Drugs on the Gonads

Following their administration, drugs are delivered to the ovaries or testes in blood flowing to these organs. Because their function in part is to produce gametes, the gonads are especially vulnerable to adverse effects of certain drugs. Additionally, both the ovaries and testes are endocrine organs that are regulated by pituitary hormones. Drugs that affect pituitary function can thus have indirect effects on the gonads and influence fertility.

Ovaries

The ovaries of small animals receive about 13% of the total blood flow to the uterus.[1] Relative to tissue weight, however, the ovaries receive an extremely high blood flow, about 4500 ml/min/kg. This can increase 10-fold during pregnancy.[2] Most of this blood flow (88%) is distributed to the corpus luteum during pregnancy and the flow to this structure is an astounding 20,000 ml/min/kg. Therefore, large amounts of a drug contained within the blood may be presented to the ovaries in a relatively short time. High concentrations of phenytoin, phenobarbital, tetrahydrocannabinol, and oxytetracycline have been found in the ovaries of animals receiving these drugs.[3-6] At equilibrium the concentration of oxytetracycline in the ovary was equal to the plasma concentration of the drug.[6] The influence of most drugs on the development of ova or on the function of the corpus luteum is unknown at this time.

Testes

The testes are vulnerable to the effects of certain drugs that may act on the vasculature or inhibit the maturation of spermatozoa within the seminiferous tubules. Blood is delivered to the testes of the dog and tomcat by the spermatic and vasal arteries. The former is tortuous and it responds somewhat differently from other arteries to endogenous mediators. This artery is constricted by catecholamines and serotonin, but does not dilate in response to heat or acetylcholine.[7] Because of this characteristic of the spermatic artery, vasopressor agents may have adverse effects on fertility by causing ischemia of the testes. Testicular degeneration has been observed following administration of serotonin.[8] Blood flow to the testes is normally low in relation to their oxygen consumption and they are threatened by anything that decreases blood flow to them or increases their metabolic rate.[9]

Diffusion barriers exist between the testicular capillaries and the fluid within the seminiferous tubules and the rete testis. These barriers may limit the penetration of substances with a high molecular weight or of drugs that are extensively bound to protein in blood plasma. The fluid contained within the seminiferous tubules and rete testis flows at a rate of 5 to 20 μl/g testis/hour; the faster rate occurs in smaller animals. This flow was observed to be constant from hour to hour and under a variety of experimental conditions.[10] Drugs contained within this fluid would bathe the germinal epithelium and be distributed from one region to another of the gonad. Many drugs will diffuse from capillaries into the testicular lymph, but not into the fluid of the rete testis. The wall of the seminiferous tubules apparently constitutes a diffusion barrier that prevents some drugs from coming in contact with the germinal epithelium.[11] It has been found that proteins don't cross this barrier and therefore protein-bound fractions of drug in plasma or lymph would not be expected to enter the fluid in the seminiferous tubules. The compound alpha-chlorohydrin that affects glycerol metabolism in the germinal cells was observed to penetrate rapidly into the fluid of the rete testis and attain equilibrium within 40 minutes.[12]

Species differences in response of the testis to different drugs and toxins present a problem to veterinarians making decisions relative to use of various drugs in breeding animals. Most studies of such drug effects have been conducted in rodents and the observations may not be applicable to the dog or tomcat. For example, cadmium salts in low concentration produce vascular lesions and severe hemorrhagic necrosis of the testes in rats, but the dog is much less sensitive to testicular toxicity of cadmium.[13,14]

Several drugs have been shown to have serious adverse effects on fertility. For example, antineoplastic drugs cause aplasia of the germinal epithelium of the testes. The ability to produce spermatocytes is regained slowly after cessation of therapy. Drugs that have this effect include methotrexate, busulfan, mustargen, cyclophosphamide, vincristine, triethylenemelamine, and procarbazine. It is not known what effect these drugs might have on the progeny resulting from matings after treated animals regain fertility. Parenteral administration of nitrofurans (nitrofurazone, nidroxyzone, and nitrofurantoin) arrests development of primary spermatocytes. This effect was reversible following withdrawal of the drugs.[15] Colchicine, a drug used for the treatment of gout, reversibly inhibits spermatogenesis, as does hexachlorophene.[16,17] Amphotericin B reversibly arrests spermatogenesis at the spermatogonial stage in dogs.[18] Griseofulvin resembles colchicine in its chemical structure and it has been reported to cause oligospermia in dogs following IP or IV administration of large doses.[19] Such effects have not been observed, however, following oral administration of the usual doses to dogs and cats.[20] This agrees with studies in men receiving up to 2 grams of griseofulvin per day for 6 months in whom no effect on spermatogenesis was observed.[21]

Follicle-stimulating hormone (FSH) from the pituitary gland is important in maintaining the seminiferous tubules and promoting spermatogenesis. Drugs that inhibit release of FSH from the pituitary gland may inhibit the conversion of primary spermatocytes to secondary spermatocytes.[22] High concentrations of androgens, estrogens, and possibly anabolic steroids suppress the release of FSH. Other drugs that disrupt spermatogenesis by this mechanism are thiophene, dimetridazole, Enheptin, and chlorpromazine.[23-25]

The clinical significance of studies concerning drug effects on testes is unclear at the present time. The groups of drugs that are most implicated in the production of infertility are used in the treatment of life-threatening diseases. Therefore, their effects on fertility are likely to be a minor concern. Long-term therapy of urologic infections with nitrofurantoin possibly should be avoided in stud dogs.

Drug Disposition During Pregnancy

Following administration of a drug, its molecules cross a series of biologic membranes to enter the blood where they are in solution in plasma water or bound to serum proteins. Blood that contains the drug circulates throughout the body and the drug diffuses into tissues, combines with drug receptors, is metabolized in the liver or other tissues, and is excreted by organs or secreted by glands (Fig 2). After fertilization occurs the distribution of a drug to the female genital tract has added significance when deciding to use it or not.

Most drugs are weak electrolytes and are composed of relatively small molecules. Factors that affect their ability to cross biologic membranes include ionization state, lipid solubility, and molecular size.[26] They affect the ability of drugs to enter oviductal or uterine fluids and to cross the placenta into the fetal circulation.

Prefertilization Period

After ovulation, the ovum enters the oviducts and is carried in the oviductal fluid in these structures. This fluid has a pH higher than that of the plasma;[27] consequently, basic drugs would attain lower concentrations and acidic drugs higher concentrations in these fluids.[28] The influence of various drugs on the unfertilized ovum is unknown and probably of little consequence.

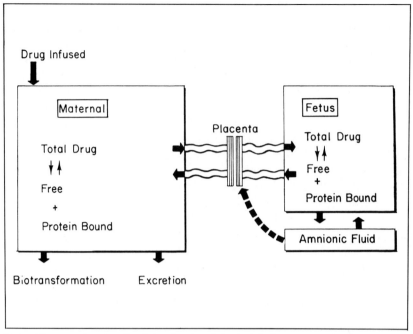

Fig 2. Diagram showing the fate of a drug injected during pregnancy.

Postfertilization Period

The ovum is fertilized in the segment of the oviduct nearest the ovary and undergoes cleavage as it moves through the duct toward the uterus. This is a crucial period in the development of puppies or kittens. Drugs or other chemicals can accumulate in the luminal fluids of the oviduct and uterus. Caffeine, nicotine, thiopental, DDT, and isoniazid attained concentrations that were 50% greater in these fluids than the concentration in blood plasma of pregnant rabbits.[29] Drugs present in luminal fluid can diffuse into the developing blastocyst during its migration and in the period immediately following implantation. This corresponds with the period of rapid development of canine and feline embryos (Table 1). Studies of the uptake of drugs by blastocysts from rabbits revealed that caffeine, nicotine, DDT, barbital, thiopental, isoniazid, antipyrine, sulfanilamide, thalidomide, and salicylate were absorbed rapidly by the blastocysts.[30] Compounds that exceeded a molecular weight of 60,000 did not penetrate the blastocyst. It has also been observed that gentamicin molecules were present in the lumen of the cow's uterus within 15 to 30 minutes after IM administration of a 4 mg/kg dose.[31]

Placental Transfer

During implantation the fetal membranes fuse with the uterine mucosa to form the placenta, which enables exchange between the fetal and maternal circulations. The transfer of drugs across the placenta is more significant from the standpoint of their pharmacologic effects on the fetus than on their potential teratogenic effects because much of organogenesis is completed by the time placentation has developed in the dog or cat.

Concepts of the placental "barrier" have been revised considerably as a result of research conducted during the past 20 years. Most drugs will readily diffuse across the placental membranes because their molecular size is relatively small and most drugs are lipid-soluble. The concentration of a drug in the fetal circulation and tissues depends on many factors, including its molecular size and lipid solubility, placental blood flow, extent of protein-binding of the drug, and disposition of the drug in the dam. The placenta may be freely permeable to a certain drug and yet the amount reaching the fetal circulation may be very low because the drug is bound to albumin in the maternal circulation. Similarly, a drug will not attain significant concentrations in the fetus if it is rapidly metabolized or excreted by the dam. Conversely, a reactive metabolite of a "safe" parent drug may be formed in the dam and passed across the placenta to the fetus. Because drug metabolism pathways differ widely among species, it is conceivable that such a metabolite could be formed in one species but not in another.[32] Generally the fetus has a limited capacity to metabolize drugs and may be exposed extensively to parent drugs or their metabolites that pass through the placenta.[33]

Table 1. Developmental Periods in the Dog, Cat, and Some Laboratory Animals

Species	Time Fertilized Ova Enter Uterus (day)	Implantation (days)	End of Embryonic Period (days)	End of Metamorphosis (days)	Birth (days)
Swine	3-4, postcoitus	11-12	20	35	112-116
Dog	5-6, postcoitus	14-21	20	30	63-68
Cat	4, after ovulation	13-17	18	22	63-66
Rabbit	4, postcoitus	7-8	10	14	32
Rat	4, postcoitus	4.5-6.5	12.5	15	22
Mouse	4, postcoitus	4.5	9	13.5	19
Hamster	4, postcoitus	4.5-5	8.5	12	16
Guinea pig	4, postcoitus	6	15	26	64-68

From Davis, LE and Stanton, HC: In *Current Therapy in Theriogenology*, p 47, WB Saunders Co, Philadelphia, 1980. Hansel, W, and McEntee, K: In *Duke's Physiology of Domestic Animals*, 9th edition, p 782, Comstock, Ithaca, 1977.

Because of the complex relationships between the drug, dam, and fetus, one cannot obtain a clear understanding of placental permeability to a given substance by merely sampling blood from the dam and the umbilical vein.[34] A valid way of measuring the placental transfer of a drug involves the maintenance of a constant concentration in maternal blood while intermittently sampling blood from the fetus.[35] By applying this method it was learned that constant blood concentrations of some drugs in dams may be hazardous to the fetus. For example, diazoxide destroyed pancreatic islet cells and caused diabetes in fetal lambs, chlorpromazine caused tachycardia and degenerative changes in the fetal liver, and phenylbutazone caused renal damage in the fetus.[36,37]

An important corollary of these experimental observations is the increased risk to a fetus when a drug is administered to a pregnant female whose ability to eliminate the drug has been reduced by disease. Drugs given to a dam with renal insufficiency or hepatic disease may be so slowly eliminated from her body that constant concentrations are established. This would greatly increase the exposure of the fetus to the drug.

Dysmorphogenesis

The action of a dysmorphogenic agent on the conceptus depends on the developmental stage of the embryo; the genetic susceptibility of the embryo; and the physiologic, nutritional, and pathologic status of the dam. The period during which chemical substances can affect development of the embryo or fetus is frequently quite short. Ontogenesis is a continuum of precisely orchestrated biochemical events that succeed one another at a rapid rate. Accordingly, each organ undergoes a "critical period" of differentiation at precise times following conception and it is at these times that the conceptus is most vulnerable to environmental influences.[38,39]

Gestation may be considered as consisting of 4 periods: blastogenesis, embryogenesis, metamorphosis, and fetal growth. Following fertilization of the ovum the zygote undergoes cleavage as it passes from the oviduct into the uterus as a free blastocyst. The blastocyst attaches to the endometrium and continues the process of embryogenesis. During this period the embryo undergoes very rapid and important transformations. These processes will be briefly described, using the pig as a model because the development of this species has been studied extensively. Although other species undergo similar changes, the temporal relationships of the transformations may be different. The comparative time intervals for the major

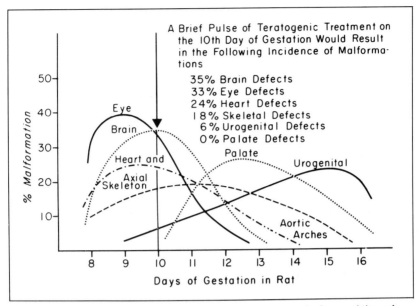

Fig 3. Association of malformations produced by a teratogenic drug and time of exposure. From Wilson, JG: In *Teratology Principles and Techniques,* p 256. University of Chicago Press, 1965.

events for different species are listed in Table 1. Comparative values for certain laboratory animals have been included because most studies of drug teratogenicity have been performed in these species.

The primitive streak is complete and the notochord is forming in the porcine embryo by the time of its attachment (11 to 12 days). The primordial nervous system; sense organs; the circulatory, excretory, and digestive systems; and limb buds are formed from the 12th to the 20th day. The period of metamorphosis (days 20 through 35) is marked by differentiation and organogenesis. The enamel organs are formed for subsequent tooth development, the nasal septum becomes complete, the chambers of the heart are separated, ossification of bone commences, skeletal muscle is formed, and the mammary and endocrine glands' primordia appear. By the 35th day the facial clefts are closed and the palate is completed. The fetal period, which extends from the end of metamorphosis to birth, is characterized by growth of the fetus. Most organs are differentiated prior to this time. During fetal life the gut is withdrawn from the umbilical hernia (36 to 50 days), the external genitalia become differentiated (39 to 95 days), and histogenesis of the nervous system proceeds.

Teratogenic agents affect the conceptus in different ways depending on the stage of gestation. Exposure of the blastocyst to certain drugs prior to attachment may interfere with implantation and terminate pregnancy. Chemicals are most likely to cause morphologic changes in the embryo during the mid-embryonic period when organogenesis is most active (Fig 3). There is increasing evidence that certain chemical substances, including methyl mercury, lead, nicotine, and perhaps some pesticides, may cause more subtle physiological changes when administered to the dam in late pregnancy after the organs are formed, but during a critical period in development of organ functions. The developing nervous system seems to be especially susceptible to injury and permanent though subtle changes in postnatal behavioral patterns may result. Impaired endocrine development may not be obvious until the animal approaches sexual maturity.

It is difficult to assess the role of drugs and other chemical substances in producing embryonic death or anomalous development in domestic animals because other factors can influence development. Such influences include genetic defects, radiation, infections, vitamin deficiencies and maternal endocrine disorders. Few studies have been made to evaluate the teratogenicity of drugs in any domestic animal. Nearly all of our knowledge has been derived from studies of chicks and laboratory rodents and in most cases we do not know the relevance of this information to other species. A number of drugs and other chemicals that are potential teratogens on the basis of studies of laboratory animals are listed in Table 2. These drugs should be used with caution in pregnant animals.

Development of Drug Receptors in the Fetus

When a drug enters the fetal circulation, several factors determine its pharmacologic effects. They include (1) the fetus' capacity to nonspecifically bind or metabolically inactivate the drug, (2) the fetus' ability to mobilize transmitter substances in the case of indirectly acting drugs or to convert inactive pro-drugs to active drugs, (3) the kinetic characteristics and density of tissue drug receptors, and (4) the capacity of the end organ to respond to stimuli to carry out its functions. There is some information on the 1st factor in a few species, but little can be said about the other factors at this time.

Both alpha- and beta-adrenergic receptors are present in the fetal lamb by the middle of gestation. Injection of isoproterenol, epinephrine, levarterenol, or methoxamine into the fetal circulation will elicit characteristic cardiovascular effects. Norepinephrine causes constriction of the ductus arteriosus and ductus venosus.[40] Blockade of these receptors by various drugs will impair the ability of the fetus to respond to stress related to hypoxia or hemorrhage.

In many ways the sympatheticoadrenal system of the newborn pig is immature. Although this neonate is capable of synthesizing and inactivating catecholamines, it may have difficulty in mobilizing a stored transmitter from the gland in response to stress. There is also some emerging evidence that the newborn pig may not be fully capable of mobilizing or utilizing its energy reserves at birth because of low adrenergic, metabolic receptor sensitivity.[41] This has also been noticed in cats and dogs.

Cholinergic receptors, acetylcholine, and acetylcholinesterase are present in embryos at a very early stage, before the innervation of developing tissues.[42] Skeletal muscle, smooth muscle, and the heart of the fetus respond to the effects of cholinergic drugs and cholinesterase inhibitors. The cholinergic system is probably important in homeostasis of the fetus and therefore drugs that modify these functions may be harmful to the fetus.

The adrenocorticotrophic hormone (ACTH), vasopressin, renin, and angiotensin II are all present in the fetus by the middle of gestation. Corticosteroid concentrations in the plasma of fetal lambs are low, but they increase sharply a few days before parturition.

Of special interest is the observation that fetal tissues contain appreciable quantities of prostaglandins. Prostaglandin E_1 causes constriction of the umbilical-placental blood vessels, dilation of the pulmonary vasculature, and maintains patency of the ductus arteriosus. Administration of prostaglandin synthetase inhibitors (such as aspirin or indomethacin) may interfere with regulation of these structures by prostaglandin E_1. Indomethacin has caused closure of the ductus arteriosus in human infants several days postpartum.[43]

The fetal thyroid gland may be affected by drugs administered to the bitch or queen during the latter half of gestation. Neonatal goiter may be produced by iodides (expectorants), methimazole, propylthiouracil, chlorpromazine, lithium, phenylbutazone, sulfonamides, theophylline, and radioactive iodine.[44] The goiter may result in respiratory distress in the newborn, a difficult delivery, or mental retardation of the offspring.

Effects on the Fetus of Drugs Administered During Parturition

Veterinarians should be aware of the possible effects on the fetus of drugs administered to the dam during parturition. It is fortunate that most births of animals are uneventful and that there seldom is

Table 2. Drugs Found to be Embryotoxic in Laboratory Animals

Drugs	Species	Defects
Acetazolamide	Mice, rats, hamsters	Forelimb abnormalities
Acriflavine	Chicks	Spina bifida
ACTH	Mice	Cleft palate
Adriamycin	Rats, mice	Cardiovascular and gut
Amantadine	Rats	Hindlimb abnormalities
Apomorphine	Chicks	Limb abnormalities
Asparaginase	Rats, mice, rabbits	Multiple
Beclomethasone	Mice	Cleft palate
Betamethasone	Rats, mice	Cleft palate
Busulfan	Rats	Cleft palate and digital
Chlorambucil	Rats	Neural and urogenital, skeletal system and palate
Chloroquine	Rats	Ocular
Codeine	Hamster	Cranioschisis
Cortisone	Mice, rats, rabbits	Cleft palate and lip
Cyclophosphamide	Mice, rats, rabbits, monkeys	Multiple
Cytosine arabinoside	Chicks, rats, hamsters, mice	Cleft palate and skeletal, cerebellar, and retinal
Daunomycin	Rats	Cardiovascular, gut, and urogenital
Dexamethasone	Rabbits	Cleft palate
Dextroamphetamine	Mice, rabbits, rats	Cardiovascular and brain, ocular and cleft palate
Diazepam	Mice	Cleft palate
Dimercaprol	Mice	Limb abnormalities
Dimethylsulfoxide	Hamster, chicks	Exencephaly, limb abnormalities and microphthalmia
Diphenylhydantoin	Mice	Multiple
E coli endotoxin	Rats	Hydrocephalus and neural
EDTA	Rats, chicks	Cleft palate, brain, and eye
Estradiol	Rats, mice	Genital and cleft palate
Estrone	Mice	Cleft palate
Evans blue	Rats	Brain and heart
Fluocortolone	Mice, rabbits	Cleft palate, and exencephaly
5-Fluorocytosine	Rats	Cleft palate and lip
Glucagon	Rats	Cataracts and microphthalmia
Gold	Rats	Multiple
Griseofulvin	Rats	Multiple
Halothane	Rats	Vertebral and costal

Table 2. (Continued)

Drugs	Species	Defects
Hydrocortisone	Mice	Cleft palate
Indomethacin	Mice, rats	Skeletal and closure of ductus arteriosus
5-Iododeoxyuridine	Mice, rats	Exencephaly, skeletal, cleft palate
Lithium	Rats	Palate, eye, ear
Meclizine	Rats, rabbits, ferrets, mice	Cleft palate, microstomia, micrognathia
6-Mercaptopurine	Chicks, mice, rats, rabbits	Skeletal
Mercurials	Mice, rats	Cleft palate and hydrocephalus
Methadone	Rats, rabbits, hamsters, guinea pigs	CNS
Methampyrone	Mice	Exencephaly
Methotrexate	Mice	Exencephaly and cleft palate
Nidroxyzone (Furadroxyl)	Mice	Limb abnormalities
Nitrogen mustard	Mice, rats, chicks	Skeletal, cleft palate, anencephaly
D-penicillamine	Rats	Skeletal
Perphenazine	Rats	Cleft palate and micromelia
Phencyclidine	Rats	Skeletal and cleft palate
Phenobarbital	Rabbits	Skeletal and aortic arch
Prednisolone	Mice, rats	Cleft palate and adrenal
Procarbazine	Rats	Ocular and skeletal
Prochlorperazine	Mice, rats	Cleft palate and anencephaly
Propylthiouracil	Rats	Thyroid hypertrophy
Quinine	Guinea pigs	Inner ear and deafness
Reserpine	Rats	Anophthalmia
Salicylate	Mice, rats	Multiple
Sulfonamides	Chicks, rats, mice	Limb abnormalities
Tetracycline	Rats	Teeth and stunting of limbs
Thyroxine	Rats	Cataracts
Triamcinolone	Mice	Cleft palate
Triethanomelamine	Rats, mice	Multiple
Trimethoprim	Rats	Cleft palate and micrognathia
Valproate	Mice	Cleft palate, skeletal, renal
Vincristine	Hamsters, rabbits, rats, monkeys	Ocular, skeletal, exencephaly, microcephaly
Vitamin A	Rats	Multiple
Vitamin D	Rats, rabbits	Aortic abnormalities

From Shepard, TH: *Catalog of Teratogenic Agents,* 3rd ed, Johns Hopkins University Press, Baltimore, 1980.

indication for use of drugs at parturition. Drugs may be given during a cesarotomy, however, and occasionally a pregnant animal may be receiving a drug(s) for a chronic condition unrelated to the pregnancy.

Most general anesthetics will cross the placenta and depress the central nervous system of the newborn. The inhalant anesthetics are subsequently eliminated unchanged from the lungs of the neonate and are the least troublesome in terms of prolonged depression. Anesthetic agents that require biotransformation (barbiturates) or renal excretion (ketamine) are likely to cause prolonged depression of the offspring following delivery and they should be avoided. Ketamine accumulates in the placenta and attains concentrations in fetal plasma and brain that are similar to those in maternal plasma.[45]

Opiates readily enter the fetus from maternal circulation and cause respiratory depression in newborn animals. Depression caused by opiates is readily reversed, however, by naloxone or nalorphine administered to an affected offspring following its delivery. Meperidine has been found to inhibit constriction of the ductus arteriosus, whereas morphine had no effect. This was attributed to the anticholinergic effects of meperidine. Its clinical significance is unknown.

Autonomic drugs administered to a dam prior to or during parturition may affect various regulatory mechanisms of the fetus during delivery. Though most adrenergic drugs are not transferred across the placenta, their administration to the dam may be harmful to the fetus because fetal asphyxia has resulted from vasoconstriction of placental vessels.[46] Atropine and several adrenolytic agents (eg, phenothiazines) readily enter the fetal circulation and may have pharmacologic effects in the neonate during and following parturition. Some anticholinesterase agents (organophosphorus compounds, neostigmine) cross the placenta and may produce myasthenia in the newborn.[47]

Tranquilizers that cross the placenta may produce undesirable effects in the newborn. For example, chlorpromazine has caused prolonged sedation and retinopathy. Diazepam, chlordiazepoxide, and phenytoin readily enter the fetus.

If absorbed rapidly into the maternal circulation, local anesthetics will cause bradycardia, acidosis, and CNS depression in the fetus. This could occur when lidocaine was given IV to control cardiac arrhythmias in the dam during parturition.

Corticosteroids administered to the dam will enter the fetus and may suppress function of the hypothalamic-pituitary-adrenal axis. Salicylates cause a tendency to bleed in newborn animals.

Certain antibiotics should not be used late in pregnancy because of their potential harm to the fetus. For example, tetracyclines may produce abnormal dentition in the offspring. Furthermore, parenteral administration of tetracycline has caused a fulminating and usually fatal hepatitis in the dam. Streptomycin may cause deafness in the neonate and nitrofurantoin can cause hemolysis.

Both digitoxin and digoxin cross the placenta and the concentrations of digoxin in the fetal heart have been twice the levels in the dam's heart.[48] The neonate will slowly eliminate a glycoside from its body, and one exposed to these drugs should be closely monitored during the 1st week or 2 of its life.

The extensive use of oxytocin in veterinary obstetrics for a long time suggests that this drug does not cause adverse effects on newborn animals. Oxytocin will cause constriction of umbilical vessels, however, and this could be harmful to an already hypoxic fetus.

Use of Drugs in Breeding Animals

Because of the many uncertainties involved, the prudent clinician will be very conservative about giving drugs to dogs and cats after they have been bred. Careful assessment of risk/benefit considerations is especially important in this circumstance and drugs should not be given for trivial reasons. If at all possible, drug therapy in bitches or queens should be avoided following breeding. It is not always possible, however, to avoid the use of drugs during pregnancy and in some cases a pregnant animal may require therapy for a medical problem. In others, there may be no history that mating has occurred. In these cases there is little that can be done to avoid the possible teratogenic effects of drugs because the most susceptible period of the embryo occurs when signs of pregnancy may not be obvious.

Clinicians should always avoid the use of drugs that are potentially teratogenic in animals following breeding. The most critical periods are 5 to 15 days following coitus in the queen and 8 to 20 days in the bitch.[50] Drugs that should be avoided during pregnancy are listed in Table 3. They are not absolutely contraindicated at all stages of pregnancy and their use can depend somewhat on the degree of fetal development. Drugs that affect organogenesis should not be administered during the first 30 days of gestation. Drugs that alter functions of the fetus should be avoided during the latter part of pregnancy and during parturition.

Drugs that have been found safe for use during pregnancy are listed in Table 4. They have not been associated with malformations in the offspring of laboratory animals. The clinical use of these drugs by veterinarians has been widespread without adverse effects in

Table 3. Drugs Contraindicated During Pregnancy.

Drugs	Adverse Effects
Acetaminophen	Methemoglobinemia
Androgens	Masculinization of fetus
Antineoplastics	Fetal death and anomalies
Bishydroxycoumarin	Fetal death and intrauterine hemorrhage
Chloramphenicol (early)	Fetal death
Chlorpromazine	Neonatal hepatic necrosis
Cholinesterase inhibitors (term)	Neonatal myasthenis
Corticosteroids (see text)	Cleft palate
Estrogens	Feminization of fetus
Iodides	Fetal goiter
Isoniazid	Retarded psychomotor activity
Lithium salts	Fetal goiter
Mepivacaine	Fetal bradycardia
Nitrofurantoin	Fetal hemolysis
Phenobarbital (high doses)	Neonatal hemorrhage
Phenylbutazone	Neonatal goiter and nephrosis
Propylthiouracil	Neonatal goiter
Quinine	Deafness and thrombocytopenia
Reserpine	Respiratory obstruction
Salicylates (near term)	Neonatal bleeding
Streptomycin	Hearing loss and congenital anomalies
Sulfonamides (long-acting)	Liver atrophy and hyperbilirubinemia
Tetracyclines	Impaired bone and tooth development
Thiazides	Fetal death and thrombocytopenia
Vitamin A (large doses)	Multiple anomalies
Vitamin D (large doses)	Hypercalcemia and mental retardation
Vitamin K analogs	Hyperbilirubinemia
Phenytoin (cats)	Congenital anomalies
Meclizine	Congenital anomalies
Diazoxide	Destruction of fetal islet cells
Iododeoxyuridine	Congenital anomalies
Griseofulvin	Congenital anomalies
Gold salts	Congenital anomalies
EDTA	Congenital anomalies
Prochlorperazine	Congenital anomalies
Prochlorperadine	Impaired growth of fetus
Propranolol	Fetal bradycardia
Indomethacin	Premature closure of ductus arteriosus
Ethoxyzolamide	Congenital anomalies
Sodium selenites	Impaired growth of fetus
Dimethylsulfoxide	Congenital anomalies
Acetazolamide	Fetal anomalies
Iodinated casein	Neonatal goiter
Amphotericin B	Congenital anomalies
Fluocytosine	Congenital anomalies
Warfarin	Intrauterine hemorrhage
Isoproterenol	Fetal tachycardia
Phenylphrine	Placental vasoconstriction, fetal hypoxia
Methoxamine	Placental vasoconstriction, fetal hypoxia
Meperidine (term)	Inhibit closure of ductus arteriosus

From Davis, LE: *Veterinary Clinical Pharmacology, WB Saunders Co, Philadelphia. In press.*

fetuses being reported. Most antimicrobial drugs, with the exceptions of tetracyclines, chloramphenicol, and long-acting sulfonamides, are safe for use in pregnant dogs and cats. This is fortunate because acute infections are the primary conditions for which therapy is indicated. There also are enough antiparasitic drugs included in the safe list to provide a choice for treatment of a dam during pregnancy. Even though these drugs are relatively safe for use in pregnant animals, the clinician should be conservative in their use. For example, high doses of atropine at term may induce uterine inertia and overzealous use of furosemide may interfere with normal lactation in the dam by causing dehydration. Barbiturates are best avoided during parturition or cesarotomy because they can cause excessive depression of the puppies or kittens.

A greater problem arises in making rational decisions about use of the drugs listed in Table 5. These agents either have not been studied in pregnant animals or they have been associated with congenital

Table 4. Drugs Found to be Safe for use During Pregnancy.*

Acetylcysteine	Disophenol	Morphine
Ammonium chloride	Doxapram	Neomycin
Amoxicillin	Doxylamine	Niclosamide
Ampicillin	Enflurane	Nitrous oxide
Atropine	Ephedrine	Oxytocin
Cephalexin	Erythromycin	Penicillin
Cephaloridine	Ethrane	Pentobarbital
Cephalothin	Furosemide	Phenobarbital
Chloramphenicol (latter half)	Gentamicin	Pilocarpine
Chlorpheniramine	Glycopyrrolate	Piperazine
Chymotrypsin	Guaifenesin	Polymyxin B
Clindamycin	Halothane	Pralidoxime
Clonazepam	Heparin	Primidone
Codeine	Kanamycin	Procaine
Colistin	Ketamine	Pyrantel
Dextromethorphan	Lidocaine	Pyrilamine
Diazepam	Lincomycin	Salbutamol
Dichlorvos	Mannitol	Spironolactone
Dicloxacillin	Mebendazole	Sulfonamides (not long-acting)
Diethylcarbamazine	Metaproterenol	Tetracaine
Diethyl ether	Methapyrilene	Theophylline
Digitoxin	Methenamine	Thiopental
Digoxin	Methohexital	Tiletamine
Dimenhydrinate	Metronidazole	Triamterene
Diphenhydramine	Miconazole	Urokinase

*Criteria: Drugs included in this table have not been teratogenic in laboratory animals. There have been no reports of deleterious effects resulting from their administration to pregnant animals.

From Davis, LE: *Veterinary Clinical Pharmacology*, WB Saunders Co, Philadelphia. In press.

Table 5. Drugs not Proven to be Safe for use During Pregnancy but not Necessarily Contraindicated.*

Acepromazine	Glycobiarsol	Procainamide
Aminopentamide	Hexylcaine	Prochlorperazine
Aminopromazine	Hydralazine	Promazine
Arsenamide	Hydrocortisone	Proparacaine
Aspirin (early pregnancy)	Iron dextran	Propiopromazine
Bithionol	Lenperone	Pyrimethamine
Bunamidine	Levamisole	Quinacrine
Butorphanol	Liothyronine	Quinidine
N-Butyl chloride	Meprobamate	Ronnel
Caffeine	Methocarbamol	Saffan
Chlorpromazine	Methoxyflurane	Spectinomycin
Chlorprothixene	Methylprednisolone	Stanozolol
Cimetidine	Neostigmine	Styrylpyridium
Colchicine	Nitroglycerine	Thiabendazole
Cortisone	Nitroprusside	Thyroxin
Cythioate	Nystatin	Toluene
Dapsone	Phenoxybenzamine	Trichlorfon
Dichlorophene	Phthalofyne	Trifluomeprazine
Dithiazanine	Physostigmine	Trimethoprim
Dobutamine	Prazosin	Xylazine
Fentanyl-Droperidol	Prednisolone	

*Criteria: Drugs included in this table have either been associated with congenital malformations in one species of laboratory animals or there is no information concerning their use during pregnancy..

From Davis, LE: *Veterinary Clinical Pharmacology.* WB Saunders Co, Philadelphia. In press.

anomalies in some, but not all, species of laboratory animals in which they were studied. An example is the corticosteroids. They cause a high incidence of cleft palates in laboratory animals. In a study of the teratogenicity of several different corticosteroids, prednisolone and cortisone caused a lower incidence of cleft palates than triamcinolone, betamethasone, dexamethasone, or methylprednisolone.[51] It would be better, therefore, to select prednisolone for animals that absolutely require a corticosteroid during pregnancy rather than one of the others. When used for certain conditions, the corticosteroid may be withdrawn during pregnancy. For example, the signs of rheumatoid arthritis may subside substantially during pregnancy due to hormonal changes in the dam. When the need for a drug is not urgent, its administration should generally be postponed until after pregnancy and lactation are completed. For example, thiacetarsamide (Caparsolate) may be toxic (though this is not known) to an embryo or fetus, and it thus would be advisable to delay heartworm treatment until after the puppies have been weaned.

In life-threatening situations, appropriate therapy for a pregnant or lactating animal should not be withheld. Even though there is a risk of damaging the fetus, the potential benefit of treatment makes the risk acceptable. The fetuses will not survive if the mother dies!

References

1. Duncan, SLB: J Physiol (London) **204** (1969) 421.
2. Abdul-Karim, RW and Bruce, N: Fertil Steril **24** (1973) 42.
3. Waddell, WJ and Mirkin, BL: Biochem Pharmacol **21** (1972) 547.
4. Waddell, WJ: In *Fundamentals of Drug Metabolism and Drug Disposition.* pp 505-514. Williams and Wilkins, Baltimore, 1971.
5. Kennedy, JS and Waddell, WJ: Toxicol Appl Pharmacol **22** (1972) 252.
6. Bretzlaff, KN *et al:* Amer J Vet Res **44** (1983) 760.
7. Setchell, BP *et al:* Circ Res **18** (1966) 755.
8. Boccabella, AV *et al:* Endocrinology **71** (1962) 827.
9. Setchell, BP and Waites, GMH: J Physiol (London) **171** (1964) 411.
10. Setchell, BP and Waites, GMH: J Reprod Fertil **30** (1972) 225.
11. Setchell, BP *et al:* J Physiol (London) **200** (1969) 73.
12. Edwards, EM *et al:* J Reprod Fertil **30** (1972) 225.
13. Gunn, SA and Gould, TC: In *The Testis,* vol 3, pp 377-48l. Academic Press, New York, 1970.
14. Chatterjee, SN and Kas, AB: Indian Vet J **45** (1968) 649.
15. Nelson, WO and Steinbergern, E: Fed Proc **12** (1953) 103.
16. Barsoum, H: J Pharmacol Exp Therap **115** (1955) 319.
17. Thorpe, E: J Comp Path **77** (1967) 137.
18. Texter, JH and Coffey, DS: Invest Urol **7** (1969) 90.
19. McNall, EG: *Antibiotics Annual, 1959-1960,* pp 674-679, Antibiotica, Inc, New York, 1960.
20. Fulvicin-U/F. Package insert, Schering Corp, 1979.
21. MacLeod, J and Nelson, WO: Proc Soc Exp Biol Med **102** (1959) 259.
22. Liddle, GW and Liddle, RA: Endocrinology. In *Pathophysiology of the Biological Principles of Disease,* p 698. WB Saunders Co, Philadelphia, 1981.
23. Steinberger, E *et al:* Anat Rec **125** (1956) 312.
24. Gretillat, S: Acta Trop **20** Suppl **9** (1966) 275.
25. Chatterjee, A: Experientia **21** (1965) 545.
26. Baggot, JD: *Principles of Drug Disposition in Domestic Animals.* WB Saunders Co, Philadelphia, 1977.
27. McLachlan, JA *et al:* Fertil Steril **21** (1970) 84.
28. Conner, EA and Miller, JW: J Pharmacol Exp Therap **184** (1973) 291.
29. Sieber, SM and Fabro, S: J Pharmacol Exp Therap **176** (1971) 65.
30. Fabro, S and Sieber, SM: The Foeto-Placental Unit. Int Cong Series 183, p 313, Excerpta Medica Found, Amsterdam, 1969.
31. Al-Guedawy, S *et al:* Disposition of Gentamicin in Blood and Uterine Fluid of Cows. J Vet Pharmacol Therap (in press).
32. Hucker, HB: Ann Rev Pharmacol Toxicol **10** (1970) 99.
33. Gillette, JR and Stripp, B: Fed Proc **34** (1975) 172.
34. Boulos, BM *et al:* Arch Internat Pharmacodyn Therap **191** (1971) 142.
35. Almond, CH *et al:* Surg Res **10** (1970) 7.
36. Boulos, BM *et al:* J Clin Pharmacol **11** (1971) 206.
37. Boulos, BM *et al:* Arch Internat Pharmacodyn Therap **194** (1971) 403.
38. Krecek, J: In *Biopsychology of Development,* pp 233-247. Academic Press, New York, 1971.
39. Stanton, HC: J Environ Path Toxicol **2** (1978) 201.
40. Owman, C *et al:* In *Fetal Pharmacology,* p 179. Raven Press, New York, 1973.
41. Stanton, HC and Woo, SK: Amer J Physiol **234** (1978) 137.
42. Karczmar, AG: In *Handbuch der Experimentellen Pharmakologie,* vol **15**, p 159. Springer-Verlag, Berlin, 1963.

CHAPTER 4

43. Brash, AR *et al:* New Engl J Med **305** (1981) 67.
44. Martin, EW *et al:* In *Hazards of Medication,* p 278. JB Lippincott, Philadelphia, 1971.
45. Mirkin, BL: In *Fetal Pharmacology,* p 15. Raven Press, New York, 1973.
46. Shnider, SM *et al:* Amer J Obstet Gynec **106** (1970) 680.
47. Mirkin, BL: In *Fetal Pharmacology,* p 12. Raven Press, New York, 1973.
48. Fouron, JC: Biol Neonat **23** (1973) 116.
49. Davis, LE: *Veterinary Clinical Pharmacology,* WB Saunders, Philadelphia. (In press.)
50. Schardein, JL: *Drugs as Teratogens,* p 17. CRC Press, Cleveland, 1976.
51. Walker, B: Proc Soc Exper Biol Med **125** (1967) 1281. Teratology **4** (1971) 39.
52. James, LF *et al:* Amer J Vet Res **27** (1966) 132.

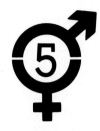

Pregnancy
and Parturition

PRE- AND POSTNATAL CARE OF FEMALE CATS
BY EMERSON D. COLBY

Prebreeding Examination

The prebreeding examination is important because it provides the opportunity to examine the queen, become informed about her diet and vaccination record, and ask pertinent questions about her previous reproductive history. Other useful information obtained at this time includes details about the queen's environment, her association and proximity to other cats, and her normal behavior patterns. Such information may be pertinent to the queen's behavior during mating, parturition, and caring for her kittens.

Queens used for breeding should have negative tests for feline leukemia virus. If the queen is in a cattery or other large colony, it would be advisable to also test her for the presence of feline infectious peritonitis virus. If there is evidence that either virus is present, the queen should not be used for breeding. Queens to be bred should be vaccinated against panleukopenia and upper respiratory disease complex at least 7 days prior to the next anticipated estrus. They should not be vaccinated during estrus or pregnancy.

The physical examination should be thorough and include palpation of the mammae. It should be performed when the owner is present so that any previous problems can be discussed. Primiparous queens should be handled gently and an attempt made to palpate the uterus. The examination should include tests and inspection for internal and external parasites. If parasite treatment is indicated, it should be given prior to estrus or pregnancy.

Breeding Procedure

The queen should be mated in the male's environment. When the male is transferred to the queen's environment, he may spend more time acquainting himself with the new surroundings than with mating. The male should be a proven stud. When purebred animals are involved, it is pertinent to ask about the male's offspring.

The queen should be bred at least twice daily for 3 or more days and preferably 3 or more times to ensure adequate release of luteinizing hormone to induce ovulation. When the queen is primiparous, her mating behavior should be observed. Occasionally a queen will not show signs of estrus until handled or exposed to the male. Queens will rarely breed only once and still produce a normal litter.

Smears of vaginal cells are often made and examined to determine the presence of estrus and the quality of the male's semen.[1,2] Material for the smears can be obtained by using a swab or by placing 2 or 3 drops of sterile saline solution into the vagina with a medicine dropper and then withdrawing the available fluid. Either technic may induce ovulation in the queen. When smears are made after mating to assess the semen, I prefer to wait for 30 to 60 minutes before using the medicine dropper method because the saline solution is frequently colder than vaginal fluids and thus damages spermatozoa. Vaginal smears can be examined when wet or they may be air-dried and stained with Wright's stain as for a blood smear. Vaginal smears cannot be used to assess the quantity of semen nor to provide evidence of pregnancy.

Examinations During Pregnancy

Queens usually require no special attention during the 1st half of gestation. They usually are palpated for evidence of pregnancy beginning 17 days after breeding. At this time the implantation sites are firm, round, and about 1 to 1.5 centimeters in diameter. As the uterus lengthens with fetal growth the firmness disappears. Fetal heads may be identified at about 50 days. Palpation of a pregnant queen can be harmful if performed roughly or otherwise improperly.

By day 25 of gestation the fetuses will be fully formed and around day 42 the fetal skeletons are visible in radiographs. Normal activity of the corpus luteum (CL) decreases after its peak on about day 21. At about day 44 to 46 the CL's function ceases. At that time, progesterone is being produced by placental tissues in sufficient quantities to maintain pregnancy.

Superovulation is infrequent except in queens in which estrus is induced with exogenous hormones. From 4 to 6 eggs are usually shed and 3 to 5 kittens comprise the average litter. When the number of fetuses is abnormally high, the uterus becomes overcrowded and fetal deaths may be related to deficient blood supply. Dead fetuses may frequently be found during a normal parturition and they often appear to have died at about 30 to 35 days of age.

Superfecundation refers to fertilization of 2 or more ova released at the same time by spermatozoa of different males. This may be common among domestic cats that roam. Ova are thought to be fertilizable for as long as 24 hours and spermatozoa are capable of fertilization for as long as 50 hours. Thus superfecundation can easily occur. Color patterns of the offspring may reflect superfecundation.

Superfetation occurs when cats are bred very early and very late during a prolonged estrus or during separate estrous periods. The reported incidence of this phenomenon is low. Cats have been known to have had an estrous cycle in which mating has occurred and then to have another estrus within 10 to 14 days. Though the 2nd estrus may be brief, mating can occur. Superfetation may be reflected by live or more often dead premature fetuses resulting from the 1st mating and a fetus born several days after others have been born. Surviving kittens may also be different in size.

Monozygotic twinning is rare in cats. It would be reflected by color patterns and markings of 2 kittens that were mirror images of each other. It is perhaps more common that twinning is confused with what is known as synchorial littermates. When synchorial littermates are found at necropsy or cesarean section, it appears that 2 ova have been implanted within the same area and are subsequently enclosed within the same placenta. When found at about 24 days of gestation, both fetuses may be alive. Later in gestation, it will be noticed that one fetus died earlier than the other and that both have died before the 50th day of gestation.

Ectopic pregnancy is fairly common in the cat. The cause may be related to injury during pregnancy or to abnormal disposition of the egg after its fertilization. Cats have been known to complete a normal gestation and show signs of queening without expelling a fetus. This usually is discovered by observing an extrauterine fetus in abdominal radiographs. The dead fetus may be a single mass or scattered throughout the abdomen. Fetal death in these cases appears to occur during mid-gestation because most of the fetuses have formed some bone. It is assumed that nidation occurs on the mesentery until the blood supply is inadequate to support the fetus.

The normal gestation period of the cat is approximately 63 days. Kittens born prior to 58 days have a less-than-average chance of survival. Gestation periods of 70 days have occurred and apparently more often in Persians and related purebreds. Queens with a higher than normal number of fetuses usually have a shortened gestation. It appears that the number, not the size, of fetuses shortens the gestation. Environmental stress may slightly lengthen gestation, especially in primigravid queens.

Care of Pregnant Queens

Stress related to shipment, change in environment, and infection is probably greatest during the period when the placenta is starting to secrete progesterone. It would thus be unwise to stress a queen during the last 20 days of her gestation. Fetuses grow significantly during the last 15 days of gestation and during this time the queen's food consumption increases. Vitamin and mineral supplements are not usually required, but additional food should be provided. Because of its higher lactose content, cow's milk will cause many cats to develop diarrhea; kitten milk replacer (KMR) is preferable.

Queens that are near parturition should be handled carefully. Their hindquarters should be supported when they are lifted. A queen with 5 or more kittens will have considerable pressure upon the diaphragm. Additional pressure created by handling the cat can result in serious respiratory distress.

A queen should be undisturbed when parturition is imminent. She usually will seek a secluded place to deliver her kittens. The queen's behavior will change and mammary enlargement will occur. One or more days prior to parturition, milk may be expressed from the mammary glands. Though it is not necessary to clip the hair of long-haired cats from the mammae and perineum, it does help the queen to clean herself following expulsion of the fetuses.

Parturition

Parturition in cats is usually not complicated. The fetuses are arranged head to head, head to tail, and tail to tail within the uterus and posterior presentation is common. Delivery of kittens is not observed often because it usually occurs during the night or another time when the cat is not disturbed. The placenta is usually eaten by the queen. The kittens may be delivered slowly, one at a time, or several may be delivered in a short period. They occasionally are delivered almost simultaneously. In other cases, the kitten(s) delivered first are already nursing when the final one is born. Retention of the placenta is rare and post-parturient bleeding is uncommon. It is helpful when the owner knows approximately when parturition started, the condition of the kittens at birth and the condition of the queen if problems should arise.

When first seen, kittens often have been cleaned and are nursing. Difficult deliveries may be alleviated by lubricating the queen's vulva and vagina with mineral oil or an antibiotic ointment and then assisting the queen to expel the fetus. When a fetus can't be expelled by the queen, help should be given as soon as possible. Occasionally the fetus can be repositioned for delivery by external manipulation of the uterus. This should be done carefully or both the fetus and uterus may be damaged. Such assistance should be provided only as a last resort for a queen with a flaccid abdomen.

Kittens may have umbilical cords tied together. When dried, the cords are extremely tough and must be cut, not pulled apart. Kittens have been found tied together in a ball when the cords become entangled. Occasionally the cords become entangled in a way that they strangulate extremities of a kitten's body.

Because nursing stimulates the let-down of milk and the release of oxytocin, this hormone is rarely needed to assist the queen in delivering kittens. If birth of a litter is observed the fetal membranes can be counted, but in the majority of cases most, if not all, of the membranes are consumed by the queen before her parturition is discovered. It is probably more important to observe the queen for evidence of fever or listlessness or for a vaginal discharge not associated with normal parturition. When the kittens are crying and restless, this may be a clue that the queen is not nursing them and that a problem has developed that may be related to retained fetal membranes. In such cases, oxytocin should be administered intramuscularly or intranasally to stimulate additional uterine contractions. Previous history of such problems in a queen should prompt closer observation during her subsequent pregnancies.

Postpartum Care and Problems

In catteries and laboratories where there are apt to be many contemporaneous litters of kittens, the litters should be isolated as much as possible. The queens and their kittens should be handled infrequently, except when a queen tends to neglect her kittens. At the same time the queen should be provided enough space to remove herself from the kittens, especially as they grow and become more active.

It should be ensured that a lactating queen is provided with adequate food. The quantity supplied and the method of providing it are started late in gestation and continued throughout the lactation period. Calcium may be added to the food or supplied through the use of KMR, which also adds to the liquid intake. Queens that are nursing kittens will appear very thin and this will be very apparent after 4 to 6 weeks. Though the drain of nutrients and fluids is considerable, it need not be detrimental to the queen if sufficient replacements are provided.

As the kittens grow older and begin to eat foods other than the queen's milk, they are given soft moist foods and milk replacements, such as KMR. When the latter is used for young kittens, it can be diluted 1 to 1 with lukewarm water. More than one food dish should be provided for a litter. When kept at room temperature, KMR ferments quickly and therefore it should be replaced frequently.

Queens normally have 5 pairs of mammary glands, but it is not uncommon to find one or a pair of glands missing.[3] Supernumerary teats are common and may be functional.

Mammary Hyperplasia

Mammary hyperplasia may occur in young queens during their 1st estrous period. Affected glands may be enlarged, warm, and sensitive when palpated. Not all of a queen's mammae may be hyperplastic and they may be affected randomly. The fluid from a hyperplastic mammary gland is often dark brown. Occurrence of mammary hyperplasia may not be discovered until after a gland(s) has ruptured. Treatment involves the administration of a diuretic and corticosteroid. A ruptured gland should be treated topically. Surgical removal of a single gland in cats is difficult because of the continuity of mammary tissue between the glands. An ovariohysterectomy is indicated because the hyperplasia tends to recur at each estrus.

Mastitis

Acute mastitis is not uncommon in cats and the posterior pair are usually affected. Staphylococci and streptococci are the most common causes. Affected glands are usually swollen, red, and sensitive. An affected queen will be unwilling to nurse and neglected kittens quickly become weak and dehydrated. Treatment of bacterial mastitis may include a systemic antibiotic for 10 to 14 days, drainage of an abscess, and topical applications to reduce inflammation. If possible, cultures and sensitivity tests should be performed to guide selection of an appropriate antibacterial drug. Kittens should be separated from an affected queen. Occasionally, the affected mammae can be covered with a bandage and the kittens allowed to nurse on unaffected glands, 2 at a time. This can be done only when the queen is cooperative and usually requires considerable patience by a human caretaker. It is usually preferable to feed KMR to the kittens. If the kittens seem to need an artificial heat source, a heat lamp or pad can be used.

Chronic mastitis is usually found incidentally during a physical examination. The affected mammary tissue becomes nodular. When nodules are palpated, neoplasia should be suspected unless the history indicates otherwise. Affected glands should be biopsied.

Agalactia and Galactostasis

Agalactia is rare in cats.[4] Behavior that suggests agalactia may be manifested by a restless queen that appears to be reluctant to nurse her kittens. She may lie as though to nurse, but get up when approached by the kittens. Oral administration of acepromazine at a dosage of 1/8 to 1/4 mg/lb may calm the queen sufficiently to enable nursing. The administration of acepromazine may have to be repeated several times until the queen will readily allow her kittens to nurse. If milk excretion appears to be slow, small amounts of oxytocin in the form of a nasal spray (Syntocin) can be instilled several times daily.

The term galactostasis refers to cessation of milk secretion. In cats this occurs most often in the thoracic mammae. When galactostasis occurs, the mammae become engorged and warm. The teats should be examined to be certain that they are capable of excreting milk. When teat inversion has occurred, gentle massage of the nipple may be corrective. After milk is being excreted again, suckling should not be interrupted. A diuretic, such as furosemide (5 mg/kg daily), may be helpful in relieving congestion, but it should not be continued indefinitely because it will reduce milk production. Use of a diuretic should be accompanied by topical treatments to relieve mammary congestion.

Lactational Tetany

Lactational tetany occurs in cats during parturition and lactation.[4] If it is untreated, the tonic convulsions may result in death. The frequency of lactational tetany is low, but when it occurs the signs are usually impressive. It occurs in cats of all ages. The incidence is greatest among queens with large litters. When the condition occurs during nursing, it is usually when there is the greatest demand for milk or between the 3rd and 4th weeks postpartum.

The signs of lactational tetany in the queen progress from ataxia and weakness to vomiting and hyperpnea. Muscle spasms develop subsequently and lead to tremors and convulsions. The body temperature of an affected queen may be as high as 108 F. Prior to death the animal appears to be in shock, the mucosae are pale and dry, the pupils become dilated, and the temperature is subnormal.

Treatment must be prompt after the diagnosis has been made. A blood sample may be drawn for future analysis to corroborate the diagnosis and a calcium level less than 7 mg % is evidence of hypocalcemia. A 10% solution of calcium gluconate should be given IV slowly to an animal in the advanced stages. When given rapidly, this drug can cause cardiac irregularities. From 2 to 5 ml may produce the 1st signs of recovery, but some cats may require twice that amount before any change is noticed. If the response is still slow when giving the larger dose, a 10% solution of dextrose may be administered slowly IV. The dextrose is given in the event that the patient has become hypoglycemic because food intake has ceased.

When an animal has recovered from the advanced stages or is presented during the early stages of lactational tetany, she can be given a calcium solution, such as Calphosan, SC in doses of 5 to 10 ml. Calphosan has also been given in 0.5- to 1.0-ml doses IM. Following recovery from the acute signs, a queen should be given 5 grains of calcium (lactate or gluconate) daily for 5 days to a week. Her diet should then be appropriately adjusted and it may be advantageous to restrict continuous nursing by periodically covering the queen's mammae with a bandage. The mammae should be examined periodically because lactation may continue due to the presence of the kittens. This can be prevented by separating the queen and kittens for periods each day. If this is done, the kittens should be removed to another room because any auditory or visual stimuli may affect the results. If it appears that the kittens would benefit from nursing and the queen could tolerate it, periodic nursing could be allowed. This should be closely watched and stopped if the queen shows any signs of hypocalcemia. When lactational tetany is recognized early and treated effectively, kittens can be allowed to nurse a few minutes at a time, but not left with the queen. The nursing interval can then be gradually extended. It usually requires 3 to 5 days before the kittens can be left with the queen uninterruptedly.

Occasionally an acid-base shift occurs with lactational tetany because of respiratory alkalosis. A blood pH of over 7.45 and an alkaline urine will reveal the alkalosis. Treatment consists of slow IV administration of physiologic saline solution. Alkalosis is most likely to develop during the late stages of lactational tetany after the animal has been hyperventilating for some time.

Postpartum Hemorrhage

Postpartum hemorrhage is minimal in cats and when it occurs the bleeding may last only 3 to 5 days. The color of the discharge should be noted. Tears in the vaginal mucosa will cause the discharge to be bright red. When the discharge is dark red, it originates in the uterus and may often be viscid. If a hemorrhagic discharge is considerable and appears to originate in the uterus, intramuscular administration of ergonovine maleate (0.1 mg) may be efficacious. Calcium gluconate (10% solution) may increase the uterine response to ergonovine. From 5 to 10 units of oxytocin may also be given to cause uterine contractions and thus control bleeding. If the hemorrhage cannot be stopped with such therapy, an ovariohysterectomy should be performed.

Orphaned Kittens

Orphaned kittens may be raised successfully by giving them KMR initially and then adding ground cat food to it to make a slurry as the kittens grow older. During the first 2 to 3 weeks the orphaned kittens should be fed from 5 to 7 times daily, providing about 8 ml of KMR per ounce of body weight daily. The KMR can be given by stomach tube if necessary. Many of these orphaned kittens can be fed with a medicine dropper or a small bottle with nipple. The KMR should be warmed to the cat's normal body temperature before it is fed. After each feeding for at least 3 weeks, the anal and genital areas of each kitten should be washed with a warm moist cloth to stimulate defecation. A gain in body weight of 7 to 10 grams per kitten daily is satisfactory. A healthy kitten that is nursing normally will usually gain about 100 grams every week. Human baby foods may be given to orphaned kittens after 3 weeks to supplement their diet of ground cat chow and KMR. Vitamin supplements are usually not needed. When feeding kittens by hand, it should be remembered that they must have time to breathe and that the feeding cannot be hurried.

Weaning

The results of recent research at our laboratory indicate that kittens are best weaned at 6 weeks of age. When weaned at this time, they rarely lose weight as they do when weaned at 4 weeks of age. Kittens weaned at 5 weeks of age usually maintain their weight and it is an acceptable time for weaning.

Some queens that have been nursing kittens for 3 to 4 weeks will appear thin and dehydrated. They usually have normal hemograms, however. Nevertheless, queens should be gradually separated from their kittens after nursing them intensively for several weeks.

The amount of food fed to a queen should be reduced gradually as she ceases to nurse her kittens. Cats usually will reduce their food intake voluntarily until they have attained a nutritional balance. If a queen that has just weaned her kittens is to be bred again, she should be given a thorough physical examination in which her mammary glands are palpated for any abnormality.

Special Care

It may be advantageous to clip the hair around the perineum of long-haired kittens to prevent formation of feces-hair mats. Such matting may interfere with a kitten's ability to defecate and thus cause a serious problem.

Vaccinations

The timing of vaccinations for kittens can be a problem when there are many litters at a cattery where the upper respiratory disease complex persists. It has been observed that SC administration of a modified-live-virus vaccine beginning at 4 weeks of age is satisfactory. The vaccine is given again at 8 weeks if deemed necessary. When the vaccine is first given at 12 weeks of age, it should be given IM in a divided dose in both hindlimbs. Subsequent vaccinations are given annually on the animals' birthdays.

Fading Kitten Syndrome

The "fading kitten" syndrome continues to be an enigma with no solution.[5,6] Studies of this condition have been made at catteries and research colonies in which the cats have had positive antibody titers to FIP virus. In most cases the fading kitten syndrome becomes recognized because of reproductive failures and/or young kitten mortality. Attempts to isolate viruses from affected kittens and sick adults have not been successful.

A fading kitten is frequently born weighing less than normal ($\pm$ 90 gm for female kittens and $\pm$ 100 gm for males). They may appear emaciated and weak when delivered and then fail to nurse or they may appear normal at birth and live normally for a few days or even weeks before dying without apparent cause. Affected kittens that live longer than a few days rapidly become anorectic, depressed, and dehydrated.

Kittens may be born prematurely when the queen suffers an acute infection caused by a virus associated with the upper respiratory disease complex. This also occurs when a pregnant queen is stressed otherwise. These kittens are also weak and resemble those with the "fading syndrome."

Cardiomyopathy

Acute congestive cardiomyopathy with severe dyspnea, cyanosis, and death may occur in kittens that have been alive for several months or longer. The percentage of kittens that die with this condition is unknown.

Recurrence of Estrus

The average queen will begin to show evidence of estrous cycling within 2 to 4 weeks after weaning. The length of the post-weaning period may be related to the frequency of nursing the kittens beyond the 4th week postpartum. If the queen is abruptly separated from the kittens when they are 4 to 6 weeks old, she will show signs of estrus in about 14 days. If kittens are weaned in the fall of the year and the queen is exposed only to sunlight, she probably will not cycle until the next breeding season. In contrast, queens exposed to sunlight and continuous artificial lighting have had estrous cycles before the natural breeding season.

About 2 litters per year are normal for the domestic cat. Females as young as 5 months old have become pregnant and had normal litters. Queens that were 10 years of age have also become pregnant and had normal kittens. Older queens have fewer kittens per litter, however.

When estrus is induced in a queen by use of exogenous hormones, it usually requires higher doses of the hormones to induce another estrus.

References

1. Cline, EM *et al:* Feline Pract **10:2** (1980) 47.
2. Herron, MA: Feline Pract **7:2** (1977) 36.
3. Crouch, JE: Text — Atlas of Cat Anatomy. pp 182, 183. Lea & Febiger,Philadelphia, 1969.
4. Stein, BS: Feline Medicine and Surgery, 2nd ed. American Veterinary Publications, Santa Barbara, CA 1975.
5. Scott, FW *et al:* Feline Pract **9:2** (1979) 44.
6. Scott, FW and Geissinger, C: Feline Pract **8:6** (1976) 31.

PRE- AND POSTNATAL CARE OF FEMALE DOGS
BY JACOB E. MOSIER

Prenatal care of the bitch logically commences at the time a female is selected for breeding. A bitch that may be used for breeding should be fed to achieve optimum, but not maximum, size and weight.[1] Overweight females should be reduced during the anestrus period. Early recognition and prompt treatment of parasitisms, especially ascariasis, prevent somatic encystment during the early growth period and subsequent activation during pregnancy.

A bitch selected for breeding should be given a thorough physical examination and her ancestry scrutinized for evidence of inherited problems. The minimum laboratory data should include information about the animal's packed cell volume, total protein level, and parasitisms. Both the hematocrit and total serum protein levels decrease during gestation and if the hemoglobin level falls below 10 g/dl or total serum protein falls below 5.5 g/dl, the survival of newborn puppies is threatened. It is also important that a breeding bitch be vaccinated periodically to maintain high antibody titers for transfer in colostrum.

Nutritional Requirements

Nutritional needs of the bitch during gestation are provided satisfactorily by a commercial dog food manufactured under quality control. Supplemental feeding is not necessary for healthy bitches. If supplemental feeding is provided, small quantities of cooked eggs, meat, milk, cottage cheese, or raw liver are acceptable. It is important that the dam's food intake not be increased above the maintenance requirement during the period from onset of estrus to implantation. Excessive caloric intake during this period may increase the incidence of embryonal deaths and result in decreased litter size. The level of food intake can be appropriately increased starting on the 5th week of gestation. An approximately 10% increase can be allowed on each of the 5th, 6th, and 7th weeks. Food intake is then held at the 8th-week level through parturition. It subsequently is increased to meet the needs for maintenance of lactation at an appropriate level for the number of puppies being fed.

Bitches should weigh approximately 10% more than their prebreeding weight at the end of gestation.[2] Most of the weight gain occurs during the last half of gestation. As the pregnancy progresses the daily ration should be given in 2 or 3 feedings to prevent some of the discomfort that may occur with once a day feeding during advanced pregnancy. Failure of the dam to gain weight during gestation should serve as a warning that the puppies will be small and lactation may be less than satisfactory. Increasing the level of the dam's protein intake by 2 to 4% may increase the newborns' vigor and the dam's milk secretion. Feeding from 0.5 to 1.0 oz of liver per 25 lb of body weight 2 to 3 times weekly is considered helpful.

Extreme obesity may complicate the dam's whelping due to clumsiness, early fatigue, and poor muscle tone. Certain bitches have a noticeable lack of appetite during the 1st month of pregnancy.[3] Giving them vitamins, especially C and B-complex, may stimulate their appetite. Dams that become quite restless may be helped by mild sedation. Though some bitches consume little or no food in the 24 hours preceding whelping, persistent anorexia after whelping usually signals serious complications. Generally the food intake during lactation will increase 25% per week so that by the 4th postparturient week, the bitch will be consuming at least twice the amount fed during the last week of pregnancy. Properly formulated vitamin-mineral mixtures fed at recommended levels may be beneficial during lactation and they are commonly used.

Diagnosis of Pregnancy

Pregnancy is best diagnosed 25 to 30 days following cessation of estrus. Abdominal palpation will reveal ovoid enlargements of the uterus. The enlargements should be uniform in size and a difference in size should alert the clinician about the possibility of embryonal death and resorption. Abdominal distention usually is apparent and the teats become larger, more turgid, and deeper in color after the 35th day of gestation.

Vaginal bleeding may occur at the end of the 7th week. Though the bleeding may reflect abortion, many affected bitches will carry their puppies to term. Restricting the dam's activity and keeping her in quiet surroundings are indicated.

Preparation for Parturition

The whelping area should be selected at least 7 to 10 days prior to parturition. Moving the bitch to a new environment immediately before whelping may result in restlessness, prolonged labor, constant pacing, scratching at an outside door, and whining. The initial labor may be brief, inhibited, and unproductive. The whelping box should be sufficiently large for the bitch to stand and turn around without disturbing the newborn. The sides of the box should be high enough to prevent drafts and on one side there should be an opening that the bitch, but not the puppies, can step over without difficulty.

The temperature of the room in which the whelping box is placed should be within a range of 60 to 75 F. Additional heat should be provided in one area of the whelping box for the puppies. An electric heating pad may be useful for this purpose. Heat lamps are also used. There should be adequate room around the heat source so that the puppies can move to or away from it.

The whelping box should have a top in case the dam wants to be secluded. Hinging the top will enable easy access to and from the box for dams that seem to desire more contact with people. Shredded paper or disposable diapers can be used for bedding.

About a week before whelping the dam's perineum should be clipped and the long hair around the mammary glands should be removed. Bathing is recommended if it is convenient and at least the bitch's mammary glands and teats should be washed. Her teeth and gingiva should be inspected for evidence of periodontitis or tartar and the owner should be advised to clean the animal's teeth and gingivae daily with a mixture of salt and baking soda.[4] The bitch should be brought to the whelping area early so that she will identify it as familiar territory. When a bitch is disturbed during parturition, labor may be delayed for as long as 4 hours.

Postparturient Care

A vigorous, healthy bitch will complete whelping in several hours. Her uterus should then involute rapidly. There usually is slight, blood-tinged discharge from the vulva for a few days. This discharge is never profuse and will become nearly colorless by the 5th postparturient day.

The postparturient environment should provide reasonable seclusion, clean bedding, and protection from temperature extremes, drafts, and excess humidity. The feeding area for the dam should be separated from the nest. Any heat sources should be placed where the bitch can move away from them if she becomes too warm.

The condition of the dam's mammary glands, character of the vulvar discharge, and her food intake and eliminations should be monitored daily. If the dam's environment is not optimal or if she is not in prime condition, consideration should be given to administering oxytocin or an ecbolic after the last puppy is delivered. Oxytocin (5 to 20 units) is frequently given, but ergonovine may be preferred because of its longer effect and ease of oral administration. A single dose of ergonovine will be effective for approximately 3 hours. A dose of 0.2 mg given 3 times daily for 1 or 2 days to a 25-lb bitch will assure involution of the uterus and the placental attachments. A long-acting penicillin preparation is commonly given immediately after whelping. There is some objection, however, to the routine administration of an antibiotic to postparturient dams. The routine use of antibiotics can lead to development of resistant strains of bacteria that cannot be treated with preferred antibiotics. This practice may also prompt the animals' caretaker to be less careful in providing a sanitary environment for the dam and puppies.

The behavior of the dam during the immediate postparturient period is critical for puppy survival. When one seems to be agitated and does not relax and care for her puppies, a single IM injection of progesterone (0.4 mg/lb) may be helpful. A restless dam should be examined for evidence of toxemia or infection, and measures taken to alleviate any abnormality. Indifference or aggressiveness toward the puppies may reflect a dam's earlier experience, improper feeding, lack of proper exercise, or discomfort. It may be necessary to supervise suckling for several days and force the bitch to lie on her side while the puppies suckle for 10 to 15 minutes. Neglected puppies should be removed to a heated area and protected from a dam that becomes aggressive. If a bitch is indifferent to her puppies, the attendant must stimulate urination and defecation by gentle massage of each puppy's perineum. Administration of a tranquilizer or analgesic at low dosage may induce a dam to accept her newborn. Oxytocin can be given to stimulate milk letdown.

In the early postnatal period the primary problems involving the uterus include retained placenta, subinvolution of the uterus or placental sites, and metritis. Daily inspection of the vulva will enable prompt detection of a discharge that is associated with placental retention. Though the placenta usually passes through the birth canal with each puppy, it occasionally will be retained briefly and pass several minutes to an hour after the puppy is delivered. Appearance of a black or dark green discharge indicates placental retention. Abdominal palpation may reveal a firm, usually fusiform mass that is characteristic of a retained placenta within the uterus. Within 12 hours the vaginal discharge will become more copious and darker. If the placenta is not expelled within 24 hours, the possibility of uterine infection is considerably increased.

When a placenta has been retained for 12 or more hours, intrauterine injection of an antibiotic is indicated to prevent or control metritis. Failure to deliver a placenta should prompt consideration of a laparotomy to remove it. When there is evidence of uterine wall necrosis, a hysterectomy should be performed.

Subinvolution of the Uterus

Involution of the canine uterus follows parturition along with gradual reconstruction of the endometrial layer. Failure of the uterus to undergo reduction in size and a delay in regression of the endometrium is referred to as subinvolution. This occurs when postparturient uterine contraction is incomplete and placental fluids and debris are retained in the uterine cavity. Subinvolution of the uterus occurs more frequently in primigravid bitches that are less than 4 years old.

Though the cause of uterine subinvolution is unknown, uterine inertia or fatigue must be considered as causal factors. The subinvolution usually occurs in both horns, but unilateral and segmented subinvolution have been observed. Abdominal palpation of the uterus will often reveal the degree of subinvolution.

Treatment is directed toward emptying the uterus, restoring uterine tone, and preventing metritis. Puppies are removed from the dam for 24 hours. From 5 to 10 ml of a Furacin-saline mixture (1:9) are instilled into the uterus through an insemination tube. Medicaments that can be given perorally include ergonovine (0.1 to 0.2 mg TID) and an antibiotic. The drugs are continued for 3 and 5 days, respectively. On the day after initiation of therapy the puppies can be allowed to nurse again.

Subsequent fertility is usually not affected by subinvolution of the uterus following a parturition. When a bitch is fed and exercised properly, normal involution can be anticipated after future parturitions.

Metritis

Acute metritis is most likely to occur within the first week following parturition or abortion. A number of organisms have been incriminated, including hemolytic staphylococci, streptococci, corynebacteria, *Proteus, E coli,* and *Hemophilus.* Retention of a fetus or placenta, introduction of infection by contaminated instruments or hands, unsanitary surroundings, tissue damage, and uterine inertia may contribute to the development of metritis.

Infection is accompanied by depression, anorexia, and toxemia. Affected bitches are febrile (103 to 105 F) and have rapid pulse rates. Milk flow is diminished and the bitch shows little interest in her puppies. As a result, the puppies are frequently restless and cry intermittently. Their growth rate decreases markedly and their ani may become red and swollen. The dam's vaginal discharge is thin, sometimes fetid, and red except when the placenta is retained. In this event the discharge is green to black. The mucous membranes of the bitch are congested and she may strain and, unless severely depressed, repeatedly lick her vulva. Either leukopenia or leukocytosis may occur and with elevated leukocyte counts there may be a shift to the left.[6]

A flaccid uterus may respond to prostaglandins, estrogen, calcium, and either oxytocin or ergonovine. Oxytocin (10 to 20 units) may be effective in emptying a uterus of fluid and debris, especially in bitches affected shortly after parturition. Ergonovine given at a dosage of 0.2 mg TID for 2 or 3 days has given more consistent results, however, than has oxytocin. Intrauterine instillation of 2 to 20 ml of Furacin in saline (1:9) is often beneficial. A broad-spectrum antibiotic should be given for at least 3 days after the patient's temperature has returned to normal. An antihistamine may be given to reduce the effect of histamine release at the site of infection. Fluids given IV will prevent or remedy dehydration and maintain renal function. Giving 5% glucose solution along with electrolytes will help to prevent serious damage to the liver as the body strives to detoxify the toxins produced by bacteria. Puppies should not be permitted to nurse a dam with acute metritis.

The course of acute metritis is usually short, ranging from 3 to 5 days. Improvement is indicated by reduction in temperature, return of appetite, reduction in vulvar discharge, drop in pulse rate, and general improvement in the dam's attitude and appearance.

Agalactia

Agalactia (absence of milk flow after parturition) can result from either lack of milk production in the mammae or failure of milk letdown. The failure of mammary development prior to whelping is generally considered the first indication of agalactia. This may be the result of hormonal deficiency or defective secretory tissue. Though estrogen activates the development of the ducts and progesterone affects development of the alveoli, their effects in the bitch are less than in ruminants.

Prolactin and growth hormone are responsible for initiation of lactation and maintenance of secretory levels. Inhibition of prolactin secretion results in reduction of milk production. Estrogen activates the lactogenic activity of the anterior pituitary gland, whose normal function is essential for milk secretion. Certain protein sources are more effective in milk production. For example, liver is more effective than egg or round steak. Nursing stimulates sensory nerve endings in the dam's teats and thus serves as a stimulus to milk letdown and production. Anesthetics and tranquilizers may alter the normal response and result in temporary agalactia. When the mammae have developed normally and milk letdown has not occurred, the administration of oxytocin will cause contraction of the myoepithelial cells and forcible expression of milk into the larger ducts and teat canal.

When mammary development has been subnormal, stimulation of milk production is less effective. Certain bitches are very nervous and they fail to provide proper care of their puppies. Giving such a dam 0.4 mg of progesterone per kg of body weight will have a quieting effect and subsequent suckling by the puppies will enhance milk flow.

When milk production is marginal, the puppies should be allowed to suckle and the dam's diet should be considered along with any signs of disease. Any treatment should be limited to specific agents for demonstrated abnormalities.

Mammary Congestion (Galactostasis)

Edema and swelling of the mammary glands are occasionally observed prior to parturition, but these changes usually occur within a few hours to 3 days following parturition. Galactostasis is most common in heavily lactating bitches that are being fed high-caloric, high-protein diet. Affected bitches are uncomfortable and sometimes anorectic. Palpation will reveal that their mammae are grossly enlarged and warm and that their teats are difficult to grasp. Milk may drip from some of the teats.

Treatment involves withholding food and administering a diuretic. Milking the glands that are grossly distended will provide temporary relief of discomfort. The judicious application of hot packs or whirlpool treatment can be combined with massage to reduce severe congestion. Failure to relieve galactostasis can result in subsequent failure of lactation in affected glands. Careful monitoring of affected animals is indicated to enable early detection of infection.

Mastitis

Mastitis may be either acute or chronic, depending on the history and the condition of the mammae at the time of their infection. Acute mastitis occurs most frequently in bitches housed in unsanitary surroundings that have recently whelped and have considerable congestion of the mammae. It also seems to occur more often during hot, humid weather.

A variety of organisms, including staphylococci, streptococci, and *E coli*, have been incriminated as causes of mastitis.[7] Trauma and mammary congestion are generally thought to be involved. Uterine infection may be the source or merely coincidental. Early signs of mastitis are swelling and erythema of the affected gland. It then becomes hot, painful, and discolored. An affected dam is anorectic, listless, and febrile. She usually shows evidence of discomfort and loses interest in her puppies. The puppies, in turn, are restless, cry frequently, and appear bloated. The dam's milk gradually thickens and becomes yellow, pink, or brown depending on the amount of blood and purulent exudate present. Cytologic examination will reveal many leukocytes and erythrocytes. Aseptically collected samples should be cultured and sensitivity tests should be performed.

Treatment is directed toward controlling the infection. Antibacterial agents given systemically are effective in early mastitis. If an infection becomes localized, the resulting abscess should be incised and drainage established. Local infiltration of an infected gland with penicillin or penicillin and streptomycin may prevent abscessation. Puppies should be prevented from suckling severely affected glands by applying a mammary bandage. When the milk is not frankly purulent, the puppies may be allowed to continue to suckle. If several glands are affected or the inflammation is severe, however, it may be best to move the puppies to an incubator and treat them as orphans. Affected glands should then be periodically milked during the day. Penicillin given at 24-hour intervals, penicillin/streptomycin given at 12-hour intervals, or kanamycin given at 12-hour intervals for at least 5 days is usually effective.

Cold packs are useful in the early stages of mammary congestion and hot packs are usually indicated after the inflammation is well-established. Hot packs will hasten localization of the infection and give relief from pain.

There is a tendency for mastitis to recur in subsequent lactations in a once-affected bitch. There is also some evidence that there is an inherited tendency for mastitis in certain families of some breeds.

References
1. Sheffy, BE: Vet Clinics No Amer **8(1)** (1978) 12.
2. Donovan, EF: In *Current Veterinary Therapy VII*, pp 1212-1213. WB Saunders Co, Philadelphia, 1980.
3. Freak, MJ: Vet Rec **74** (1962) 1325.
4. Vine, LL: *Feeding, Whelping and Natal Care of Dogs.* Arco Publishing Co, New York.
5. Foy, MW: *Guidelines to Behavior in Dogs.* Gaines Res Prog, Spring, 1968.
6. Lipowitz, AJ and Larson, RE: In *Current Veterinary Therapy VII*, pp 1214-1215. WB Saunders Co, Philadelphia, 1980.
7. Trainor, E: In *Current Veterinary Therapy III.* WB Saunders Co, Philadelphia, 1968.

NORMAL AND ABNORMAL PARTURITION
BY JACOB E. MOSIER

Introduction
Gestation in the dog and cat averages 63 days, with a range of 59 to 67 days. Apparently "normal" births have occurred in both species as many as 7 days before or after the average 63 days. The greater the deviation from the 63-day average, however, the greater is the probability of an abnormal parturition. The common practice of breeding bitches at 2-day intervals and the variation in time of ovulation

hinder precise determination of the gestation period. Likewise in the cat, estrus may last from 4 to 10 days and queens may breed on 2 or 3 consecutive days.

Preparturition

The exact mechanism that initiates parturition in the dog and cat is unknown. At the end of gestation, a change in the progesterone:estrogen ratio is one important factor in the initiation of parturition. Estrogen sensitizes the myometrium to oxytocin. A relative increase in estrogens and adrenocorticosteroids is thought to result in release of prostaglandins from the placenta.[1] Prostaglandins, in turn, inhibit the production of progesterone, increase uterine contractility, and trigger the release of oxytocin.

Approaching parturition is characterized by the dam's anxiety, restlessness, and intermittent nest-making. A decrease in her activity and appetite may occur as soon as 7 days before whelping. A queen may become more vocal and seek a dark, dry area where she can remain relatively undisturbed. Other queens will seek human companionship. The dam's rectal temperature usually is slightly depressed (0.5 to 1.0 F) during the final week of pregnancy. Milk may be present in the mammary glands 2 to 3 days before stage 1 of parturition in the primiparous bitch. In the multiparous bitch it is not uncommon for milk to be present as early as 7 days before birth of the 1st puppy.

Normal Parturition

Stage 1

The dam's general activity becomes more intense 12 to 24 hours before onset of labor. A bitch may shiver, pant, refuse food, and sometimes vomit. A queen becomes restless, somewhat anxious, and makes frequent trips to her box where she may display nesting behavior. The rectal temperature of the dam usually declines 1 to 2 degrees within 8 to 24 hours prior to parturition. During this period the dam enters the 1st stage of parturition with accompanying dilation of the cervix and relaxation of the vagina. This stage can last from 1 to 36 hours and it averages 6 to 12 hours. Uterine contractions occur intermittently without visible contraction of abdominal muscles. The bitch may glance occasionally at her flank area and the queen may vigorously lick the mammary and perineal areas. Both the bitch and queen appear to be uncomfortable.

Active contractions of both longitudinal and circular muscle fibers of the uterus are most intense just anterior to the most caudal fetus. Dilation of the cervix begins at the external os, the pelvic ligaments relax, and mucus may pass through the cervix during the 12 hours preceding the end of the 1st stage. Uterine contractions then occur at progressively closer intervals. Near the end of the 1st stage, the most caudal fetus will rotate on its long axis and extend its head, neck, and limbs. Four hours before the end of the 1st stage, the dam's cervix will have dilated to approximately 8 mm in diameter.[4] The allantochorionic membrane appears in the vagina near the end of stage 1. Its rupture will result in some discharge of fluid. Shortly after the rupture of the allantochorionic membrane, the amnionic sac will pass through the vagina and may protrude as a water bag between the lips of the vulva. This signals the start of stage 2.

Stage 2

The 2nd stage of parturition usually lasts 3 to 6 hours depending on the number of fetuses and the health of the dam. A dam will usually lie on her side during labor although it is not uncommon for her to stand intermittently, strain, and occasionally deliver a fetus while standing. Some bitches and queens will lean against a wall. It is during this stage that the dam's abdominal muscles are used in expulsive efforts. The 1st fetus is usually delivered within 20 to 30 minutes after onset of the 2nd stage.

The presence of a fetal head in the vaginal canal increases the intensity and frequency of muscle contractions. Distention of the cervix and vagina results in a feedback stimulus for the hypothalamus to release oxytocin. In an average birth from 2 to 3 strong contractions will propel a fetus through the pelvic canal. In primiparous bitches the lips of the vulva may be insufficiently relaxed to permit easy passage of the 1st puppy. The resultant pressure can result in enough pain to temporarily inhibit straining. Especially during birth of the first puppy or kitten by a primigravid dam there may be a sharp cry due to pain as the head of the puppy or kitten is forced through the lips of the vulva.[5,6] An episiotomy should be performed when manual assistance is ineffective.

A fetus may be delivered within the amnionic membrane. Normally the dam will first remove the membrane and then proceed to thoroughly cleanse the newborn by licking. This seems to stimulate circulation and respiration. The umbilical cord is severed by the dam and the placenta may be ingested. Some bitches will continue to nibble at the umbilical cord until it is quite short. Normal puppies are suckling within a few minutes after their birth. Most kittens begin to suckle within 1 to 2 hours after delivery of the last fetus.[7]

Stage 3

The 3rd stage of parturition consists of delivery of the placenta and partial involution of the uterus after delivery of each puppy or kitten. The placenta may be eliminated with the newborn or retained for a variable period. Sometimes 2 placentas are expelled together after delivery of 2 puppies or kittens. In any event the placenta should be eliminated within 45 minutes after birth of a newborn. Involution occurs in that portion of the uterus from which the fetus and placenta have been expelled. The period of rest may vary from 10 minutes to several hours.

The number of cycles of 2nd and 3rd stages depends on the number of puppies or kittens in the uterus. Length of parturition varies considerably depending on the breed, individual, and environment. Examination is recommended for any dam that has been in labor for more than 2 hours without delivering a fetus. This also applies to a dam that has had slight and nonproductive straining for more than 1 hour following delivery of a fetus. Dams that are resting comfortably while caring for puppies or kittens already born are not in trouble, but are in a resting phase. Small amounts of warm water or milk should be offered during a resting phase when the parturition is extended. Gathering the newborn animals in front of the dam during labor will enable the dam to position herself for delivery and care of the next fetus.

Abnormal Parturition

The term, abnormal parturition, refers to extended labor, gestation that is either too long or too short, or to parturition in which the possibility of death of a newborn or the dam is increased.

Signs suggesting abnormal parturition include the presence of green to black, bloody, or otherwise abnormal discharge; unusual odor; ineffective labor; cessation of labor; depression and obvious fatigue of the dam; excessive pain; and stillbirth. The cause may be complicated and an astute clinician will consider the various possibilities before initiating any treatment.

Abnormalities of Onset or Duration of Parturition

Early Parturition: Though the average gestation period is considered to be 63 days, many dogs and cats will deliver their offspring prior to the 63rd day. Whelping or queening between the 56th and 63rd day of gestation may be normal for an individual dam. In such cases, however, the newborn will usually be small and immature. When early parturition occurs in a bitch or queen, the owner should be questioned about the dam's prior gestations and the birth record of the dam's mother. Certain males may be associated with early parturition. Parturition prior to 56 days is not normal and should be considered a late abortion.

Delayed Parturition: Though parturition as late as the 70th day of gestation has occurred with normal delivery of live fetuses, it is reasonable to classify any gestation beyond 67 days as being abnormal. When the dam is normal insofar as can be determined by clinical examination and her behavior is consistent with prolonged gestation, the unborn animals may be in no danger. Because of repeated breedings and the inability to determine the precise time of ovulation it is difficult to determine the exact day of conception, and therefore a prolonged gestation may not be as extended as the owner has calculated. Delayed parturition does occur and it has been associated with dams bred in late middle age or older, the presence of only 1 or 2 fetuses, and the occurrence of *in utero* death of fetuses. Other factors associated with prolonged gestation are injection of progestogen, hypothyroidism, and delayed involution of corpora lutea. Fetuses with defective or abnormal heads may be responsible for a prolonged gestation.[1]

Prolonged Parturition: Length of the whelping period may be affected by several factors, including the dam's age, muscle tone, metabolic rate, and the number of fetuses. A dam that labors vigorously for more than 2 hours following the onset of parturition and fails to deliver a fetus should be examined by a veterinarian.[4] This general rule can be altered when the owner knows the pattern of parturition of a particular dam.

Live offspring have been delivered 36 hours following an earlier delivery. Survival of an *in utero* fetus depends on the placental attachment and an adequate supply of oxygen. If a dam has delivered one or more fetuses and then fails to deliver others present in the uterus within the next hour, she should be examined.[8] In such cases it may be helpful to take the bitch for a short walk, offer her warm milk, allow the previously delivered newborn animals to nurse for 5 to 10 minutes, feather the vagina, or administer calcium and oxytocin. Some dams become anxious if isolated from the owner, while others are restless in the owner's presence.

Newborn animals removed from the dam during parturition should be allowed to suckle for a short period every 2 hours.

Dystocia

The term dystocia refers to a painful, slow, or difficult delivery of fetuses. Dystocia may be classified as fetal, maternal, or placental.[9] A fetal dystocia is due to the shape, size, or position of the fetus. Maternal dystocia results from a deformity or inadequacy of the dam. Placental dystocia results from difficulty in delivery of the placenta.

A diagnosis of dystocia is based on the history, results of a physical examination, and observation of the bitch in labor. The history should include information relative to previous whelpings, breeding dates, behavior during gestation and especially during the 24 hours preceding the examination, time of onset of labor, the frequency and intensity of labor, condition of previously delivered newborn, and the time interval between deliveries.

The examination should include consideration of the possibility of hypoglycemia, hypocalcemia, and uterine inertia. The abdomen should be palpated to assess uterine tone, relative distention of the abdomen, and location of the fetus(es), especially the most caudal one. The perineal hair is clipped, especially in long-haired dogs, and the perineum and vulva are thoroughly cleansed. If the bladder is distended, an attempt should be made to express the urine. If feces are present in the rectum, an enema should be given. Attention should be paid to the relaxation of the dam's vulva and pelvic ligaments. Digital examination may reveal hypertrophy of the posterior vaginal sphincter, contracture of the vagina, or pelvic abnormalities that may be congenital or the result of an injury. The diameter of the dam's pelvis may be flattened dorsoventrally, especially in Scottish Terriers and Sealyhams.[10]

Maternal dystocia can result from failure of the vulva to dilate adequately, vulvovaginal strictures, a flattened or narrow pelvic inlet, incomplete dilation of the cervix, uterine torsion, or uterine inertia.

When the cervix is dilated and a fetus is present at the cranial opening of the birth canal, it may be possible to determine that the fetus is abnormally large, otherwise abnormal, or malpresented. Fetal oversize is more common in the bitch than in the queen and it may be associated with small litters.[9] Disproportionate size may be due to a large fetus or a smaller than normal birth canal.

Common fetal abnormalities include anasarca, extra limbs, hydrocephalus, and chondrodystrophy. A large head is common in brachycephalic breeds.[11] Most fetal dystocias are the result of abnormal position, presentation, or posture.[5] Presentation refers to the relation of the long axis of the fetus to that of the dam and the part of the fetus closest to the pelvic canal. It may be anterior or posterior, longitudinal or transverse. Fetal position refers to the surface of the uterus to which the fetal vertebral column is applied, such as dorsal, ventral, lateral, and oblique. Posture refers to the position of the head and limbs of the fetus. The presentation, position, and posture of the fetus may be determined by abdominal palpation, digital palpation through the vagina, or radiography. Correction of malposition or abnormal posture may be attempted by repulsion of the fetus, digital manipulation of a fetus, or by use of instruments to manipulate a fetus.

Death of fetuses can result in failure of parturition to occur and thus be perceived as a dystocia.

Uterine inertia may be primary or secondary. Primary inertia is generally attributed to lack of tone or to a degenerative change in the uterine muscle.[10] It may also occur with hypocalcemia and/or hypoglycemia and when the dam is in poor condition. Overstretching of the uterine muscle by a large number of fetuses or placental fluids may result in inertia. Occasionally, posterior presentation of the 1st fetus may delay dilation of the cervix and be confused with inertia. The wedge effect of the fetal nose and head seems to stimulate cervical dilation. Secondary uterine inertia results from exhaustion or prolonged labor. With all causes, uterine inertia is characterized by feeble muscle contractions and no movement of the fetus. When parturition is prolonged, fatigue of the uterine muscle may result in segmental contraction or retraction rings (Bandl's rings).[12] These muscular contractions around or caudal to a fetus can impede its movement toward the birth canal.

Administration of oxytocin, calcium, and glucose may be combined to convert weak, irregular contractions of the uterus to regular and forceful contractions. Administering meperidine hydrochloride (2-5 mg/lb IM), calcium gluconate (5-30 ml/dog and 1-3 ml/cat of 10% solution IV), and 20% glucose solution (5-30 ml IV) 30 minutes prior to injection of oxytocin may be beneficial when inertia is suspected. Failure of drugs to produce the desired results or their contraindication should prompt initiation of other measures to relieve the dystocia.

Retention of the placenta may accompany mild uterine inertia in the bitch. This is rarely a problem in the cat. When inertia is due to exhaustion, the fetal membranes will usually pass within 12 hours.[5,13] The presence of a black or dark green discharge is indicative of a retained placenta. Massaging the uterus through the abdomen may stimulate its passage. In another method of removing retained membranes, a gauze pledget is grasped with a narrow-shanked forceps and inserted into the uterus through the vagina. By twisting the forceps in 1 or 2 complete turns the membranes may become attached to the gauze and then removed with gentle traction combined with massage of the uterus through the abdomen.

The measures taken to relieve dystocia will depend on the dam's physical condition, the number of fetuses involved, the cause of the dystocia, the available facilities and assistants, the owner's preference, and the veterinarian's judgment. The options range from use of oxytocin to delivery of the fetuses by cesarean section. Each option may be exercised with variable success, depending to some extent on the experience and judgment of the clinician.

Use of Oxytocin

Prior to administering oxytocin, the clinician should be certain about the position and presentation of the most caudal fetus; that there are no pelvic, vaginal, and vulvar abnormalities; that the cervix is dilated; and the size of the most caudal fetus. Oxytocin is used to reinforce weak uterine contractions provided that the cervix is open and the uterine muscle is not under tension.[14]

Weak, ineffective labor and primary uterine inertia may be remedied by giving oxytocin when there are no contraindications to its administration. The presence of obstructions to delivery through the birth canal, mouth-breathing by the dam, evidence of prolonged uterine fatigue, or a vigorously contracting uterus contraindicate the use of oxytocin. The clinician should assess the uterine tone and vigor of the contractions by abdominal palpation, noticing the length and frequency of contractions. Injecting calcium and/or glucose IV may be helpful when uterine contractions are short, infrequent, or ineffective and there are no obstructions to delivery of a fetus.

Undesirable side-effects associated with the use of oxytocin may result from excessive dosage, too frequent administrations, and its administration when the uterus is already contracting vigorously. When given under these circumstances, oxytocin may prolong compression of the placental vasculature and thus cause fetal stress or death.

The dose of oxytocin ranges from 5 to 20 units in the dog and 3 to 5 units in the cat. It can be given SC or IM. The effects of one dose will last approximately 15 minutes. When repeated doses are given, there should be a minimum of 30 minutes between doses. Oxytocin should not be given solely to accelerate labor.[15]

Digital Manipulation

"Feathering" the vagina may initiate a strong vigorous contraction of the uterus and propulsion of the fetus through the birth canal (Ferguson's reflex). This manipulation is especially useful after the position or posture of a presenting fetus is corrected. The procedure involves using a gloved finger to stretch the vaginal wall in a dor-

resulting in labor of variable intensity depending on the degree of fatigue.

The caudal fetus can sometimes be manipulated through the abdomen, especially in small and thin dams. Such manipulation is most effective when the fetus is in anterior presentation. When performing it, the clinician is positioned behind the patient with a hand on either side of the dam's abdomen. The clinician's fingers are then placed on the back of the fetal occiput to direct the fetal head into the birth canal. External pressure can be exerted with the hands or a sling made of bandage material to assist the contraction of the abdominal muscles.

Manipulations made through the vagina should be preceded by preparing the perineum. Long hair is usually removed with a clippers or scissors to prevent entanglement and contamination. The perineum and vulva are then thoroughly washed with a mild soap and thoroughly rinsed with water. This can be done conveniently with the dam standing on a table.

When a fetus is being manipulated with a gloved finger inserted into the vagina, it is helpful to place the other hand over the dam's abdomen to stabilize the fetus. Manipulating the fetus through the vagina is indicated when the posture or position of the caudal fetus is abnormal and when the finger can be used to assist passage of the fetus through the birth canal.

A fetus stalled in the birth canal can sometimes be delivered by applying traction to the fetal feet or legs. This manipulation is especially useful with a posterior presentation and when the fetal feet are at the vulva. Covering the fetal feet with thin gauze will help to secure a grasp of them. Traction on a fetal head must be applied very carefully. Such traction is applied only as the dam strains to expel the fetus.

Traction can sometimes be applied by placing fingers on the skin overlying the dam's vagina and grasping the head or pelvis of the fetus through the vaginal wall. Occasionally, mild digital pressure can be exerted through the rectum.

Use of Instruments

A variety of instruments, including the clam shell or sponge forceps, an obstetrical hook, and a Roberts' snare, can be used to assist delivery. The relative small size of the queen restricts the utilization of instruments. Their use should be preceded by adequate preparation of the perineum. The Rampley sponge-holding forceps is especially useful because of its narrow shanks.[4] A forceps should not be used if the fetus is beyond the reach of a finger because of the danger of lacerating the uterine wall or birth canal.

The forceps is inserted in a closed position until contact is made with the fetus. At that point it is opened sufficiently to grasp the fetal head or pelvis and advanced until the desired grasp on the fetus is made. An index finger is inserted beside the forceps to assure that neither the uterine or vaginal wall is grasped by the forceps.

A forceps may be used to move a fetus through the birth canal, if there is adequate space for the instrument without exerting harmful pressure on the fetus. When a fetus enters the caudal end of the birth canal, traction should be exerted downwards and backwards and in concert with the dam's straining. After the fetal head or pelvis is through the vulva, the delivery can be completed with fingers. Slight rotation and traction should be applied alternately to facilitate passage of the fetal shoulders or pelvis through the birth canal.

The need to use a forceps to deliver more than one fetus should cause the clinician to consider cesarean section. Delivery by forceps is especially indicated when the presenting fetus is dead or slightly oversized and unassisted delivery of the rest of the litter is likely after the presenting fetus is removed. Delivery by forceps is also suitable for the last fetus of a parturition. A forceps can be used with greater force when there is little concern for the life of the fetus.

Obstetrical Hooks: A hook fashioned from a spay hook shaped into a short sharp point is useful in some deliveries. It is especially useful when the nose or lower jaw of a fetus becomes wedged under the brim of the pelvis. In such cases the hook may be inserted into the intermandibular space of the fetus and traction applied carefully as the dam labors. Blunt hooks may be used to move the fetus to a better position for delivery or to manipulate retained legs or deviated heads.

Obstetrical Snares: Though not commonly employed, Roberts' snare forceps can be useful in small dogs and cats.[11] After a fetus is stabilized at the pelvic brim, a closed forceps carrying the snare is passed into the uterus and over the fetal head until the tip of the forceps lies above the neck of the fetus. The jaws are then opened as widely as possible, turned downward until they are ventral to the fetal neck, and then closed. The encircling noose is thus applied and traction can be employed.

Use of Lubricating Gels
Sterile lubricating gels are essential in most dystocias because the lack of lubrication will result in excessive injury to the birth canal and cause swelling and reduction in its diameter. Loss of fetal fluids may result in a dry vagina and increased friction between the vaginal wall

and fetal hair. Lubricating gel should be forced around the body of a fetus before applying traction.

Episiotomy

Occasionally the vulva fails to relax sufficiently to permit passage of the fetus. In such cases an episiotomy will facilitate delivery. The technic for episiotomy is described in Chapter 6.

Cesarean Section

A decision to perform a cesarean section is based on the clinician's judgment and the owner's acquiescence. The indications and a technic are discussed in Chapter 6.

General Care

Throughout dystocia the dam should be constantly monitored for evidence of shock, toxicity, and fatigue. Parenteral fluids and analgesics should be given as indicated and the dam should be handled gently and kept clean.

References

1. Bennett, D: In *Current Therapy in Theriogenology.* p 595. WB Saunders Co, Philadelphia, 1980.
2. Wilkinson, GT: Diseases of the Reproductive System. Refresher Course on Cats, p 39. Proc #53-55, University of Sydney, 1980.
3. Freak, MJ: Vet Rec **96** (1975) 303.
4. Bardens, J: Personal communication.
5. Freak, MJ: Vet Rec **60** (1948)295.
6. Schneck, S and Norris, N: *Cat Care,* p 16. William Collins Sons and Co, Glasgow and London, 1975.
7. Hart, BL: *Feline Behavior.* A Practitioner Monograph, p 18. Veterinary Practice Publishing Co, Santa Barbara, 1978.
8. Buckner, RC: In *Canine Medicine,* 4th ed, vol 1, p 501. American Veterinary Publications, Santa Barbara, 1979.
9. Dorland: *The American Illustrated Medical Dictionary.* WB Saunders Co, Philadelphia, 1942.
10. Donovan, EF: In *Current Veterinary Therapy VII,* p 1212. WB Saunders Co, Philadelphia, 1980.
11. Arthur, GH: *Wright's Veterinary Obstetrics,* 3rd ed, p 161. Williams & Wilkins, Baltimore, 1964.
12. Roberts, SJ: *Veterinary Obstetrics and Genital Diseases,* p 231. Published by the author, Ithaca, NY, 1971.
13. Whitehead, JE: In *Feline Medicine and Surgery,* p 227. American Veterinary Publications, Inc, Santa Barbara, 1964.
14. McDonald, LE: *Veterinary Pharmacology and Therapeutics,* 53rd ed. Iowa State University Press, Ames, 1968.
15. Ebert, J: Deutsche Tierarzt Woch **83** (**2**) (1976) 74.

FALSE PREGNANCY
BY JAMES H. SOKOLOWSKI

Introduction
False pregnancy (pseudocyesis) in the bitch is a clinical condition in which physiologic and psychologic (behavioral) changes occur.[1] The condition occurs in nonpregnant females during diestrus. Affected animals are usually presented to a veterinarian because they have been mothering inanimate objects, have enlarged mammary glands, are lactating, and may be nursing themselves. Although many affected bitches recover without treatment, the behavioral changes are of concern to the owner and affected mammary glands may be more susceptible to becoming inflamed. This complex condition is not generally recognized in the queen.

It has been reported that most bitches that have estrous cycles and do not have overt pseudopregnancies do have uterine changes. It is not known that uterine pseudopregnancies can result in uterine disease. Spontaneous mammary secretion of milk or clear liquid must also be considered in any discussion of false pregnancy.

Tissue Changes
Corpora lutea (CL) are commonly present in animals with false pregnancy and production of progesterone by CL was once thought to be the cause of false pregnancy. The CL in affected animals are not atypical, however, and they generally appear to be composed of typical luteal tissue.[2]

The uterus of a pseudopregnant bitch is usually enlarged and with extreme uterine pseudopregnancy there are annular bands of hyperplastic endometrial tissue. These bands often resemble the endometrium associated with the placenta of a pregnant bitch. The endometrium may vary histologically from normal hyperplastic endometrium of a pregnant bitch to the cystic dilation, polymorphic infiltration, and other changes associated with severe hyperplastic endometritis.[2]

The ovaries and uterus thus do not have prominent changes that are characteristic of false pregnancy. The tissue changes reflect a progestogen-stimulated endometrium and the clinical signs are related to normal hormonal influences.

Hormonal Factors

The precise mechanisms associated with development of clinical pseudopregnancy are unknown. Retained or persistent corpora lutea have been considered the cause of false pregnancy, but recent information indicates that elevated progesterone levels are not associated with this condition.[3,4]

Development of mammary glands can be induced in several species (including primates and rodents) by administering various combinations of estrogen, progesterone, prolactin, and growth hormone.[5,6] Prolactin plus a corticosteroid (of either endogenous or exogenous origin) has been given to stimulate lactation. High levels of progestogens and/or estrogens will inhibit prolactin and thereby prevent continued lactation. Mammary changes that occur after administering progestogen are probably caused by growth hormone rather than prolactin. Low levels of estrogen, however, will result in release of prolactin. Maintenance of elevated levels of prolactin stimulates lactation.

Prolactin has been found to be elevated during false pregnancy in rodents and with galactorrhea in women.[7] Because the bitch may have post-ovulatory rise in serum estrogens and lactation can be stimulated and/or maintained by prolactin alone, it thus is possible that clinical signs of false pregnancy result from elevated prolactin stimulated by the post-ovulatory rise in estrogen in conjunction with other unknown factors.

Treatment

The treatment for false pregnancy has been largely empirical, involving the use of male or female hormones at relatively high dosages.[9,10] As will be discussed, these treatments have caused problems. Though treatment of false pregnancy is sometimes necessary because of behavioral changes or the ill effects on the mammary glands, many cases are unnoticed by the animal's owner or are so mild that treatment is unneeded. In many overt cases there is spontaneous remission, which should be considered before instituting treatment.

Because the drugs used in treating pseudocyesis may alter a normal pregnancy or possibly mask a pyometra, these conditions must be considered before instituting treatment. It is also important to recognize that false pregnancy or galactorrhea may be caused by pituitary neoplasms. Galactorrhea alone has been associated with primary hypothyroidism without pituitary dysfunction.[11] In such cases, replacement therapy is indicated.

Table 1. Products Used to Treat False Pregnancy and Suppress Lactation

Generic & Trade Names	Use	Route of Administration	Dosage	Side Effects/Comments
Current Products:				
Megestrol acetate (Ovaban, Megace)	False Pregnancy	Oral	1 mg/lb for 8 days	Side Effects — Mammary enlargement, lactation, listlessness, increased appetite, temperament changes. Not to be used in dogs with mammary tumors or in pregnant dogs. Prolonged use may result in mammary nodules and cystic hyperplasia of the uterus.
Methandriol dipropionate (Probolic)	Suppress Lactation	IM	5 to 25 mg daily on alternate days	Monitor blood calcium and sodium and water retention with prolonged use.
Estrone (V-estrovarin)	False Pregnancy	IM	1 to 5 mg	Side Effects — Uterine hypertrophy and bleeding. Extreme sensitivity or overdose may result in blood dyscrasias.
Testosterone propionate (Repotest)	False Pregnancy Suppress Lactation	IM	1 mg/lb repeated in 8 to 10 weeks as needed	Monitor blood calcium and sodium and water retention with prolonged use. Excessive clitoral enlargement and inflammation will result with prolonged use.
Previously Marketed:				
Medroxyprogesterone acetate	False Pregnancy	IM	250 mg	Side Effects — Endometrial hyperplasia, pyometritis.

Table 1, continued

Testosterone	False Pregnancy	IM	0.25 to 0.5 mg/lb every second or third day (duration not stated)	see Testosterone propionate
Hydroxyprogesterone acetate	False Pregnancy	Oral	0.9 to 4.0 mg/lb daily — duration not reported	see Megestrol, Medroxyprogesterone
Diethylstilbestrol	False Pregnancy	IM	0.5 to 1.0 mg/lb as a single injection	see Estrone
Progesterone	False Pregnancy	IM	10 to 50 mg daily until signs subside	see Megestrol, Medroxyprogesterone
Reported Previously:				
Mibolerone	False Pregnancy Suppress Lactation	Oral	18 mcg/lb for 5 days	Side Effects — Clitoral enlargement, vaginal discharge, mounting behavior, musky body odor, epiphora. Do not use in pregnant bitch.
Delmadinone acetate	False Pregnancy	Oral	0.25 to 0.5 mg/lb daily 6 days	see Megestrol, Medroxyprogesterone
		SC	1.25 to 2.5 mg/lb daily 2 days	
Methyloestronolore	False Pregnancy Suppress Lactation	Oral	0.5 to 1.5 mg/lb daily for 3-5 days	Side Effects — Endometritis see Megestrol
		SC	2.0 to 3.5 mg/lb daily for 1-2 days	
Bromocriptine	False Pregnancy Suppress Lactation	Oral	Not given	Unsuitable for dog due to emetic properties.

Current Treatments

A progestogen (megestrol acetate), an androgenic/anabolic steroid (methandriol dipropionate), an estrogen (estrone), and an androgen (testosterone) are the only products that currently carry a label indication for treatment of false pregnancy and/or suppression of lactation in the bitch (Table 1).

Short-term administration of megestrol, methandriol, and testosterone has not caused any life-threatening side effects. Megestrol acetate has resulted, however, in mammary enlargement, lactation, and other minor effects typical of progestational activity. In addition, relapses have been reported after administration of this hormone. This rebound phenomenon should be expected because short-term, low-level administration of progestogen often results in an increase of endogenous estrogen that would trigger release of prolactin and result in recurrence of pseudopregnancy. In a progestogen-stimulated uterus, estrone may cause hypertrophy, bleeding, and (in extreme cases) suppression of bone marrow.

Although no side effects have been reported when methandriol dipropionate has been given in massive doses, this steroid can alter serum calcium levels and, with prolonged use, influence retention of sodium.

Previously Used Drugs

Progestogens (hydroxyprogesterone acetate, progesterone, medroxyprogesterone acetate) and estrogens (estradiol cypionate, diethylstilbestrol) have been used in the past to treat false pregnancy. With all of these hormones there have been problems related to efficacy or safety and they are no longer recommended as treatments for false pregnancy.

Medroxyprogesterone acetate has been associated with mammary development, overt lactation, cystic endometrial hyperplasia, pyometra, mammary nodules and tumors, and maintenance of pregnancy when given to both pregnant and nonpregnant females. Hydroxyprogesterone acetate and progesterone have been marginally effective. Though not as severe, the side effects of these hormones were similar to those reported for medroxyprogesterone acetate.

Estrogens have produced uterine and vaginal hypertrophy with bleeding, prolongation of sexual receptivity, pyometra, and blood dyscrasias. Their short-term use usually resulted in minor side effects other than serum electrolyte imbalances. With long-term use of androgens there have been reports of hepatic damage, excessive clitoral enlargement and inflammation ("tail-lighters"), vaginal discharge, and urinating patterns of males.

Other Treatments

An androgenic/anabolic steroid, mibolerone, has been reported to be effective in the treatment of false pregnancy,[12,13] suppression of lactation and therefore reduction in mammary gland size. Behavioral aspects of false pregnancy are also reduced following mibolerone administration. Its short-term administration has not resulted in side effects, but its long-term use may result in clitoral enlargement, vaginal discharge, mounting behavior, musky body odor, and epiphora. Care should be taken to differentiate false pregnancy from a true pregnancy before giving mibolerone because this drug can cause fetal abnormalities.

Other progestogens (delmadinone acetate and methyloestrenolone) have been reported to be effective in treating false pregnancy and suppressing lactation.[14] These compounds have the same potential for causing uterine side-effects as reported for other progestogens.

A specific antiprolactin drug (bromocriptine) has been given to pseudopregnant bitches, but because of its potency as an emetic it is unsuitable.[10]

False Pregnancy and Other Diseases

False pregnancy is related to other reproductive disease only through its occurrence during the luteal phase of the estrous cycle.

With the possible exceptions of vaginal hyperplasia and pituitary dysfunction, female reproductive disorders occur in response to cyclic estrogen and then progesterone. They therefore are manifested during the luteal phase of the estrous cycle. Though the occurrence of pseudopregnancy in relation to uterine inflammation, mammary tumors, pituitary tumors, and other conditions has been studied, no consistent correlation is apparent. It thus must be concluded that naturally occurring pseudopregnancy results from the release and responses to prolactin.

Conclusion

Although spontaneous remission of false pregnancy may occur, the owner of a bitch with physiologic and psychologic signs of the condition is usually interested in prompt relief of the clinical signs. On the basis of the clinical response and minimal side effects, the androgenic/anabolic steroids seem to be the drugs of choice.

References
1. Voith, V: Mod Vet Pract **6** (1980) 75.
2. Whitney, JC: J Small Anim Pract **8** (1967) 247.

3. Hadley, JF: Vet Rec **96** (1975) 545.
4. Smith, MS and McDonald, LE: Endocrinol **94** (1974) 404.
5. Archer, DF: Fertility and Sterility **28** (1977) 125.
6. Knight, PJ *et al:* Vet Rec **101** (1977) 202.
7. Meites, J: J Invest Dermat **63** (1974) 119.
8. Stoye, M: Zbl Vet Med **B20** (1973) 1.
9. Johnston, SD: In *Current Veterinary Therapy* VI, p 1240. WB Saunders Co, Philadelphia, 1977.
10. Allen, WE and Stockman, V: Vet Rec **104** (1979) 220.
11. Chastain, CB and Schmidt, B: JAAHA **16** (1980) 851.
12. Sokolowski, JH and Geng, S: Amer J Vet Res **38** (1977) 1371.
13. Sokolowski, JH: Canine Pract **9** (1982) 6.
14. Gerber, HA and Sulman FG: Vet Rec **76** (1964) 1089.

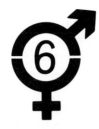

Surgical
Procedures

ANESTHESIA FOR CESAREAN SECTION
BY G. JOHN BENSON & JOHN C. THURMON

Introduction

Cesarean section in animals is often an emergency procedure. Veterinary assistance has often been delayed and the physical condition of the dam and fetuses has suffered. When the fetuses are determined to be dead, the veterinarian can direct full attention to the dam. If the fetuses are alive and their survival is desired, the veterinarian must consider the welfare of both the neonates and dam.

The anesthetic protocol used for cesarean section should ideally provide adequate muscle relaxation, analgesia, and narcosis or sedation for optimal operating conditions and safety to the dam. Fetal depression and decreased viability are directly proportional, however, to the degree of maternal depression. Thus, the veterinarian is faced with the dilemma of having to anesthetize a dam that may already be depressed without further stressing the fetuses.

Drugs that depress the dam, such as anesthetics, narcotics, tranquilizers, and sedatives, must cross the blood-brain barrier. It therefore is impossible to anesthetize the dam and not expose the fetuses to the anesthetic drugs because properties that allow drugs to cross the blood-brain barrier also promote their placental transfer.

No anesthetic agent or protocol is ideal for all dams at parturition. When selecting the anesthetic protocol, the obstetrical problem and the skill and experience of the veterinarian must be considered. The choice of anesthetic must also be based on knowledge of the physiologic alterations caused by pregnancy and labor, the pharmacology of the anesthetic agents when administered in the perinatal period, the direct and indirect effects of the anesthetic on fetuses and neonates, the advantages and risks of the technics chosen, and the significance of obstetrical complications on management of anesthesia.

Physiologic Changes During Pregnancy

Gestation and parturition place metabolic demands on the dam that must be met by physiologic adjustments. Most of the data concerning these adjustments have been obtained from women and ewes. Though little is known about comparable changes in the dog or cat, their magnitude in these species should be comparable. Birth weight expressed as a percent of maternal weight for humans, sheep, dogs, and cats is 5.7%, 11.4%, 16.1%, and 13.2%, respectively.[1] Thus the physiologic burden appears to be greater for the dog and cat than the woman or ewe and one might expect the needed physiologic adjustments to be equal or greater in dogs and cats.

Cardiovascular Changes

Cardiac output increases during pregnancy, reaching 30 to 50% above normal near parturition.[2] This increased cardiac output results from an increase in circulating placental and ovarian hormones.[3] Further increases in cardiac output occur during labor and immediately postpartum. During labor, blood is extruded from the contracting uterus into the general circulation, increasing cardiac output an additional 10 to 25%.[4] Cardiac output during labor is also influenced by the dam's body position, pain, apprehension, and administration of analgesic or anesthetic agents.[5] During pregnancy, blood volume increases by approximately 40%; plasma volume increases more than red cell volume, resulting in decreased hemoglobin concentration and packed cell volume.[5] Systolic and diastolic blood pressures remain unchanged during pregnancy, but during labor the systolic pressure increases 10 to 30 mm Hg.

The pulse rate increases during pregnancy, but central venous pressure does not because the increase in blood volume is offset by increased distensibility of veins and increased capacity of the uterine, renal, skeletal, and skin vasculature. Central venous pressure increases slightly (4 to 6 cm H_2O) during labor, but it can increase by 50 cm H_2O during painful deliveries.[6]

Dorsal recumbency of the dam can result in compression of the vena cava and aorta by the enlarged uterus and its contents. This can lead to decreased cardiac output due to decreased venous return and decreased uterine and renal blood flow. Though the effect of dorsal recumbency is not as great in the bitch as in women, we still recommend that the bitch should not be kept in dorsal recumbency for prolonged periods.[7,7a,8]

Because cardiac work is increased during pregnancy and at parturition, the heart's reserve is decreased and pulmonary congestion and heart failure may result in patients with cardiovascular disease. Any additional stress related to pain and anxiety should be avoided in such patients. Care is also required to avoid severe cardiac depression induced by excessive doses of analgesic, sedative, or anesthetic agents.

Increased cardiac output tends to decrease the induction rate of anesthesia with inhalation agents. Nevertheless the induction of anesthesia with inhalation agents is often more rapid in pregnant patients because respiratory alterations (discussed later) more than offset the effects of increased cardiac output on uptake and distribution of inhalation anesthetics.[5]

Because venous engorgement decreases the size of the epidural space, the dosage of local anesthetics required for epidural anesthesia should be reduced by approximately 33% of the dosage needed for nonpregnant patients.[5]

Administration of ecbolic agents during or following parturition can adversely affect cardiovascular function. For example, oxytocin in large or repeated doses induces peripheral vasodilation and hypotension that can adversely affect both the dam and fetuses because of decreased tissue perfusion. Ergot derivatives directly cause vasoconstriction and hypertension. If given following delivery when cardiac output is highest, severe hypertension and cardiac failure can occur.[9]

Pulmonary Changes

During pregnancy the respiratory center becomes more sensitive to carbon dioxide tension ($PaCO_2$), resulting in an increase in minute volume of ventilation to 50% above normal at term. This effect is due to increased levels of serum progesterone. During gestation, the $PaCO_2$ decreases and is near 30 mm Hg (normal is 36 to 44 mm Hg) at parturition. Because of long-term renal compensation, this respiratory alkalosis does not affect arterial pH. Though oxygen consumption increases 20% due to the needs of the developing fetus, placenta, uterine muscle, and mammary tissue, oxygen tension in arterial blood is maintained. Ventilation may be further increased during labor by pain, apprehension, and anxiety.[5]

Pregnancy also affects the mechanics of ventilation. Airway conductance is increased and total pulmonary resistance is decreased as a result of hormone-induced relaxation of bronchial smooth muscle. Lung compliance is unaffected. Functional residual capacity (FRC) is decreased because of cranial displacement of the diaphragm and other abdominal organs by the gravid uterus. In addition, FRC decreases further during labor due to increased pulmonary blood volume subsequent to intermittent uterine contraction. Due to the decrease in FRC, airway closure at end exhalation develops in approximately 33% of parturient dams during tidal ventilation.[5] Total lung capacity and vital capacity are unaltered.

Because of the decreased FRC, hypoventilation results in hypoxia and hypercapnia more readily in pregnant than nonpregnant patients. This tendency for hypoxia is exacerbated by increased oxygen consumption during labor. Therefore, induction of anesthesia must be smooth and rapid. Excitation and struggling associated with excessive restraint and poor technic must be avoided. Intubation should be accomplished quickly and ventilation should be supported to ensure adequate oxygenation. Adequacy of ventilation may be assessed by observing rate of respiration, excursion of the chest wall and/or reservoir bag, and color of the mucous membranes.

Induction of anesthesia with inhalation agents is more rapid in pregnant than nonpregnant patients. The rate of equilibration between the partial pressure of the inspired and alveolar anesthetic agent is increased by an increase in alveolar ventilation and a decrease in FRC.

Pregnancy decreases the dosage requirements for anesthetic agents. The minimum alveolar concentration value is reduced 25% for halothane, 32% for methoxyflurane, and 40% for isoflurane in pregnant compared to nonpregnant animals. Induction of anesthesia with inhalant agents may therefore be very rapid and require as little as 20 to 25% of the time required for nonpregnant patients.[10] One must be careful, therefore, to prevent over-anesthetization of pregnant animals.

Gastrointestinal Function

Pregnancy delays gastric emptying due to physical displacement of the stomach by the gravid uterus and also due to the stomach's response to increased serum progesterone. In addition, gastric motility and lower esophageal sphincter tone are decreased. Gastric motility is further decreased by pain and anxiety during labor.[5] Acid, chloride, and enzyme concentrations in gastric secretions are increased and intragastric pressure is increased.

As a result of altered gastric function, the risk of regurgitation and aspiration of regurgitated material is increased for dams at parturition. Animals presented for cesarean section have often been fed recently or the time of their last feeding is unknown. In all cases the dam should be regarded as having a full stomach. Induction of anesthesia and tracheal intubation should be achieved rapidly to prevent aspiration of foreign material. In some cases epidural anesthesia would be appropriate.

The incidence of vomiting is increased by administration of narcotics and xylazine, hypotension, hypoxia, and use of local anesthetics. The incidence can be decreased by the judicious use of antiemetic drugs, smooth induction of general anesthesia, and prevention of hypotension during epidural anesthesia. Silent regurgitation can occur when intragastric pressure is high and this emphasizes the need for placement of a cuffed endotracheal tube. Positive-pressure ventilation with a face mask or succinylcholine-induced fasciculations can increase intragastric pressure and initiate passive regurgitation. Atropine given IV may increase the gastroesophageal sphincter tone and thus help to prevent regurgitation.[6]

Hepatic and Renal Function

Pregnancy causes minor alterations in hepatic function. Plasma protein concentration decreases slightly, but total plasma protein is increased due to the increase in blood volume. Bilirubin concentration is unaltered. Serum concentrations of SGOT and LDH are slightly increased and BSP retention time is increased. The cholinesterase concentration in plasma decreases. Despite these changes the liver function is generally adequate during gestation and parturition.[5]

Renal circulation and glomerular filtration rate are increased approximately 60% in pregnant patients. As a result of the increased renal blood flow and glomerular filtration rate, blood urea nitrogen and creatinine concentrations are less than in nonpregnant patients.[6] Sodium and water balance are unaffected.

Decrease in plasma cholinesterase may result in prolongation of succinylcholine's action in pregnant animals, especially if they have been exposed recently to organophosphate parasiticides. Normal or slightly elevated BUN or creatinine levels may reflect renal disease or insufficiency. Nephrotoxic drugs (tetracyclines, aminoglycoside antibiotics, methoxyflurane) should not be given to pregnant animals with renal disease.

Uterine Blood Flow

Fetal and maternal homeostasis and neonatal survival are dependent on maintenance of uteroplacental circulation. Uterine blood flow is directly proportional to perfusion pressure and inversely proportional to uterine vascular resistance. Anesthesia may decrease uterine blood flow and thereby contribute directly to reduced fetal viability. In addition, uterine vascular resistance is indirectly increased by uterine contractions and the hypertonia induced by uterine contractions (oxytocic response). Arterial hypotension is induced by hypovolemia or sympathetic blockade. Vasoconstriction is induced by endogenous sympathetic discharge or by exogenous sympathomimetics, such as epinephrine, norepinephrine, methoxamine, phenylephrine, and metaraminol.[5,11,12] Hypotension induced by anesthetic agents and increased uterine tone induced by ecbolics should be avoided if possible.

Summary of Physiologic Changes

Because cardiac reserve diminishes during pregnancy, cardiac decompensation or failure can occur. Likewise, pregnant patients are prone to hypoventilation, hypoxia, and hypercarbia due to altered pulmonary function. Because the required dosage for inhalant anesthetics becomes less than normal, the likelihood of overdosing these agents increases. Vomiting or regurgitation and aspiration can occur if induction of anesthesia and intubation are not performed quickly. Because of the physiologic alterations induced by pregnancy, therefore, parturient patients are at greater risk when anesthetized. The physiologic changes associated with pregnancy and labor are summarized in Table 1.

Perinatal Pharmacology

The uptake, distribution, and excretion of anesthetic agents are altered in pregnant animals. The concentration of free drug in maternal plasma, which is the portion of the administered dose that affects the dam and fetuses, depends on several complex processes that occur simultaneously. These include uptake from the site of administration, protein binding, distribution to maternal tissues, uptake and biotransformation by the dam's liver, maternal excretion, placental transfer, and fetal distribution and metabolism.

Quantitative studies of drug disposition in pregnant patients are sparse and the effects of physiologic changes associated with pregnancy on drug disposition are generally unknown.[13] For example, an increase in cardiac output results in a decrease in the percentage of

Table 1. Physiologic Alterations Associated with Pregnancy

Parameter	Change
Heart rate	Increased
Cardiac output	Increased
Blood volume	Increased
Plasma volume	Increased
Packed cell volume, hemoglobin, and plasma protein concentration	Decreased
Arterial blood pressure	Unchanged
Central venous pressure	Unchanged-increases during labor
Minute volume of ventilation	Increased
Oxygen consumption	Increased
Arterial blood gases and pH	pH and oxygen tension unchanged, carbon dioxide tension decreased
Total lung capacity and vital capacity	Unchanged
Functional residual capacity	Decreased
Gastric emptying time and intragastric pressure	Increased
Gastric motility and pH of gastric secretions	Decreased
Gastric Cl and enzyme concentration	Increased
SGOT, LDH and BSP retention time	Increased
Plasma cholinesterase concentration	Decreased
Renal plasma flow and glomerular filtration rate	Increased
BUN and creatinine	Decreased
Na^+ and water balance	Unchanged

cardiac output that perfuses the central nervous system. Because of the increase in blood volume, the plasma concentration of a given dosage of a drug given IV would be reduced. As a result, the required dosage of an injectable anesthetic agent, such as thiamylal, for induction of anesthesia would appear to be increased. This effect is partially offset, however, by the reduction in concentration of plasma protein and thus less drug being protein-bound. A larger percentage of the administered dose would then be active and exert an effect on the central nervous system.

The effects of pregnancy on drug biotransformation and excretion are variable and not fully understood. The dosage of inhalant anesthetics is reduced due to an unknown mechanism. Hepatic biotransformation of barbiturates appears to be decreased in pregnancy.[13] As a result of the decreased concentration of plasma cholinesterase, the metabolism of succinylcholine and procaine is decreased, although usually not significantly.[13] The increase in renal blood flow and glomerular filtration should favor renal excretion of drugs.

At one time the placenta was regarded as a barrier to passage of drugs from dam to fetus. It is now recognized as being quite permeable to anesthetics and anesthetic adjuncts. Any drug given to the dam will cross the placenta at a rate unique to each drug and then affect the fetus. The effect will be proportionate to that observed in the dam. Factors that affect placental transfer of drugs and their distribution into and ultimate removal from fetal tissues include the physiochemical properties of the drug; structure of the maternal circulation, the placenta, and fetus; and the hemodynamic and pharmacokinetic events that occur within them.[13]

Medicaments administered at parturition affect the fetus either directly as a result of placental transfer or indirectly through their effects on the dam. Placental transfer of drugs can occur by several mechanisms: simple diffusion, facilitated diffusion via carrier systems, active transport, and pinocytosis. Simple diffusion is by far the most important. The amount of a drug crossing the placenta and entering the fetal circulation is measured by the Fick equation:

$$Q/t = K\frac{A(Cm\text{-}Cf)}{D}$$

In this equation, Q/t = amount of diffused substance per unit of time, K = diffusion constant of a given material, A = surface area available for diffusion, D = thickness of the placenta, Cm = concentration of material in maternal blood perfusing the placenta, and Cf = concentration of drug in fetal blood perfusing the placenta.

Surface area and thickness of the placenta vary among species of animals. The common farm animals have thick epitheliochorial placentas with relatively small areas for diffusion. The dog and cat have thinner endotheliochorial placentas with somewhat larger zonary areas of implantation. Women and rodents have the thinnest type of placenta.[14,15]

The diffusion constant (K) is unique to each drug and it is affected by the conditions present in the dam at the time of the drug's administration. K is determined by molecular weight, degree to which the drug is bound to maternal plasma proteins, lipid solubility, and degree of ionization. Drugs that are poorly ionized and have a low molecular weight (<500), a low degree of protein binding, and high lipid solubility have high K values and diffuse rapidly across the placenta. Drugs that cross the placenta slowly have a high molecular weight (>1000) and low lipid solubility, and are highly protein bound and ionized. Most anesthetics and anesthetic adjuncts have high K

values. The muscle relaxant drugs are an exception; they are highly ionized and have low lipid solubility. Their K value is therefore low and, while they can be recovered from fetal blood, muscle relaxants are generally regarded as having minimal placental transfer and a few direct effects on the fetus.[13,16]

The degree to which a drug is ionized in the body is determined by its pKa and the pH of the patient's body fluids. The pKa is the pH at which the ionized and nonionized forms of the drug exist in equal proportions and it is unique to each drug. Drugs that are weak acids will be less highly ionized as the pH decreases.[16] For example, thiopental is a weak acid with a pKa of 7.6. When it is administered to a patient with pH of 7.4, 61% of the drug is nonionized and active. In patients with a pH less than 7.4, a greater proportion of the administered dose will be nonionized. Therefore, acidemia decreases the required anesthetic dosage of thiopental. As the degree of ionization decreases so does the fraction of the dose that is protein-bound and thus not able to exert its effect. Weakly basic drugs, such as narcotics and local anesthetics, are more highly ionized at pH's below their pKa.[17]

The distribution of drug between dam and fetus is influenced by their blood pH and drug pKa. The fetal pH is normally 0.1 units less than that of the dam. Therefore, weakly basic drugs, such as narcotics, will be found in higher concentration in fetal tissues and plasma than in the dam due to "ion trapping." The nonionized form can cross the placenta but due to the maternal-fetal difference in pH, ionization occurs in the fetus. This decreases the concentration of fetal nonionized drug and more nonionized drug can cross the placenta to the fetus.[18]

Concentration of a drug in maternal blood is dependent on the total dose, site and route of administration, rate of distribution and uptake of the drug by maternal tissues, and maternal metabolism and excretion. Thus, drugs with a rapidly declining plasma concentration, such as thiopental and succinylcholine, have a high maternal blood concentration for only short periods. This is in contrast to the sustained maternal blood levels of inhalation anesthetics that results in continuous placental transfer of the drug to the fetus.[13,18]

Drug concentration in the fetus is the result of passive diffusion across the placenta and it is altered by redistribution in the fetus, fetal metabolism, and protein-binding. The concentration of a drug in the umbilical vein is not the same as that available to fetal target organs (brain, heart, and other vital organs). As much as 85% of umbilical venous blood initially passes through the fetal liver, where a drug may be sequestered or metabolized. In addition, umbilical venous blood containing the drug enters the inferior vena cava via the ductus venosus and mixes with drug-free blood returning from the lower extremities and pelvic viscera. In this way the fetal circulation buffers vital fetal tissues from sudden high concentrations of the drug. Binding of drug to fetal proteins may limit the amount of available drug and thus reduce toxicity.[13,16]

Metabolism of drugs in the fetus is not as efficient as it is in adults because the fetal liver microsomal enzyme system is not as mature nor as active as it is in adults. Drug concentrations and effects in the fetus can therefore be considerably greater and of longer duration than in the dam. Finally, drug toxicity in fetuses can be enhanced by a drug's transformation to more toxic metabolites and by drug interaction.[18]

Clinical Implications

Anesthetic and anesthetic adjunct drugs should be carefully chosen and properly administered to avoid undue maternal and fetal depression. No agent should be used unless it is distinctly indicated.

Drugs that induce sedation and/or tranquilization include the barbiturates, phenothiazines, butyrophenones, benzodiazepines, and xylazine. All of them rapidly cross the placenta and cause depression in neonatal animals. Barbiturates cause neonatal respiratory depression, sleepiness, and decreased activity. Suckling is decreased and has been reported to be depressed for 4 days in human neonates.[18]

Phenothiazine and butyrophenone tranquilizers are frequently used as preanesthetic agents and are often used in conjunction with narcotics. The former potentiate narcotic depression and add little to narcotic-induced analgesia. In addition, they induce hypotension via alpha-adrenergic blockade and depress the central nervous system. This results in respiratory depression and decreased ability to regulate body temperature. The duration of action of phenothiazines is long, lasting up to 8 hours.[5,18] Tranquilizer-sedative drugs should be given only to very apprehensive or excited dams at parturition, and then only in dosages sufficient to induce a calming effect. There is little indication for the routine use of these agents in parturient animals.[18]

When diazepam (Valium) is used to induce sedation of a dam, it can induce neonatal lethargy, hypotonus, and hypothermia.[13] These effects are avoided by administering less than 0.14 mg/kg IV.[18]

Xylazine (Rompun) is a potent sedative-hypnotic drug with significant analgesic properties. It rapidly crosses the placenta, however, and depresses both maternal and fetal respiration and circulation.

When xylazine is used in conjunction with ketamine HCl, there are significant and potentially life-threatening cardiopulmonary changes that result in decreased tissue perfusion in healthy dogs.[19] Therefore, use of xylazine or xylazine-ketamine combinations should probably be avoided in animals being prepared for cesarean section. Similar effects have been reported recently for ketamine-acepromazine mixture in cats.[20]

Narcotics cross the placenta rapidly and can cause respiratory and CNS depression in neonates that may last as long as 24 hours.[18,21,22] In addition, elimination of the drug may require 2 to 6 days. It appears that the depression is proportional to the degree of analgesia and thus the choice of a narcotic agent is based partly on the duration of action desired.

The most commonly used narcotics are fentanyl, meperidine, and oxymorphone. They are listed in the order of increasing duration of action.[18] Other drugs with narcotic agonist and antagonist activity have recently been used to induce analgesia. They include nalbuphine and butorphanol. These drugs reportedly cause less respiratory depression than pure narcotic agonists. In addition, a narcotics license is not required for use of these drugs. One of the advantages of narcotic agonists is that direct antagonists are available to reverse their action. Among the antagonists, naloxone at a dosage of 0.04 mg/kg appears to be one of the most effective. It is a pure antagonist and has no narcotic agonist action. Because nalorphine and levallorphine have narcotic activity, they can increase depression induced by other nonnarcotic agents, such as barbiturates and phenothiazines.

Because all narcotic antagonists rapidly cross the placenta, their administration to the dam prior to delivery has been advocated to reverse narcotic-induced depression of neonates. Such use deprives the dam of analgesia when it is needed most, however, and these agents should be administered directly to the neonate.

Because naloxone has a shorter duration of action than most narcotic agonists, narcotization may recur after naloxone is metabolized and excreted.[18] Dams and neonates should therefore be carefully monitored following the administration of naloxone. If signs of narcosis recur, more naloxone should be given.

The most commonly used drugs to induce anesthesia by IV injection are the ultrashort-acting barbiturates, such as thiopental, thiamylal, and methohexital. When administered in low doses (less than 4 mg/kg) to women, they cause minimal fetal depression.[18] Ketamine can also be given IV to induce anesthesia for intubation. Because effective dosages for these agents are higher in dogs and cats than in humans, some neonatal depression has been associated with their use.

Other injectable nonbarbiturate anesthetics are currently being used in England and Europe. Though these agents are not approved for use in the US at this time, they may become available. One of them (Althesin) is a combination of 2 progesterone-like steroids. This drug can be administered both IV or IM to cats. It induces anesthesia smoothly and rapidly. Cardiovascular depression is proportionate to dosage and it is similar to the depression caused by equivalent doses of thiopental or methohexital. Althesin causes less respiratory depression than barbiturates and it is compatible with the commonly used preanesthetics, muscle relaxants, and inhalation anesthetics.[23] Due to its short duration of action, this drug is best suited for induction of anesthesia for cesarean section. It does cross the placenta, however. Its use in the dog is limited because the solubilizing agent causes release of histamine. Althesin has been used to induce anesthesia in dogs pretreated with antihistamines.[24]

Etomidate is a short-acting, nonbarbiturate anesthetic. In dosages suitable for induction of anesthesia it has produced anesthesia with no significant cardiovascular effects in dogs. On this basis, etomidate has been judged superior to thiamylal for induction of anesthesia in the dog. In women, etomidate induces anesthesia more rapidly and recovery from it is more rapid than from thiopental.[25] Enhanced perfusion of fetal tissue is reflected by more rapid initiation of the neonates' spontaneous breathing and greater vitality than with thiopental.[26] Other drugs with similar action include propanidid and metomidate.

Skeletal muscle relaxants cross the placenta to a limited degree and induce little effect on the neonate when used in reasonable dosages.[16] These agents are thus very useful when used in combination with other drugs for cesarean section.[23,24] The most commonly used relaxants are succinylcholine and pancuronium. Due to its rapid onset and short duration of action, the former is especially useful when combined with an ultrashort-acting barbiturate for induction and when muscle relaxation of short duration is desired. Pancuronium can be used to induce muscle relaxation of longer duration (45 minutes). Though gallamine may also be used, this drug appears to cross the placenta more quickly than the other muscle relaxants and it has no distinct advantages. For this reason, its use in obstetrics has diminished.[18]

Inhalation anesthetics readily cross the placenta and achieve fetal and maternal equilibration rapidly. The degree of fetal depression is thus proportional to the depth of anesthesia induced in the dam. Deep levels of anesthesia in the dam cause maternal hypotension, decreased uterine blood flow, and fetal acidosis. Due to the rapid induction and recovery of dam and neonate, the less soluble inhalants (halothane, enflurane, isoflurane) are preferable to the highly soluble ones, such as methoxyflurane. Nitrous oxide can be used to supplement the more potent inhalants and thus decrease the total amount administered. If nitrous oxide is administered at a 60% level, fetal depression is minimal and neonatal hypoxia does not occur.[18,24,25]

Administration of oxygen to the dam is not accompanied by a significant decrease in uterine blood flow or fetal acidosis.[18] The concentration of 2, 3 diphosphoglycerate is relatively low in fetal red blood cells. This anion competes with oxygen for binding on the hemoglobin molecule. Fetal hemoglobin can carry more oxygen at low oxygen tensions than can adult hemoglobin (Fig 1). This is important because it ensures a higher level of hemoglobin saturation at normally low oxygen pressures in fetuses.[26] Because administration of oxygen to dams can result in a significant increase in fetal oxygen, this is indicated regardless of the anesthetic protocol. Oxygen concentrations of 50% or greater during general anesthesia will result in more vigorous neonates.[18]

The total effect of CO_2 on the fetus is not clear, but passive hyperventilation of the dam results in hypocapnia and decreased flow of blood in the uterine artery. This decrease in placental perfusion

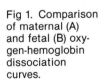

Fig 1. Comparison of maternal (A) and fetal (B) oxygen-hemoglobin dissociation curves.

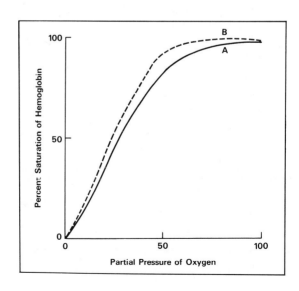

causes fetal hypoxia, hypercapnia, and acidosis. Active hyperventilation by dams may have the same effect. With adequate arterial oxygenation a modest increase in CO_2 is tolerated by the fetus.[18]

Local anesthetics are frequently used in combination with other drugs or as the sole agent for regional anesthesia. Because the esters of para-aminobenzoic acid (procaine, tetracaine) are metabolized by maternal and fetal pseudocholinesterase, there is little accumulation of these agents in the fetus when they are infiltrated locally or given epidurally. Amide derivatives (lidocaine, mepivicaine, bupivicaine, and etidocaine) are metabolized by hepatic enzymes. Following their absorption from the site of injection, the blood levels of these drugs decrease slowly, but they can reach significant levels in the fetus. Fetal blood concentrations of lidocaine or mepivacaine in excess of 3 μg/ml can cause neonatal depression at delivery. Such concentrations rarely occur following epidural administration of these drugs, but they can occur with excessive doses given locally.[18] These drugs can indirectly affect the fetus. Sympathetic blockade resulting in maternal hypotension and decreased uteroplacental perfusion may follow an epidural injection. This can be controlled by judicious administration of intravenous fluids to compensate for increased capacity of the vascular system.[25] Vasopressors can also be used to treat maternal hypotension resulting from sympathetic blockade. Because ephedrine acts centrally and has minimal vasoconstrictor properties, it is used to treat maternal hypotension and thus restore uterine blood flow. Mephentermine acts similarly. Other agents with alpha-adrenergic activity increase maternal blood pressure by increasing systemic vascular resistance. This results in a decrease of uterine blood flow and often fetal deterioration. These agents also stimulate hypertonic uterine contractions and further decrease uteroplacental perfusion.[18,25]

Anticholinergic agents (atropine, glycopyrrolate) should be administered to most dams at parturition to decrease salivation and to inhibit excessive vagal tone that may occur when traction is applied to the uterus. Many dams have eaten recently, increasing the likelihood of regurgitation, which is also enhanced by hypoxia or hypotension. The influence of anticholinergics on vomiting is controversial.[6,29] Atropine has not decreased the incidence of vomiting by women at parturition.[28] Glycopyrrolate increases gastric pH and thus decreases the severity of signs associated with regurgitation and aspiration of vomitus.[30] Because glycopyrrolate does not readily cross the placenta, it does not affect the fetus to the same extent as atropine. Therefore, it may be a more appropriate anticholinergic.[31]

Technics for Cesarean Section

Satisfactory anesthesia for cesarean section can be induced in a number of ways. The choice of anesthetic protocol is based on safety to the dam and fetus, comfort of the dam, convenience to the surgeon, and familiarity with the technic. The drugs used should cause minimal depression of the fetuses. Likewise, the time from induction of anesthesia to delivery should be minimal because its prolongation is associated with decreased neonatal viability.[25] Therefore, the surgical site should be prepared prior to induction of anesthesia and the surgery should be performed rapidly and efficiently.

Cesarean section can be performed with either regional or general anesthesia. The advantages of the latter include speed and ease of induction, reliability, and controllability. General anesthesia provides optimum operating conditions with a relaxed, immobile patient. Tracheal intubation ensures control of the dam's airway and thus prevents aspiration of vomitus. It also provides a route for administration of oxygen. When general anesthesia is properly administered, the dam's cardiopulmonary function is maintained.[23,25] In addition, most veterinarians are more confident of their ability to induce general anesthesia safely than to induce regional anesthesia successfully.

General anesthesia is not without disadvantages, however. It causes greater neonatal depression than regional anesthesia. If the plane of anesthesia is too light, catecholamine release by the dam can result in hypertension and decreased uteroplacental perfusion, leading to both maternal and fetal stress and deterioration of cardiopulmonary function.[11,12,21] Problems of airway management during general anesthesia are more likely to occur when the trachea is not properly intubated. Aspiration of foreign material and inability to intubate the trachea are the leading causes of maternal mortality associated with cesarean section in women.[23,25] Fortunately, dogs and cats are relatively easy to intubate. General anesthesia may be more appropriate than regional anesthesia in certain circumstances, including the occurrence of maternal hypovolemia, exhaustion of the dam, maternal heart disease or failure, morbid obesity, unusual resistance by the dam, upper airway obstruction in brachycephalic dogs, and when the veterinarian is inexperienced in regional anesthetic technics.

A variety of technics have been found satisfactory for induction of general anesthesia for cesarean section.[24,27,32] The following example can be used as a guideline to establish a protocol to meet the requirements of individual patients:

1. Premedicate with atropine (0.044 mg/kg) or glycopyrrolate
   (0.011 mg/kg) given IM or IV 10 to 20 minutes prior to induction
   of anesthesia. Avoid tranquilizers, sedatives, hypnotics, and
   narcotics unless they are indicated because the animal is overly
   apprehensive or aggressive.
2. If possible, give oxygen 3 to 5 minutes by mask prior to inducing anesthesia.
3. Induction of anesthesia should be smooth and rapid. Tracheal
   intubation should be performed rapidly to gain control of the
   airway, ensure adequate oxygenation, and to prevent aspiration of foreign material. Spraying the larynx with lidocaine will
   help to prevent laryngospasm and coughing; it will also ease
   tracheal intubation. Drugs used to induce anesthesia include:

Thiamylal Na	6-8 mg/kg IV
Thiopental Na	6-8 mg/kg IV
Methohexital Na	5 mg/kg IV
Droperidol-Fentanyl	1 ml/20-30 kg IV
Diazepam	0.2-0.5 mg/kg IV
+	
Ketamine HCl	4-8 mg/kg IV
(not approved for dogs)	
Acepromazine-Oxymorphone	0.1 mg/kg to maximum
(not suitable for cats)	of 4 mg acepromazine
	given IM or IV and 0.11
	mg/kg oxymorphone
	given IV

Succinylcholine (0.3 mg/kg) can be administered IV with any of
the induction drugs to facilitate tracheal intubation. When this
drug is used, intubation must be rapid and ventilation controlled until spontaneous breathing resumes.
4. Following intubation, oxygen should be administered. If
   available, nitrous oxide can be administered in a 50-50 mixture
   with oxygen.
5. Halothane, methoxyflurane, enflurane, or isoflurane can be administered to induce additional analgesia and narcosis as needed. Prior to delivery of fetuses the vaporizer concentration
   should be low (0.5-1%; 0.5% to 0.75%; 0.8 to 1.7%; 0.7 to
   1.39%, respectively). After delivery the concentration can be
   increased as needed for surgical closure. Muscle relaxants may

be given to induce relaxation at light planes of anesthesia and thus avoid excessive depression. These agents include:

	Dosage	Duration of Action (min)
Succinylcholine	0.2 to 0.4 mg/kg	15
Gallamine	0.4 mg/kg	20 to 40
Pancuronium	0.06 to 0.14 mg/kg	30 to 60

Muscle relaxation induced by gallamine or pancuronium may be reversed with neostigmine (0.06 to 0.2 mg/kg) or edrophonium (0.1 to 0.2 mg/kg). Either of these agents should be preceded by administration of atropine (0.04 mg/kg) to prevent bradycardia.

Following completion of surgery, the dam is allowed to recover in a quiet area and the tracheal tube is removed. Because vomiting and aspiration of vomitus can occur during recovery from anesthesia, removal of the tube should be delayed until the dam can protect her airway and maintain sternal recumbency.

Regional anesthesia for cesarean section is a well-established technic.[24,27,33] Local infiltration or a field block is possible, but both procedures have disadvantages compared to epidural anesthesia. Infiltration requires larger amounts of the anesthetic agent, which are absorbed and depress the fetus. Muscle relaxation and analgesia are not as satisfactory or uniform as they are with epidural anesthesia. Therefore, a field block is often supplemented with heavy sedation or tranquilization, which can result in deep maternal and fetal depression. For these reasons, either general anesthesia or epidural anesthesia is preferable to regional anesthesia.

Because the spinal cord terminates at the level of the 6th lumbar vertebra in the dog and cat, subarachnoid (true spinal) injection of an anesthetic agent is not common when made at the lumbosacral junction. Epidural anesthesia has the advantages of being simple to induce, causing minimal exposure of the fetus to drugs and less intraoperative bleeding, and allowing the dam to remain conscious. In addition, muscle relaxation and analgesia are optimal. Disadvantages of epidural anesthesia include the occurrence of hypotension secondary to sympathetic blockade. Nausea and vomiting can occur during epidural anesthesia due to hypotension and visceral manipulation. Because the dam remains conscious, movement of the forelimbs and head often occur.[33] This precludes the use of epidural anesthesia in highly excited or fractious dams. Finally, the successful induction of epidural anesthesia requires that the veterinarian be well acquainted with the technic. The skill required is well within the reach of any clinician, however, and it can be quickly acquired.

The hypotension induced by epidural anesthesia can be readily controlled by giving fluids and catecholamine. Lactated Ringer's solution, normal saline solution, or half-strength saline solution mixed with equal volumes of 5% dextrose solution can be administered at a dosage of 20 ml/kg over a 15 to 20 minute period to maintain arterial blood pressure. When hypotension is severe, ephedrine can be administered IV (0.3 mg/kg). Drugs and dosages for epidural anesthesia in the dog and cat include 2% procaine (1.0 ml/1.5-2.5 kg), 2% lidocaine (1.0 ml/3-5 kg), and 2% mepivacaine (1.0 ml/6-10 kg).

As with general anesthesia, anticholinergic agents may be used to prevent bradycardia.

Care of the Newborn

Following its delivery, the newborn's head should be freed of membranes and the oropharynx should be cleared of fluid. The umbilical vessels should be milked toward the fetus to empty them. They are then clamped approximately 2 cm from the body wall and severed from the placenta. The newborn animal can then be gently rubbed with a towel to dry it and to stimulate its breathing. The pup or kitten may be cradled in the hands and gently swung in a head-down position to help clear the respiratory tract of fluid. When doing this the fetal head and neck should be supported to prevent injury.

Doxapram can be used to stimulate breathing in a neonatal pup or kitten. For puppies the dosage is 1 to 5 mg (approximately 1 to 5 drops from a 20- to 22-gauge needle) and in the kitten the dosage is 1 to 2 mg (1 to 2 drops) administered orally or injected IM or SC.[34] Newborn animals are susceptible to chilling and should be kept warm. Ideally, the ambient temperature should be 85 to 90 F.[35] After the dam has recovered from anesthesia, the newborn animals can be placed with her. If regional anesthesia has been used, the newborn animals can be placed with their mother as soon as the surgery is completed.

References

1. Dawes, GS: Foetal and Neonatal Physiology, p 15. Year Book Medical Publishers Inc, Chicago, 1968.
2. Kerr, MG: Brit Med Bull **24** (1968) 19.
3. Ueland, K and Parer, JT: Amer J Obstet Gynecol **96** (1966) 400.
4. Ueland, K and Hansen, JM: Amer J Obstet Gynecol **103** (1969) 1.
5. Shnider, SM: The Physiology of Pregnancy. Paper presented at annual refresher course lectures, ASA annual meeting, 1978.

6. James, FM III: Physiologic Changes During Pregnancy. Paper presented at annual refresher course lectures, ASA annual meeting, 1980.
7a. Probst, CW and Webb, AI: Amer J Vet Res **44** (1983) 1963.
7. Marx, GF: Physiology of Pregnancy — High Risk Implications. Paper presented at annual refresher course lectures, ASA annual meeting, 1979.
8. Kerr, MG and Scott, DB: Inferior Vena Caval Occlusion in Late Pregnancy. In *Clinical Anesthesia*, FA Davis, Philadelphia, 1973.
9. Lipton, B *et al:* J Amer Med Assn **179** (1962) 410.
10. Palahniuk, RJ *et al:* Anesthesiology **41** (1974) 88.
11. Wright, RG *et al:* The Effect of Maternal Stress on Plasma Catecholamines and Uterine Blood Flow in the Pregnant Ewe. Abstract of Scientific Papers, Ann meet of Soc of Obstetric Anesthesia and Perinatology, 1978.
12. Morishema, HO *et al:* Effects of Maternal Pain and Hyperexcitability upon the Fetus — Possible Benefits of Maternal Sedation. Paper presented at scientific session of ASA annual meeting, 1977.
13. Alper, MH: Perinatal Pharmacology. Paper presented at annual refresher course lectures, ASA annual meeting, 1979.
14. Ramsey, EM: The Placenta of Laboratory Animals and Man. pp 73, 142, 154, 160. Holt, Rinehart and Winston, 1975.
15. Nalbandov, AV: Reproductive Physiology, p 196. WH Freeman, San Francisco, 1958.
16. Finster, M: Perinatal Pharmacology. Paper presented at annual refresher course lectures, ASA annual meeting, 1980.
17. Collins, VJ: Principles of Anesthesiology. 2nd ed, p 199. Lea and Febiger, Philadelphia, 1976.
18. Gutsche, B: Perinatal Pharmacology. Paper presented at annual refresher course lectures, ASA annual meeting, 1978.
19. McDonnell, W and Van Gorder, J: Cardiopulmonary Effects of Xylazine/Ketamine in Dogs. Paper presented at annual scientific meeting, ACVA, 1982.
20. Becker, M and Beglinger, R: Effects of Ketamine and Its Combination With Acepromazine on the Cardiovascular System of the Cat. Paper presented at 1st International Congress of Veterinary Anesthesia, 1982.
21. Palahniuk, RJ: Obstetric Anesthesia in the Healthy Parturient. Paper presented at annual refresher course lectures, ASA annual meeting, 1979.
22. Hodgkinson, R *et al:* Canad Anaesth Soc J **25** (1978) 405.
23. Hall, LW: Postgrad Med J **48** (Supp 2) (1972) 55.
24. Corbet, HR: Aust Vet Pract **7 (3-4)** (1977) 184.
25. Nagel, ML *et al:* Amer J Vet Res **40** (1979) 193.
26. Downing, JW *et al:* Brit J Anaesthes **51** (1979) 135.
27. Gibbs, CP: Anesthesia for Cesarean Section: General. Paper presented at annual refresher course lectures, ASA annual meeting, 1981.
28. Goodger, WJ and Levy, W: Vet Clinics No Amer **3 (1)** (1973) 85.
29. Datta, S and Alper, MH: Anesthesiology **53** (1980) 142.
30. Guyton, AC: Textbook of Medical Physiology. 4th ed, p 978. WB Saunders, Philadelphia, 1971.
31. Sawyer, DC: The Anesthetic Period: Predictable Problems in the Practice of Small Animal Anesthesia. Vol 1, p 194. WB Saunders, Philadelphia, 1982.
32. Ratra, CK *et al:* Brit J Anaesth **44** (1972) 1208.
33. Dow, TGB *et al:* Obst Gynecol **51** (1978) 426.
34. Baraka, A *et al:* Anesth Analg (Cleve) **56** (1977) 642.
35. Proakis, AG and Harris, GB: Anesthesiology **51** (1978) 339.
36. Soma, LR: Textbook of Veterinary Anesthesia. pp 303-309. Williams & Wilkins, Baltimore, 1971.
37. Klide, AM: In Textbook of Veterinary Anesthesia, pp 450-467. Williams & Wilkins, Baltimore, 1971.
38. Reports on File. Pharmacology Department, AH Robins Company, Richmond.
39. Mosier, JE: In Nutrition and Management of Dogs and Cats. Ralston Purina Company, St Louis, 1981.

SURGICAL TECHNICS
BY THOMAS R. CHRISTIE

Episioplasty

Surgical repair of a vulvar or perivulvar defect is referred to as an episioplasty. The most common indication for this procedure is severe perivulvar dermatitis related to obesity or a defect in conformation that results in a recessed vulva. The resultant cleft between the vulva and adjacent skin is warm, moist, and contaminated with microorganisms that thrive in this environment.

Perivulvar dermatitis can result in contamination of the interior female genitalia during breeding and thus cause a poor conception rate or abortion. Because the vulva is recessed, insertion of the penis is also more difficult. Episioplasty, therefore, increases the chances for successful mating.

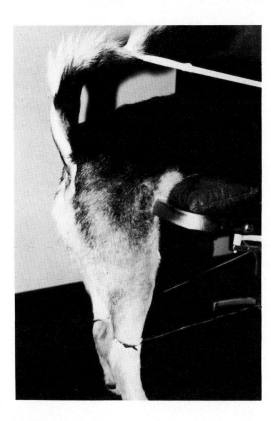

Fig 1. This standard position for perineal surgery is suitable for episioplasty.

The perivulvar cleft is readily inspected by retracting the skin laterally. The cleft can be removed by excision of the redundant skin.

Technic: Following induction of general anesthesia, the entire perineum is prepared for surgery. Preoperative preparations also include emptying the urinary bladder by catheterization and flushing the vagina repeatedly with a diluted povidone-iodine solution.

A pursestring suture is placed around the anal orifice and the animal is positioned for surgery as shown in Figure 1. Care should be taken to place the animal in an absolutely straight position prior to draping because it is important that the surgical site is properly aligned.

Prior to making the initial skin incision, a decision should be made about the amount of skin to be removed. Somewhat less skin than anticipated may be excised initially because it is always possible to extend the excised area later. Removal of too much skin will result in tension on the sutures and possible dehiscence.

The initial incision is made through the skin in the shape of an inverted U dorsal and lateral to the vulva (Fig 2a). The 1st incision is repeated with a 2nd one made parallel to the 1st (Fig 2b). The 2 incisions are joined ventrally and the resultant island of skin is undermined and dissected free. The 2 edges of skin are then approximated with an Allis forceps to determine whether or not enough skin was removed. If necessary to correct the defect, more skin can be removed. The cutaneous incision is then closed with a soft, nonabsorbable suture material (Fig 2c). Monafilament nylon is too rigid for this closure; sutures with this material are irritating and cause postoperative licking. An Elizabethan collar can be used to prevent licking.

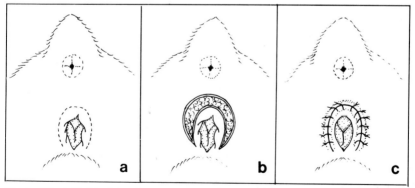

Fig 2a. The initial incision forms an inverted U around the vulva. 2b. A 2nd incision is made parallel to the 1st one and the 2 incisions are joined ventrally. 2c. After removing the island of skin between the 2 incisions the incised edges of skin are apposed with nonabsorbable sutures.

Topical application of diphemanil methylsulfate (Diathal Aqueous Suspension) or Variton Cream is also useful for this purpose. For animals in which obesity was a factor in causing the problem, an appropriate diet should be recommended.

Episiotomy

This surgical procedure is useful in increasing the exposure of the vaginal vestibule, urethral orifice, and clitoris. It is performed prior to excision of congenital vaginal septa, excision of the clitoris, reducing a vaginal prolapse, and removing vaginal tumors. The procedure may also assist manual delivery of fetuses.

Technic: The perineum from the anus to below the vulva is prepared for surgery and a pursestring suture is placed around the anus. The vagina is flushed repeatedly with diluted povidone-iodine solution. Though general anesthesia and positioning on a perineal stand are usually recommended for episioplasty, the procedure can be performed with local anesthesia in some cases.

A full-thickness incision is made through the skin and into the vagina on the midline dorsally from the junction of the vulvar labia. If the size of the vulvar orifice permits, a gloved finger can be inserted into the vagina to serve as a guide for the incision. By applying trac-

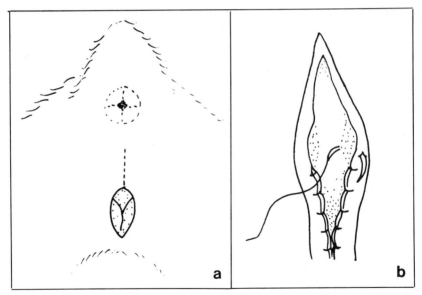

Fig 3. EPISIOTOMY. a. Enlargement of the vulvar cleft with a full-thickness incision directed dorsally. b. In closing an episiotomy the vaginal mucosa is opposed first with simple interrupted sutures.

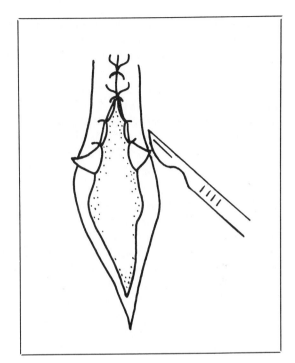

Fig 4. Permanent en-
largement of the vulvar
cleft.

tion dorsally and caudally with the inserted finger, folds in the
vaginal mucosa are removed and making an even full-thickness incision is facilitated. If the vulvar orifice is too small to permit insertion
of a finger, a Foley catheter with the bulb inflated may be used for the
same purpose.

While making the initial incision, arteries to the vulvar labia will
be seen and they should be ligated. The incision is extended through
the constrictor vestibuli muscle in the vaginal wall through the vaginal mucosa and dorsally toward the anus until the desired exposure
of the vagina is obtained (Fig 3a). Care should be taken to avoid incising the anal sphincter muscles, but this usually is not a danger
because the vulvar cleft can be enlarged more than twice its original
length before the incision reaches the anus.

An episiotomy is closed with 3 layers of sutures. In the 1st layer
the vaginal mucosa is apposed with simple interrupted, 3-0 or 4-0
chromic gut sutures (Fig 3b). The knots are tied on the submucosal
surface. The severed constrictor vestibuli muscle is then apposed
with 2-0 chromic gut. The skin is closed with a layer of simple interrupted sutures of nonabsorbable material. The 1st suture of the last 2

suture lines is preferably placed at the ventral end of the episiotomy to ensure proper anatomical apposition.

To facilitate breeding or parturition it may be desirable to keep the vulvar cleft larger than it was originally. In such cases the suture line in the vaginal mucosa is begun at the most dorsal point and continued ventrally to the level desired. The defect is then closed from the dorsal end with full-thickness sutures of nonabsorbable material to the level desired (Fig 4). This closure will leave small triangles of unsutured labia on either side that can be excised. The full-thickness sutures can be removed in 5 to 7 days.

Repair of Caudal Vaginal Strictures

Hypertrophy or fibrosis of the constrictor vestibuli muscle is fairly common and it results in strictures that can interfere with breeding. Such strictures may also cause dystocia. They can be treated surgically by performing an episiotomy as described earlier except that the vaginal mucosa is not incised. Following the myotomy the skin is closed with simple interrupted sutures of a nonabsorbable material. Because the vaginal mucosa has not been incised, the area can be dilated digitally following surgery. This should be done daily for 7 days and then on alternate days for another week. When a stricture is severe, the vulvar cleft can be enlarged in conjunction with the myotomy.

Removal of Uterine and Vaginal Tumors

Neoplasia of the uterus and vagina is uncommon in dogs and cats. Most tumors in this area are benign leiomyomas and fibromas.[1] They occur with increasing frequency in older animals.

Uterine tumors usually do not cause clinical signs and often are discovered incidentally. Occasionally, however, a uterine tumor will become large enough to partially obstruct the colon, impinge the urinary bladder, or displace other abdominal viscera (Figs 5a,b). Liposarcomas, leiomyosarcomas, and fibrosarcomas apparently are rare. These tumors may metastasize. The preferred treatment for uterine tumors is ovariohysterectomy. If a valuable breeding animal has a benign tumor in one uterine horn, a unilateral ovariohysterectomy can be performed.

Vaginal tumors are usually found when they protrude from the vulvar orifice. They may cause stranguria and recurrent cystitis if most of the tumor or its attachment to the vaginal wall is close to the external urethral orifice. Intermittent vaginal bleeding is also associated with tumors of this organ. The area at the junction of the vagi-

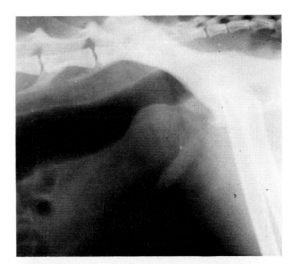

Fig 5a. Radiograph of female cat that was straining to eliminate.

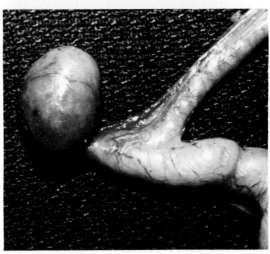

Fig 5b. Tenesmus seen in cat in Figure 5a was caused by this leiomyoma of the cervix.

nal wall and tumor is often inflamed. Older bitches with signs of vaginitis should be examined with an endoscope. Most vaginal tumors are pedunculated and easily excised after they are ligated near their origin.

An episiotomy is often needed to expose the pedicle of a vaginal tumor and to remove most of it. When the tumor is close to the urethral orifice, the pedicle must be carefully dissected or electrocautery may be needed to sever it. If tissue close to the urethral orifice is damaged, subsequent formation of scar tissue may result in stranguria. Because most vaginal neoplasms are benign, it is preferable to leave a small portion of its pedicle rather than risking normal patency of the urethral orifice. When recurrence of a tumor causes a clinical problem, the new growth can always be excised.

Cesarean Section

This procedure is preferred for dystocia of any origin. It should not be considered, however, until more conservative measures have been tried. A cesarean section should also be considered prior to other measures when several fetuses remain *in utero* and their survival is valued highly. The procedure is indicated in cases of uterine inertia, pelvic canal abnormalities, difficult presentations of a fetus, and when there has been a history of difficult parturitions. If performed properly, cesarean sections can be done repeatedly on the same animal.

Technic: A ventral midline incision is made in the abdomen from a point just caudal to the umbilicus to one just cranial to the pubis. The uterus is withdrawn from the abdominal cavity and retracted caudally to expose the dorsal surface of the uterine body (Figs 6a-e). After covering the cut edges of the abdominal incision with saline-moistened packs, the dorsal surface of the uterine body is incised over a fetus. The fetus and its amniotic sac are then removed through the incision.

After a fetus is removed from the uterus, steady pressure is applied on the fetal membranes by pulling on a forceps attached to the umbilical cord. The newborn animal is then given to an assistant who should remove the fetal membranes from its face and rub the puppy or kitten briskly with a towel to stimulate respirations. Skin over the newborn's back can be pinched to stimulate crying. The airway can be cleared by using a suction apparatus or by gently swinging the newborn while supporting its neck. The clamped umbilical cord is severed about ¾ inch from its attachment. Bleeding from it can be controlled with a hemostat or gut ligature.

Oxytocin can now be given slowly IV at a dosage of 5 to 20 units to facilitate removal of any remaining fetuses. Each fetus is successively "milked" toward the incision in the uterine body and freed from its placental attachment. After all of the fetuses have been removed from the uterus, the uterine wall should be inspected for evidence of tearing. If the uterine contents appear to have been contaminated, the cavity should be flushed liberally with Ringer's solution containing a broad-spectrum antibiotic.

The incision in the uterine body is closed with 2-0 chromic gut, using a continuous Cushing's pattern overlaid with a Lembert pattern (Fig 6). The sutured incision is then flushed with Ringer's flush

Figs 6a-e. CESAREAN
          SECTION.

a. The gravid uterus is
withdrawn from the ab-
dominal cavity and re-
tracted caudally to ex-
pose the body.

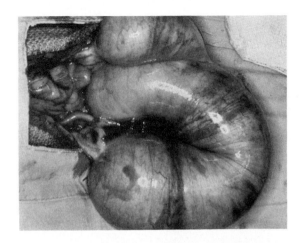

b. An incision is made
on the dorsal surface of
the uterine body.

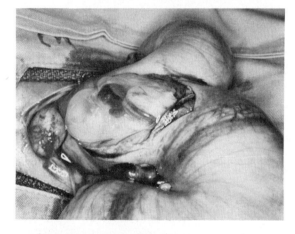

c. Fetus is being re-
moved through the uter-
ine incision.

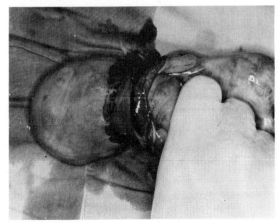

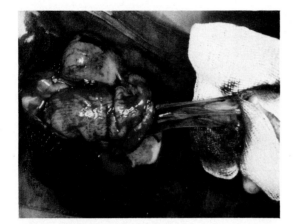

d. The umbilical cord is used to free the fetal membranes.

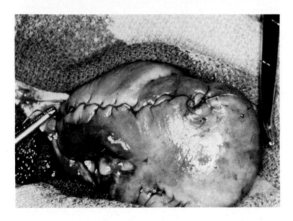

e. Uterine incision is closed with continuous Cushing sutures overlaid with a continuous Lembert suture pattern. Courtesy of RW Greene.

solution. Unless contamination has been considerable, insertion of a drain is not advisable because of the enlarged mammae. If drainage is indicated, the drain can be brought from the abdominal cavity caudal to the midline incision. The abdomen is closed in the usual way.

Subtotal Prostatectomy in the Dog

Chronic infections and neoplasms of the prostate gland are difficult to treat medically. This has been attributed to poor perfusion of drugs into prostate tissue.[2-4] As a consequence, total prostatectomy has been performed for several decades to remove infected and neoplastic glands. The technic for total transurethral prostatectomy has been described as the only way to remove the entire gland.[5,6] Total prostatectomy is difficult and has several potential complications.

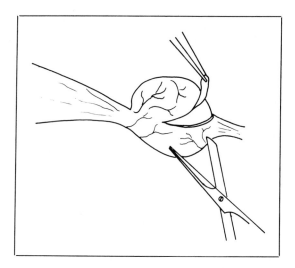

Fig 7. Incision and retraction of the prostate's capsule to preserve as much of it as possible.

Subtotal prostatectomy enables removal of the diseased portion without the risks associated with total removal of the gland.[7] By altering the technic, from 5 to 95% of a gland can be removed. Though an animal's fertility can be retained after total prostatectomy, prostatic fluid is a valuable component of semen, having both a bacteriostatic and buffering effect.[8]

Technic: To perform a subtotal prostatectomy the gland is exposed through an incision through the parapreputial skin and midline abdomen. The bladder is drawn cranially to expose the prostate gland. Fat covering the prostate is incised along the median prostatic raphe and reflected cranially. If a relatively small portion of a prostate lobe (less than 20% is to be excised, the major blood vessels to the lobe need not be ligated. Care should be taken to preserve the prostate's capsule so that it can be sutured over the defect made in the parenchyma (Fig 7). The diseased portion of prostate parenchyma is then removed. The capsule is closed with 3-0 chromic gut sutures after applying digital pressure briefly to control hemorrhage. If the surrounding tissues are contaminated during surgery, a drainage tube should be used.

When a large portion of the prostate gland must be removed, the blood supply to the gland should be carefully isolated and ligated. To locate these vessels the gland is rolled to the opposite side and the overlying fat is reflected dorsally. The urogenital artery will be seen extending in a caudal to cranial direction. Arteries that branch from the urogenital artery should be ligated where they enter the gland's parenchyma. Care should be taken to preserve the caudal vesicular artery that extends cranially to the trigone area of the bladder as a continuation of the urogenital artery. When parts of both prostatic lobes must be excised, arterial ligation should be performed on both sides of the gland.

Following ligation of the blood vessels to a lobe, the diseased portion can be removed. Care is required to avoid entering the urethra when excising prostatic tissue. Inserting a catheter will aid identification of the urethra. Nearly all of the prostatic tissue can be removed from the urethra if needed. Following excision of the diseased tissue, the surgical area is flushed and a drain is placed. The drain(s) should be brought outside the body through a separate "keyhole" incision.

Complications: Postoperative hemorrhage can be minimized by giving careful attention to ligation of blood vessels. If it persists, the surgical site should be re-entered to perform the needed ligation(s).

If the prostate's parenchyma is excised too close to the urethra the latter may be inadvertently damaged. In some cases it may not be possible to separate diseased tissue from the urethra. When the urethra is cut or part of it is excised, it should be closed if possible with 3-0 or 4-0 monofilament sutures. A stent should be used for 5 to 7 days to provide a conduit for urine while the urethral wound is healing. A large Brunswick catheter is a suitable stent.

If a fistula develops in the 1st few days after prostate surgery, placement of a large, soft catheter from the bladder to the external penile orifice will usually enable the urethral defect to heal. If necessary, a perineal urethrotomy can be performed to pass the catheter into the bladder.

The possibility of peritonitis following prostate surgery can be reduced by using Ringer's flush solution liberally before closing the incised tissues. A broad-spectrum antibiotic should be given if the patient becomes febrile or has a purulent discharge from a drain. In severe cases a peritoneal lavage system can be used.[9]

Repair of Phimosis

Phimosis is narrowness of the preputial opening that prevents withdrawal of the prepuce from the glans penis. The condition may be congenital or result from neoplasia or trauma. Surgical correction involves enlarging the external preputial orifice and severing any adhesions between the visceral and parietal layers of prepuce (Figs 8a,b).

To enlarge the external preputial orifice, a full-thickness incision is made through the ventral midline of the prepuce from the orifice caudally for 5 to 10 mm. The parietal layer of the prepuce is then sutured to the skin with simple interrupted sutures placed close together.

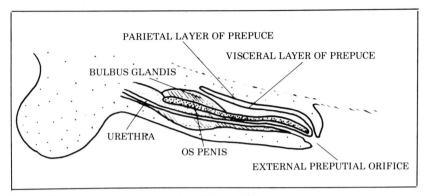

PARIETAL LAYER OF PREPUCE

VISCERAL LAYER OF PREPUCE

BULBUS GLANDIS

URETHRA

OS PENIS

EXTERNAL PREPUTIAL ORIFICE

Fig 8a. Phimosis prevents protrusion of the penis.

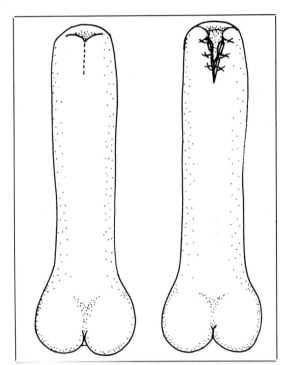

Fig 8b. Correction of phimosis involves enlargement of the preputial orifice by incision and suturing the parietal layer of prepuce to the skin.

Soft, nonabsorbable material, such as 4-0 silk, is used for suturing. Care is required to obtain precise apposition of skin and parietal prepuce and thus minimize postoperative scarring that could result in recurrence of the phimosis. Any adhesions between the visceral and parietal layers of prepuce should be severed by blunt dissection from the preputial orifice to the bulbus glandis.

Postoperatively, the penis should be extruded through the prepuce twice daily for 2 weeks. An antibiotic-corticosteroid ointment should be infused into the surgical area daily to prevent formation of new adhesions.

Correction of Persistent Penile Frenulum
This lesion occurs congenitally as a thin band of connective tissue on the ventral surface of the penis that prevents its protrusion. A frenulum will occasionally be disrupted spontaneously during the 1st 9 months of an affected dog's life. If it doesn't and the dog is to be used for breeding, the frenulum can be severed with a sharp scissors to its reflection at the junction of the penis and prepuce.

Postoperatively, an antibiotic-corticosteroid ointment should be instilled daily for several weeks at the surgical site and the penis should be extruded daily at the same time.

References
1. Morrow, DA: Current Therapy in Theriogenology, p 644. WB Saunders Co, Philadelphia, 1980.
2. Christie, TR: Pathophysiology in Small Animal Surgery, pp 447-454. Lea & Febiger, Philadelphia, 1981.
3. Barsanti, JA and Finco, DR: Vet Clin No Amer 4 (1979) 679.
4. Stamey, TA et al: J Urol 103 (1970) 187.
5. Annis, JR and Allen, AR: An Atlas of Canine Surgery, pp 150-153. Lea & Febiger, Philadelphia, 1967.
6. Howard, DR: Current Techniques in Small Animal Surgery, pp 255-261. Lea & Febiger, Philadelphia, 1975.
7. Knecht, CD: Comp Cont Educ for Small Anim Pract 1 (1979) 427.
8. Greiner, TP and Betts, CW: Textbook of Veterinary Internal Medicine, pp 1274-1305. WB Saunders Co, Philadelphia, 1975.
9. Hoffer, RE et al: JAAHA 6 (1970) 182.

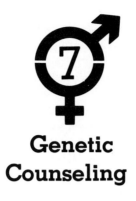

Genetic
Counseling

BY FRANCES O. SMITH

Modes of Inheritance

A basic problem for veterinary clinicians and dog breeders is determining whether an undesirable defect is heritable or congenital (present at birth but not necessarily hereditary). To address this problem, the clinician must be aware of the different modes of inheritance and the common defects associated with each mode.

Simple Dominant Traits

A simple dominant trait is transmitted by at least one parent affected with the undesirable trait. Affected animals are heterozygotes with the risk to male and female being equal. Breeding an affected animal to a normal one produces 50% affected puppies. Breeding an affected animal to another affected animal results in 75% affected offspring.

Examples of dominant traits include congenital hereditary lymphedema in dogs, hereditary cataracts in German Shepherds, and persistent pupillary membrane in the Basenji. Diseases inherited as dominant traits are easy to recognize and may be eliminated by removing all affected dogs from the breeding pool.

Incompletely Dominant Traits

Incomplete dominance results in 3 types of dogs: normal, slightly abnormal, and severely abnormal. Normal and severely abnormal animals produce similar offspring. Slightly abnormal animals produce ¼ normal, ½ slightly abnormal, and ¼ severely abnormal offspring. Abnormal animals should be eliminated. An example of an incompletely dominant trait is von Willebrand's disease in German Shepherds, Golden Retrievers, Doberman Pinschers, and Scottish Terriers.

Simple Recessive Traits

Somatic expression of a recessive gene may occur with a related pair of mutant genes, 2 alleles at a single locus, or one recessive gene inherited from each parent. The offspring is homozygous with respect to the gene. With a simple autosomal recessive gene, there are 2 phenotypes (normal and defective) and 3 genotypes (homozygous normal and heterozygous or homozygous abnormal). A normal homozygote bred to another normal homozygote can only produce normal offspring. A normal homozygote bred to a heterozygote will produce only phenotypically normal offspring. Two normal animals (phenotypically) with a recessively inherited defect should produce 25% defective offspring, and 75% that are phenotypically normal. Two of 3 normal-appearing dogs, however, will carry the hidden abnormal gene. In this way the defect may not appear in a generation before reappearing from a mating of 2 carrier animals.

The simple autosomal recessive pattern of inheritance is the most common pattern in the inheritance of congenital defects. This inheritance is difficult to control because carriers are only identified when the defect occurs. By eliminating defective dogs, recessive defects can be held to a low incidence.

Some recessive genes are lethal when they occur in homozygous form, such as cranioschisis in the Cocker Spaniel. This results in a 2:1 ratio in living pups instead of 3:1 as expected. Other examples of simple autosomal recessive traits are cyclic neutropenia in gray Collies and umbilical hernia in the Cocker Spaniel.

Sex-Linked Recessive Inheritance

Sex-linked recessive conditions also occur in dogs. In these conditions, affected males are hemizygotes. Affected offspring (usually male) are the result of matings between carrier females and normal males. From such a mating, half of the males are affected and half of the females are carriers. Affected females result from matings of affected males and carrier or affected females. Examples of sex-linked recessive conditions are hemophilia A and B in dogs.

Polygenic Inheritance

Polygenic inheritance results from the combined actions of an undetermined number of genes. Polygenic traits represent continuous variation and the frequencies in each class form a curve of normal distribution. To form a standard curve, however, the number of puppies in a single litter is not sufficient. Information on 100 members of the same breed will provide a more reliable picture of the inheritance pattern. Examples of polygenetic traits include body weight, conformation, hip dysplasia, and patellar luxation. Such traits can be influenced by environment. Heritability, which is designated as h^2, measures on a scale between 0.1 and 1.0, indicating how much of the variation in a polygenic trait is of genetic origin. For example, hip dysplasia has been given an h^2 value of from .25 to .75, with .50 being the commonly assigned number. Values greater than .25 are considered highly heritable and by appropriate selection the prevalence of a polygenic trait may be decreased. Dogs affected with polygenic defects should not be bred.

Epistasis

Epistasis refers to the suppression of one gene (dominant) by another gene at a different locus. An epistatic gene (A) is the cause of the rich red burgundy color in the Irish Setter. These dogs also carry a gene for black as evidenced by this color on the nose and footpads. The black color is prevented from being expressed in the haircoat by the gene for red.

Determining Heritability of Undesirable Traits

Clues to the heritability of a trait may be discovered in the following ways:

1. Noting the occurrence of 2 or more affected animals in the same litter, in a repeat breeding, or in breedings between closely related animals.
2. Noting a significantly greater frequency of a defect within one breed or strain.
3. Determining whether or not the pedigree has ancestors common to both parents.
4. Referring to textbooks on genetics to see if the defect is known to be heritable in certain breeds.
5. Performing test breedings to see if the defect recurs.

Test Breeding

When homozygosity is lethal, it may be difficult to identify carriers of an undesirable recessive gene. In these cases, a test breeding should be made to a known carrier female. Males are used as the suspect animal because they can have a greater numerical impact on a breed than females. Test breedings of affected individuals may also confirm that an undesirable trait is hereditary (Table 1).

Test breeding can also be used to disclose parental status by traits like hair color that may be controlled by a single gene (Table 2). For example, it can be shown how many offspring are needed from a known homozygous yellow Labrador Retriever bitch and a black male of unknown genotype to determine the probabilities that the male is homozygous (BB) for black or heterozygous (By). If the male sires even one yellow puppy, he carries the yellow gene and is genotypically By and phenotypically black.

Veterinary Cytogenetics

Cytogenetics may be used to identify intersex states or chromosomal causes of infertility, such as Klinefelter's syndrome. Males with small testes, hypospadias, and aspermatogenesis are good candidates for chromosomal evaluation. Complete anestrus or abnormal genitalia in females may reflect an intersex state.

Chromosomal analysis is performed on lymphocytes in peripheral blood. A 10-ml sample is collected in a sterile syringe containing 0.1 ml of heparin. The sample must be kept cool (not frozen) and the analysis should be begun within 24 hours.

Table 1. Test Breeding to Detect Suspected Carriers of Undesirable Genes When Bred to a Known Carrier

Offspring All Normal	Probability That Suspect Is a Carrier	
Number	Expressed as Numeral	Expressed as Chance
1	0.75	3 in 4
2	0.56	1 in 1.77
3	0.422	1 in 2.37
4	0.316	1 in 3.10
5	0.237	1 in 4.22
6	0.178	1 in 5.55
7	0.1335	1 in 7.7
8	0.100	1 in 10
9	.075	1 in 13.3
10	.056	1 in 17.7
11	.042	1 in 23.7
12	.032	1 in 31.5
13	.024	1 in 42
14	.018	1 in 56
15	.013	1 in 74
16	.01	1 in 100

Modified from F. B. Hutt in *Genetics for Dog Breeders*

Table 2. Test Breeding to Determine Parental Genotype

Offspring All Black	Probability the Male is not By*	
Number	Expressed as Numeral	Expressed as Chance
1	0.50	1 in 2
2	0.25	1 in 4
3	0.125	1 in 8
4	0.0625	1 in 16
5	0.0313	1 in 32
6	0.0156	1 in 64
7	0.0078	1 in 128
8	0.0039	1 in 256
9	0.0020	1 in 512
10	0.0010	1 in 1024

*By — Heterozygous for dominant black gene (B) and recessive yellow gene (y).

Sex chromosome studies may be done in the dog and cat by using oral epithelial cells (buccal scraping). In all species, polymorphonuclear leukocytes may be used to evaluate sex chromosomes.

Selection of Breeding Animals

Most dogs and cats are bred on the basis of the appearance preferred by individual breeders. This is referred to as mass selection.

Mass selection on a large scale is called natural selection. It results in foxes with inherent resistance to diseases that kill other foxes. Likewise, a wolf with a sound pelvis (without hip dysplasia) is more likely to live to reproduce than is a dysplastic wolf.

Progeny Testing

Progeny testing evaluates breeding stock from the standpoint of genotype. For this reason, it is the offspring that are carefully evaluated. It is easy to assess the genotypes of animals with recessive genes, but this assessment is not easy for polygenetic traits.

The basic procedures involved in progeny testing are as follows:
1. Test males rather than females because of their greater numerical influence on a breed.
2. Select young males as sires on the basis of pedigree, breed type, freedom from heritable defects, soundness, and good littermates.
3. Breed the males to unrelated females while trying to give each stud females of comparable quality so that differences in the males can be determined.

4. Evaluate many offspring so that proportions of desirable and undesirable traits can be calculated as percentages that are significant.
5. Include all progeny.
6. Record all stillbirths and neonatal deaths. Perform necropsies.
7. Use the male with the best production record.

Inbreeding/Linebreeding

Inbreeding refers to the mating of closely related animals. It is commonly considered that a brother-sister or a parent-offspring breeding is inbreeding and that breeding among more distant relatives is linebreeding. Inbreeding and linebreeding accomplish the same goal (increase homozygosity), but linebreeding takes longer to do so. Inbreeding does not cause undesirable genes, but it results in homozygosity of undesirable recessive genes.

The effects of inbreeding include uniformity of conformation and color. Inbred animals also have increased risk of infertility, small litters, fading puppies or kittens, and physical defects.

Ethics Guidelines

The clinician or breeder faced with the sudden appearance of a defect should assemble all available information to predict the likelihood of the defect's heritability. Defective dogs should not be bred. Though a dog that started to have seizures at 2 years of age may not have heritable epilepsy, it is better to not use the animal for breeding than to risk the possibility that his offspring may be affected or carriers.

Both the American Veterinary Medical Association and the American Kennel Club have specific guidelines on the repair of heritable defects.

The 1980 opinion of the AVMA:

Performance of surgical procedures in all species for the purpose of concealing genetic defects in animals to be shown, raced, bred, or sold as breeding animals is unethical. However, should the health or welfare of the individual patient require correction of such genetic defects, it is recommended that the patient be rendered incapable of reproduction.

Rules Applying to AKC Registration and Dog Shows (amended to Sept 9, 1980):

A dog which is blind, deaf, castrated, spayed, or which has been changed in appearance by artificial means except as specified in the standard for its breed, or a male which does not have two normal testicles normally located in the scrotum, may not compete at any show.

References

1. Burns, M & Fraser, M: Genetics of the Dog, 2nd ed. JB Lippincott, Philadelphia, 1966.
2. Erickson, F et al: Congenital Defects in Dogs. Veterinary Practice Publishing Co, Santa Barbara, CA, 1978.
3. Hutt, FB: Genetics for Dog Breeders. WH Freeman & Co, San Francisco, 1979.
4. Little, CC: The Inheritance of Coat Color in Dogs. Cornell Univ Press, Ithaca, NY, 1957.
5. Patterson, DF: In Current Veterinary Therapy VII. WB Saunders, Philadelphia, 1980.

Index

Pages numbers in *italic* refer to illustrations; numbers followed by "t" indicate tables.

393

Megace, 348t
Megestrol acetate
  contraceptive effect, 219
  estrus control, 197-198, *199*, 200, 201,
    201t
  treatment for vaginal hyperplasia, 230
  treatment of pseudopregnancy, 48,
    348t, 350
Meningitis, 271
Meperidine, 310, 363
Meperidine hydrochloride, 341
Mepivicaine, 366
Metabolic disorders, 80
Metestrus
  canine vaginal smears, 110-111, 111t,
    119, 120
  endocrinology of, *26-27*
  felines, 15, 16
  physiology of, *24*, *39*, 46-48, 34
Methandriol dipropionate, 348t, 350
Methimazole, 307
Methohexital, 363, 364
Methohexital Na, 368
Methotrexate, 300
Methoxyflurane, 356, 357, 365, 368
Methyloestrenolone, 349t, 351
Methylprednisolone, 221, 314
Metritis
  canines, 332-333
  clinical signs, 281-282
  felines, 132
  occurrence, 280
  treatment, 259, 282-283
  uterine horn, *170*
Mibolerone, 48, 202-205, 256, 349t, 351
Milk let-down. *See* Lactation
Mismating, 217
Mismating management. *See* Abortion
Monozygotic twinning, 319
Morphine, 310
MPA, 50-51, *53*, 68, 196, 348t, 350
Mucometra, 56
Mucoprotein, 109
Mustargen, 300
Myasthenia, 310
Myelosuppression, 218
Myotomy, 376

N-desacetyl thiocolchicine, 221, 222t
Nalbuphine, 363
Nalorphine, 310, 363
Naloxone, 310, 363

Naproxen, 225
Narcotics, 363
Nasal speculum, 93, *94*
Neomycin, 278
Neonates. *See* Kittens; Puppies
Neoplasia
  male genitalia, 172
  mammary glands, 197, *199*, 200, 323
  prostate, *175*, 177, 178
  reproductive effects, 80
Neostigmine, 310
Nephrotoxic drugs, 357
Neutrophils, 107, 108, 109, 111
Newborns. *See* Kittens; Puppies
Nidroxyzone, 300
Nitrofurans, 300
Nitrofurantoin, 300, 301, 311
Nitrofurazone, 300
Nitrous oxide, 365, 368
Nursing. *See* Lactation

Obesity
  canines, 327, 328
  perivulvar dermatitis caused by, 372,
    374
  radiography, 169
  reproductive effects, 83
Obstetrical hooks, 343, 344
Obstetrical snares, 343, 344
Oleandomycin, 291
Oncovirus, 264, 267t
Oocytes, *29-32*
Opiates, 310
Orchidectomy, 241
Orchitis, 239, 240-243, 246, 270, 271, 294
Organophosphorus compounds, 310
Os penis, 178, 245-246. *See also* Penis
Osseous deformities, 83
Osteomyelitis, 178
Otoscope(s)
  penis examination, 85
  vaginal examination, 85
  vaginoscopy, 95
Ovaban, 348t
Ovarian agenesis, 232
Ovarian cycle
  canines, 24-37, 49-57
  endocrinology of, *61*
  environmental factors, 37
  follicular phase, 24-28, *24-27*, *29-33*
  intervals between, 36-37
  luteal phase, *24*, 34, 47-48
  new follicular phase, 34-36, *35*
  physiology of, 24-37